WHEN
CANCER
HITS

Published by:

Cinco Vidas Press
12 Desbrosses Street
New York, NY 10013

ISBN: 978-0-9829175-0-3

Printed in the U.S.A.

Library of Congress information on file with the publisher.

Cover and Interior Design by:
*the*BookDesigners

For more info or to contact the author, please go to
www.cincovidas.com

WHEN CANCER HITS

YOUR COMPLETE GUIDE TO TAKING
CARE OF YOU THROUGH
TREATMENT

Britta Aragon

with Colleen M. Story

CINCO VIDAS PRESS
New York, NY
www.cincovidas.com

PRAISE FOR *WHEN CANCER HITS*

"An incredible insight for all those on the cancer journey. Britta has used her own experience to provide incredible knowledge on how to take care of yourself during your journey. She's incredibly inspiring and is committed to providing hope and guidance to those needing it during this time."

—MORAG CURRIN, *Founder of Touch Cancer Online and author of* Oncology Esthetics: A Practitioner's Guide

"Battling cancer is a Herculean task that requires courage, fortitude and many, many decisions. There are lots of experts in the field, but advice from one who went through it herself is invaluable. I wish this book had existed during my own battle."

—FRAN DRESCHER, *Cancer Survivor, Health Advocate, President of Cancer Schmancer*

"Britta Aragon arms her readers with information to help them nurture their bodies and protect themselves from chemicals linked to cancer and other serious health problems, just when they need it most. *When Cancer Hits* is an invaluable resource that offers facts and advice, without being overwhelming."

—MIA DAVIS, *Organizing Director, Campaign for Safe Cosmetics*

"Thank you to Britta Aragon for this beautiful, powerful book. *When Cancer Hits* is full of vital information about healing, hope and protecting our health and our families. This is a must-read for anyone who is healing from cancer or who has a loved one dealing with the disease."

—STACY MALKAN, *Co-Founder of Campaign for Safe Cosmetics and author of* Not Just a Pretty Face: The Ugly Side of the Beauty Industry

"*When Cancer Hits* is the perfect gift for any and every cancer patient...really for anyone looking for guidelines for preventing cancer in addition to in-depth and specific tools to help anyone in their cancer journey."

—DR. DONIELLE WILSON, *Naturopathic Doctor*

"This is the book I wish I had for every patient diagnosed with cancer. It fills the void between the diagnosis and the journey onward. A great blueprint for how to cope with the journey from choosing safe personal care products, addressing all the changes that your skin and body will go through to managing side effects."

—DR. MADELINE KRAUSS, *M.D.*

For my father, Javier Aragon.

Your courage, strength, and heart inspire me,
and remind me to always live my best life,
no matter what.

And for all those on the cancer journey:
This book is for you.
We are all beautiful.
We are all one.
You are not alone.

CONTENTS

CHAPTER ELEVEN 219
Treatments Are Over, but Things Aren't Normal

CHAPTER TWELVE....................................... 239
Your Prevention Plan: *Tips to Lower Risk of Recurrence*

Forward by Donald F. Richey, M.D.

Yes, You Have Cancer, But You Can Still Enjoy Life

YOU…HAVE…CANCER.

When the doctor says those three little words, your mind tends to black everything else out. *Am I going to live? Am I going to die? How mutilating are my treatments going to be?*

Every person I've known who's experienced cancer remembers that moment. Everything changes after that.

The good news is your chances of surviving are much better today than they used to be. Cancer treatments are much improved, even more than they were only ten years ago. I've witnessed amazing advancements in surgeries, chemotherapy, and radiation, and the end result is that more people are living longer, and many enjoy the rest of their lives cancer free.

The problem is that with these improved treatments come unpleasant consequences. I'm speaking mainly about the side effects. Most people know that cancer treatments can cause nausea and hair loss, but I recently came across a survey in which more than 350 cancer survivors were asked to rank their most bothersome side effects. Would you be surprised to learn that the top two reported were skin irritations and dry skin?[1]

What we may not realize going into cancer treatments is that the side effects that alter our appearance and how we feel "in our own skin" can be the most difficult to manage. Today's more potent and often more effective chemotherapy agents are often very taxing to the body's fast-growing cells, causing hair loss, dry skin, fragile nails, and even skin conditions like rashes, rosacea and dermatitis. In fact, oncologists sometimes measure the success of the treatment by the severity of the skin reaction! More rosacea? Great. That means the treatment is working.

Good news if you're trying to get rid of a tumor.

Not so good if you're trying to enjoy the quality of your day-to-day life.

What can you do? How can you prepare yourself for these sorts of challenges? In my work with cancer patients and survivors, I've discovered one thing—people are hungry for more information on how to deal with these cutaneous side effects. That's why I'm excited to be writing the forward for this book. What you need to get through this experience, to maintain your sense of control over your life, and to actually feel a little bit better and a little more comfortable, are tools like those supplied in this book. You need information, instruction, and suggestions for what to do if your face breaks out in a rash, for example, or your skin becomes so dry and irritated that it stings and burns with the usual products you apply. This book provides solutions for hair loss, missing eyebrows and eyelashes, thinning nails, dry skin, radiation dermatitis, and so much more.

If you're new to this journey, you may be a little skeptical. *I'm fighting for my life*, you may say. *Why would I care about missing eyelashes?* One thing that cancer survivors know is that the disease can wreak havoc on your appearance. If you take all these effects together—hair loss, thinning eyebrows and eyelashes, dark and fragile nails, and dry, dull skin—what you have is an assault on your identity. You look in the mirror and no longer see the same person. That experience can be emotionally devastating to a lot of people. You're right—you're fighting for your life. But while you're in the middle of that battle, you still have to function in your world. Perhaps you have a job, a family, or people who rely on you. If you start to look different, beaten down, and ill, it can negatively affect your confidence, which ultimately, can inhibit your ability to heal.

I started a program called "Brighter Days" about eight years ago. It's a simple program that allows me and other dermatologists to reach out and help people living with cancer to feel just a little bit better. Over the course of about one to two hours, I provide, free of charge, an in-person seminar where I a) explain the effects of chemotherapy and radiation on the hair, skin, and nails (*TALK*); b) personally attend to each member of the class, assess the condition of his or her skin and nails, and offer several personalized suggestions for better care (*TOUCH*); and c) invite all participants to share their stories (*TELL*). Now, in my nearly forty years of practicing dermatology, I've participated in many programs that benefit the community, but never have I experienced the deep sense of joy and fulfillment that I get from interacting with these individuals who come to my lectures. They are just so grateful and happy to have someone who cares enough to sit down and discuss their challenges with them, and then provide solutions they can use during the course of their treatment.

I would love to be able to somehow meet individually with every person who is diagnosed with cancer. As that is impossible, I'm recommending the next best thing—Britta's complete guide to navigating the challenges of everyday life during and after cancer treatments. It provides you with many of the instructions and tools I would present in my seminars, only you have access to it in the comfort of your own home. Inside these pages you'll find information on why certain side effects happen, and more importantly, what you can do to help alleviate the discomfort.

Not too long ago, I read an article in the *Journal of American Academy of Dermatology* that was very informative about current chemotherapeutic medications and their effects on the skin.[2] I was disappointed, however, to find that it provided no therapeutic suggestions. This points to another reason I'm so pleased with this book—it helps to fill that gap by delivering several options for dealing with these troublesome side effects.

I have no doubt that tending to what may seem like the "little things" of your cancer treatments will have a huge effect on the success of those treatments, on the quality of life you enjoy while you're going through them, and on how quickly and easily you recover afterwards. In fact, one recent study showed that having a good quality of life and low levels of depression during treatment improved survival time.[3] You can't keep your spirits up, however, if your skin is dry and covered with rashes, or you feel like you look "sick" when you go out of the house.

My daughter-in-law's mother was a very tall, elegant, and intelligent schoolteacher named Kristine. Everyone in the family admired her, and we were all stricken when she received her cancer diagnosis. She fought a valiant fight for fifteen years, undergoing multiple surgeries, chemotherapy and radiation. During her last few days here on Earth, I got a chance to talk to her. I asked her then what she thought. If I could have somehow developed a program that would have helped her care for her hair, skin and nails and thus, feel better about her appearance—even though I couldn't have changed the course of her illness—did she think that would have been helpful?

She didn't hesitate. She told me that would be a wonderful idea, and encouraged me to do it, the sooner the better.

Her answer taught me one thing—no matter what happens with the disease, we need to think more seriously about *quality of life* during treatment.

We've been used to believing that a patient should just hang on by his fingernails in a sort of limbo between "okay" and "not okay" until that final day of chemotherapy or that final radiation appointment. We're missing something with that line of logic. A patient continues to live, work, relate to loved ones, and experience life during treatment. Enhancing those experiences is vitally important. First, because it keeps hope alive and spirits strong, which has been shown in studies to boost the immune system and facilitate healing. Second, none of us ever knows what's going to happen tomorrow, so we must take full advantage of today. If, by helping you find a new way to fix your hair, moisturize your dry skin, tone down the redness of rosacea, or calm that rash, we can help you experience a better day, that's huge!

After that last talk with Kristine, I started Brighter Days. Since then I have experienced firsthand the benefits that this sort of program—and this sort of book—can have on people living with cancer. You can trust me when I say that the tools you need are here, and that you'll feel better as soon as you start reading about them and incorporating them into your life.

At the beginning of each of my seminars, I give out hats to the attendees. Most of them have lost their hair, or have thinning hair, or are only months out of treatment with the hair just starting to grow back. They all put on their hats, and it helps them to realize they're all in the same boat.

These aren't just any hats, however. Imprinted on the brim are the words "Life is Good." They're donated by the Life is Good Kids Foundation, and come in fun colors. I hand these out as an icebreaker, but also as a reminder to each individual: Yes, you have cancer, but that doesn't mean you can't still experience good things in life. It's all about your point of view and how you approach the situation. There *are* things that can make you feel better. There *are* things that can make you look more like yourself, and boost your self-confidence. There *are* ways to get through this experience with hope, optimism, and several good days to go along with the not-so-good ones. If you can maintain your positive attitude and keep your spirits up during this period of time, I guarantee it will help you in so many ways.

There are brighter days ahead. You just need the tools in this book to get there. Happy reading.

Dr. Donald F. Richey
Board Certified in Dermatology and Histopathology
Life Member, American Academy of Dermatology

Introduction

My Journey Through Cancer to a Meaningful Life

MY JOURNEY WITH CANCER STARTED IN 1992. I was sixteen years old, and I had Hodgkin's disease.

No big deal, I thought. I had volleyball games to play, friends to hang out with, and shopping to do. I'd get this "cancer" whatever-it-was taken care of and get on with more important things.

Little did I know: Cancer would change my life.

We lived in North Vancouver, Canada. I was the daughter of a successful businessman from Mexico and a strong German woman who had immigrated west after surviving the aftermath of World War II. I had an older brother and a very close-knit family of aunts, uncles, and cousins who lived nearby.

Life was good for me. I had switched from a Catholic high school to join my friends at public school, and my sophomore year seemed as though it was going to be the best yet. I was starting for the senior volleyball team, and the season looked to be a promising one. With my long dark hair and slim figure, I was getting attention from the boys, and I had many dear girlfriends. I felt young, carefree, and full of life, and couldn't wait to get started on each new day.

I don't remember when I first saw the lump. I just remember it was there, out of the blue, on the left side of my neck, near the collarbone. I asked Mom: What do you think this is? It didn't look particularly worrisome— just a little raised skin. Mom thought surely it would disappear in time. We didn't have any health issues in the family, so she wasn't worried.

1

Meanwhile, my volleyball team was set to play in the finals, and I had started dating a senior guy on the football team. I put the lump in the back of my mind. It would go away on its own, I figured.

It didn't. As the weeks went by, it got bigger. And it started to hurt. Worse, I got night sweats—episodes so bad I would have to get up in the middle of the night and change my pajamas. On top of that, my legs itched. I would wake up with my skin red and irritated from scratching so hard.

I went to see my family doctor. She referred me to a specialist. Being a self-sufficient girl, I went by myself after school. The specialist took a biopsy. Then, while I waited, he went into another room, out of earshot, and called my mother. Unbeknownst to me, he told her I had Hodgkin's disease, or Hodgkin's lymphoma.

Mom was like, "What's that?"

He told her. Cancer.

My parents were devastated. My mother later told me she couldn't believe it. Her sixteen-year-old daughter, with cancer? I'd had no prior serious health problems, and we had no history of the disease in our family. Nothing could have prepared them for this.

The doctor came back into my room. He didn't tell me about the cancer. He didn't share with me that he thought it would be best for my parents to tell me. Instead, he said he needed to operate, to remove the lump

Made sense to me. Let's get it out and get on with life.

He said he needed to do it right away.

I balked. I had a game the next day. Our volleyball team was playing for the western championship. I was starting, as middle blocker. Couldn't this wait?

No. It had to be done immediately.

"Why?" I asked.

It needed to be done right away. That was it. End of story.

I arrived home, confused as to why this had to "interrupt" my volleyball season. Mom and Dad, struggling with the enormity of my condition, had decided not to tell me right away. They didn't want to worry me. Besides, how do you tell your daughter something like that? They had to deal with their own emotions first, so they could be as supportive as possible for me.

The next day I went to the Lion's Gate Hospital to have the lump removed. To me, being unable to be with my teammates was a tragedy. My parents, however, were struggling with bigger problems.

When we emigrated from Mexico to Vancouver in 1986, my father was working at a business he owned with his brothers. By the 1990s, the business was failing, and he'd decided to leave it. For the first time in his life, he was out of a job. We were moving to a smaller home to save money. And now his daughter had cancer.

I can imagine the stress he must have gone through. He had to take care of his family, find a new career, and worry about me fighting for my life. Of course, at that time, I knew little about the load he was carrying. For me, October 1992 became the beginning of my new journey—as someone with cancer.

Will I Lose My Hair?

When I woke up from surgery, I remember seeing my dad and mom in the room. A new doctor came to me and said they were going to take care of me and get me the treatments I needed. I was still heavily drugged and didn't really understand. I did get the idea the surgery had been successful, so I figured everything was going to be fine.

I was released from the hospital the same day. I went home and slept, and when I woke up, I felt so happy! The lump was gone, and I could get back to doing all the things I wanted to do.

The next day I went to my boyfriend's house with my girlfriend, Becky. My mom called me, concerned. Shouldn't I come home and rest? I didn't think so, I told her. I had gone through a minor surgery with ten stitches. What was the big deal?

My parents were confused. They thought that when the doctor had told me I needed treatments, I had finally understood how sick I was. After that phone call, however, my mom realized I had no idea. How were they going to break the news?

Fortunately, I had a great friend named Kelly, whose mother was a nurse. My parents arranged for us all to have Thanksgiving dinner together a week after my surgery. (For those of you who don't know, Thanksgiving occurs in October in Canada.) After the meal, the adults wanted to talk, so we all sat down. Kelly's mom, Gaye, tried to explain it to me.

"You know, Britta," she said, "you have cancer. You're going to need treatments. Chemotherapy, and probably radiation. But don't worry. You have a great doctor. His name is Dr. Klimo, and he's one of the best. You're going to be in good hands."

Somewhere in my mind I understood what she was saying, but on the other hand, I didn't get the gravity of it. It was only a word. *Cancer*.

Everyone looked at me. They were waiting for my response. The clock ticked. I sat on the couch, hands in my lap.

"Can Kelly sleep over?" I asked.

You can imagine the looks they gave each other. My parents were like, well, sure, um, Kelly can stay. Then everyone grew quiet again. And still, they were watching me.

"Is my hair going to fall out?" I asked.

Gaye said it probably would.

I sat with that a minute. So did everyone else.

"Okay," I said, and shrugged.

And that was it. End of conversation.

Clearly I had no idea of the severity of my condition. I assumed I'd have the treatments and that would be that. Not once did it enter my consciousness that I would die. Not once!

My parents, meanwhile, were freaking out.

Reality Sets In

They say cancer changes you, and it's true—even if you don't realize it at the time.

That was the case for me. I was moving forward in a fog of ignorant bliss.

At first, everything went fine. I would take my chemo treatment, go home and sleep it off, and wake up the next day ready to go to the mall or to a dance or to whatever was going on. I wanted to be out. I wanted to see my friends. I wanted to be *normal*. Oh, how we all want to be normal!

For a while, cancer cooperated with me. But after the second treatment, things started to change.

I was a teenage girl. You may remember or imagine what that's like. We all want to fit in, and we want to be liked. For me, my long, shiny hair was an important part of my identity—a trait I truly liked about myself. I flushed with pride when people complimented me on it. When my hair looked good, I felt I did, too.

Then my doctor told me to cut it. It was going to fall out anyway, he said. It would be easier for it to come out in short strands rather than longer locks. I felt like he was telling me to cut off my hand.

Gaye went with me to a hair salon. I wasn't happy. I believed I had to do this against my will, even though somewhere in my mind I knew they were right—especially if my hair was going to fall out anyway.

I got a variation on the bob, with one side shorter than the other. It was perfectly stylish, but I felt naked. Who was that person in the mirror? I didn't recognize her. She looked diminished, *different*. For the first time, I was afraid of what else this disease might do to me.

I never went bald, but my hair did get really thin. I remember waking up every morning and collecting strands and clumps from my pillow that had fallen out the night before. One day while I was riding the bus home, a couple of kids noticed the bald spots on my crown.

"Where's your hair?" they asked, and started laughing.

Oh my God, I thought. *Does it look that bad?* I wanted to disappear into the seat cushion.

My dad shaved my hair, and I went wig shopping. Surprisingly, it was such a fun experience that I felt a lot better afterward. The wigs gave me back a part of myself I felt I had lost. I made them part of my new style, along with some hats and scarves. Confident again, I shoved the shame out of my mind and got back into life.

Things would soon be back to normal, for sure.

Is That What Boys Want?

But cancer wasn't finished with me. Another side effect of my chemotherapy was—contrary to what most people would expect—weight gain. I retained water from the chemotherapy drugs, and it made me look puffy. On top of that, the skin on my face swelled up as though I had inflated it, and became dry and dull.

I had covered my thinning hair with stylish wigs, scarves, and hats. But nothing could hide the cancer showing up on my face and figure.

I didn't feel pretty anymore. I was bald, overweight, bloated, my skin had lost its radiance, and I wasn't getting the attention I was used to. Don't get me wrong—everyone was very supportive, but it felt as though they were feeling sorry for me. That was the last thing I wanted. I didn't want to be "that girl with cancer" who everybody pitied.

But there was no getting around it. I didn't look the same, and the boys weren't noticing me like they used to. *Is that all boys care about?* I wondered. *Long hair and slender figures?* For the first time in my life, I felt insecure.

We want to think we're more than our appearance. And we are. But we don't realize how much we identify with what we see in the mirror until it starts to change. Cancer has a way of stripping everything down to its naked reality, and we must face what can seem a stark, unattractive, and strange reflection.

For me, despite my challenges, I never had any doubt I was going to get better. The cancer was going to go away, my hair was going to grow back, and my figure would return. In my teenage mind, it just had to be so, and I believe to this day that I was so focused on getting better that my cells listened to my commands.

I made it through my sophomore year, treatment and all, having to take only one summer class for math. I passed everything else with flying colors and won my battle against cancer. My original prescription included a year of chemotherapy with some radiation. I ended up taking six months of chemotherapy and no radiation. Dr. Klimo was surprised and thrilled at my progress, as was my family. Today, I am cancer free!

I was lucky. I had a lot of support. Encouragement flowed from my family, friends, and my friends' parents. And my general ignorance about cancer helped my attitude—I absolutely knew I would get better.

Still, cancer left its scars. To this day I fear cutting my hair too short, and I pamper my once dried-out skin. My recovery after cancer was difficult, as I felt pressured to just "move on" and get back to normal, yet I had all those overwhelming feelings and didn't know what to do with them. To cope, I turned to the one thing I could control—what I ate—and ended up with anorexia. Eventually I got over that, but I still battle with my body image, particularly surrounding weight. Fortunately, the disease also came with blessings, things I would realize as I matured. But first, I would have to face cancer again.

Cancer Returns

Surviving cancer—and my sophomore year in high school—left me feeling jubilant. The experience made me a stronger person and gave me a free spirit. After all, I had faced this disease and beaten it. Bring it on, world!

My hair grew back, my weight returned to normal, and life was good again. I came to believe my positive outlook had helped me heal, and I trusted from that moment on that no matter what life dealt me, everything would turn out all right.

Perhaps in some way the experience prepared me for the future, as about seven years later, in 1999, my father was diagnosed with colon cancer. Now, I know relationships between fathers and daughters come in all shapes and sizes, so let me tell you a little bit about mine.

My father was my hero and my best friend. I adored him. He was everything I wanted to be. Successful, optimistic, strong, smart, and a go-getter with a huge heart, he had a powerful drive to make things happen. His confidant personality was obvious in the way he approached everything he did.

After he left the failing business in 1992 and faced the world without a job, he pursued a solution with all his energy. When he found out I had cancer, his motivation doubled. He bought several books and read them all in a week. I remember titles like *Think and Grow Rich* by Napoleon Hill, *Feel the Fear and Do it Anyway* by Susan Jeffers, and *How to Win Friends and Influence People* by Dale Carnegie.

Emerging from a sort of personal soul-searching, he hit the streets. He applied for many positions within his field of finance, but it was when he saw an ad for Investor's Group that he felt a tingle of recognition. He walked into the interview and asked, "Can I make $200,000 in my first year?" The man across the desk answered that he could, so my dad asked where to sign.

He got the job. Within two years he was promoted, and by the fourth year he was regional manager.

This was my father. Strong, determined, and successful. So when he was diagnosed with colon cancer, I knew—he would defeat it.

But again, cancer had a lot more in store than I realized.

My Rock Crumbles

It was 1999. My dad was full of strength and confidence. He had optimism, determination, and faith. He was my rock. He would emerge victorious.

And he did. Four times. He would beat the cancer, but before he could truly enjoy the triumph, the disease would return for another fight. Once it came back in his liver. Then it moved to his lungs. Then it traveled into his bones, and finally it formed a tumor in his brain. Over a period of eight years, he battled the disease like a true warrior. He became a role model and an inspiration for everyone around him.

Still, as the cancer returned and returned and returned, I watched my father with growing concern. We were so alike, I had expected his experience would be similar to my own—he would take treatments for a year and then be fine. But his cancer was different. His treatment was different. As the years went on, this became more and more clear to me.

Whereas I had suffered hair loss, some skin dryness, and weight gain, my father suffered much more. In the last two-and-a-half years of his battle, his side effects became serious. He lost his hair too, but he also had blotchy and sensitive skin, neuropathy, acne rashes, peeling and cracked hands and feet (hand and foot syndrome), constipation, metal mouth, and loss of appetite. Some of his toenails even fell off. He was exhausted, and somewhere along the way he suffered Bell's palsy, which affected the nerves on one-half of his face, making him look even more tired and much older than his years.

I wanted to help. I went to the department store and bought expensive creams for dry, sensitive skin. But the solutions we tried often made things worse. The creams irritated and reddened his skin, almost as though they had burned him. Later, when he got a rash on his face, he asked me to get him a top-selling acne product. He still had to meet with clients and conduct business and support our family. How could he do that when his appearance was suffering so? I hesitantly bought him the product, but it burned his skin. It was a disaster. I felt so bad!

I had gone on from high school to study skincare and nutrition, and had become a makeup artist. Surely, I thought, I should be able to help my dad deal with these side effects that were ravaging his hair, skin, and nails. But I couldn't figure it out. I paid a lot of money to get the best products, and they were hurting him. I realized then just how sensitive his skin was—how much it had thinned from the drugs and how much nurturing it needed. I also started to understand that a lot of the alcohols and other chemicals in these products were much too harsh.

The process was so frustrating. Surely there had to be solutions to help him feel better!

What are All These Chemicals?

While I searched for safer products to help my father, he began to lose his appetite. Eventually, he was barely eating. I sought help from an amazing healer, Ora Abel-Russell, who soon became a very close friend of mine. She started working with Dad and implemented a cancer-fighting diet that called for whole grains, nuts, juices, and lots of vegetables. She knew all about fighting disease with the body's natural defenses, and she tried to fortify my dad's diet with healthy foods that would boost his immune system and starve the tumors. At the same time, she confirmed my findings about conventional cosmetics and the danger of chemicals in most of our daily products.

"Don't get him any deodorants, creams, or moisturizers that have chemicals in them," she said. "His body is too fragile for that."

Emboldened, I started reading the labels on all his products (and mine too!). Half the things I couldn't even pronounce. What was this *toxic* stuff Mom and I had been applying to my father's tender skin? I dove into the research and gradually educated myself about chemicals with the potential to irritate skin, cause allergic reactions, and even make certain side effects worse. I was especially surprised to find that some of the chemicals in common products we're exposed to every day—and that my father and I had been using—were potentially carcinogenic!

Immediately, I changed our approach. I began to seek out all-natural brands of creams, toothpastes, deodorants, hair-care products, anti-rash solutions, and more. It wasn't easy. There weren't many products that really targeted the dermatological side effects of cancer therapies or that offered nontoxic solutions. But with a little digging, we did the best we could to help increase my father's comfort.

A Legacy in My Life

I will forever remember my father's courage. He wrestled cancer valiantly for eight years, but in July 2007 it returned with a vengeance in his liver and lungs. By that time, he was tired. He had fought a long battle and he was ready to stop. He passed away on August 7, 2007.

A lot of you reading this book know what it's like to lose a loved one to cancer. It's devastating. Not only do we feel the sorrow of the loss, but anger at the disease that caused it. It seems so senseless. Why should this be allowed to happen?

I went through my own dark days after my father's death. I had spent some quality time with him before he passed, and I was grateful for that. We had shared some tender moments, and I got the chance to ask him questions I might never have asked had I not known he would soon be gone.

But once he was no longer physically with me, I suffered. I had crying spells that seemed uncontrollable. I felt as if I were in some other world between the here and there, and not really present in my day-to-day life. And I was angry. Why should cancer have taken him, when it didn't take me? I really didn't know how my family and I were going to go on without him.

But my father would not have wanted me to continue suffering. I could almost hear him telling me to get back up and make something of my life. I still had so many years to live. *Make a difference!* he might have said.

I started seeing a therapist, to help me heal. I began to express my emotions in a journal, and I found ways to celebrate my father's memory. At my wedding, which took place only two months after he passed, we released white doves in his honor. I bought a white candle just for him, and I still use its light by which to meditate. His last gift to me—an engraved jewelry box—I still keep close to my bed.

As time passed and the pain began to ease its sharp grip, I found myself remembering some of my last conversations with my dad. As best friends, we had shared so much while I was growing up, and in the end, we shared cancer as well. We both felt grateful to our cancer community—those who supported us during treatment—and we wanted to give back.

Now that he was gone, a new voice spoke louder and louder in my mind. It said that it was time to put what I had experienced to work. It was time to create something positive out of the challenges we had faced. But how was I to do that? I didn't know.

How Can I Give Back?

The answer came when I revisited the challenges my father and I had both faced during cancer treatment—from all the different side effects to attitude to perseverance. We had both struggled, trying to find natural, safe solutions, and our doctors weren't much help. They knew how to prolong our lives, how to perform surgery and administer drugs, and how to monitor our progress; but when it came to the discomforts and humiliations involved with the treatment process, they weren't the best resources.

The more I researched the subject, the more I realized that thousands and thousands of people were suffering as a result of chemotherapy and radiation, but few had access to information detailing nontoxic, gentle solutions that actually worked.

Worse, as I became obsessed with reading labels and finding out what I was really applying to my body, I became more and more concerned. We all use at least ten products on a daily basis, and most of these contain at least one chemical that can be potentially dangerous—many are linked to cancer. In fact, a study by Bionsen, an aluminum-free deodorant maker in the United Kingdom, found that the average woman applies about 515 chemicals to her face every day![1] As I became more and more alarmed, I recognized my new purpose.

I had to let people know. I had to help other cancer patients deal with these troublesome and painful side effects in ways that wouldn't further compromise their bodies. I had to get the information out about everyday chemical exposure, and I wanted to find safer and gentler solutions. Finally, I wanted to share my dad's courage in facing this disease.

I'm no medical doctor. I'm not a scientist. But I experienced firsthand the effects of cancer treatment—as both a fighter and a caregiver—and I can read what the scientists are saying. Besides, I'm passionate about skin and body care, and I can't stand the idea of people suffering so from these treatments.

Cancer has been on the rise for decades now, and we're still not sure exactly why. But the more I learn the more I'm convinced—the chemicals in our daily products, food, and environment are not helping us, and for many, they may be doing significant harm.

Cinco Vidas is Born

Convinced of my new purpose, I went to work. First, I created the business that would be the vehicle for delivering my new message: Cinco Vidas, which means "five lives" in Spanish. My heritage is Mexican, and my father endured cancer five times. Five times he renewed his commitment to life. It fit.

Next, I created the Cinco Vidas blog (www.cincovidas.com). This blog is my way to bridge the gap between the doctor's office and everyday life with cancer. Articles on nutrition, toxins in our environment, holistic therapies, natural and organic beauty care, personal growth, safe skin care, and more are available for reading and comment. My hope is that fighters, survivors, and caregivers will use the blog to find information and resources, and to share experiences and gather encouragement from the published posts.

I felt, however, that the blog wasn't enough. I wanted to reach more people, and provide a handy, accessible guide for navigating the effects of cancer treatment. I wanted to ease the pain and frustration so many cancer patients experience. And I wanted to create awareness about how we can live our lives without exposure to dangerous chemicals—and thereby feel much better!

If cancer taught me one thing, it's that we're strong, but we're also fragile. We can overcome a lot, but if we overload the body with stress and toxins, it's going to buckle under. When you think about it, there are a lot of things we can't control: the pollution in the air we breathe, the toxins around us at work, and the hidden chemicals in some of the foods we eat. Why not take charge in our own bedrooms, bathrooms, and kitchens, where we *can* reduce our risk of disease and increase our chances of staying healthy? Why not help the body fight its daily fight?

The Book I Wish We'd Had

Whether you are living with cancer, a cancer survivor, or a caregiver, or even if you just want to do everything you can to prevent cancer, I trust you'll come to the same realization I did: We can boost our immune systems, help ourselves feel better during treatment, and take positive steps to reduce our risk of recurrence.

If you've just been diagnosed, don't despair. You're not alone. There are so many of us on this journey. If you're in the middle of treatment, I'll show you some things that will help with your side effects. You'll also hear from real cancer survivors and glean advice from experts in healthcare and alternative medicine.

If you're a survivor and want to do all you can to prevent cancer from coming back, you'll find lots of tips for you throughout the book. If you're a caregiver, the following chapters will help you learn how best to ease your loved one's pain and discomfort, without making it worse.

Cancer changed me, not once, but twice. It made me realize how precious life is, and that we should be doing more to protect it. But truly, cancer has changed our world. So many people worry, at one time or another, about getting or surviving the disease. We *must* do more to prevent it. We must be more careful about how we treat ourselves, about how we deal with stress, and about what we apply to our bodies. Ultimately, we must change the environment that surrounds us to be one that is more loving, nourishing, and safe.

Let's get started with *your* world, and how you can make it more nurturing, healthy, safe, and ultimately, cancer-free. I hope this will be your first step toward a new attitude of tender and gentle self-care. Remember—in the end, the best friend you can find to walk beside you on this journey is looking at you in the mirror.

1

Cancer Changes You—How is Up to You

"I discovered you can't take care of other people until you take care of yourself first. I hadn't quite gotten that. I figured that out the hard way."

—Karen, two-time thyroid cancer survivor

NO MATTER OUR AGE, RACE, GENDER, OR PERSONAL BELIEFS, we all feel the world crack under our feet when we hear the word "cancer." I remember—and I'm sure you do, too—exactly where I was and who was around me when the word was first applied to me. I was too young to really understand all that it meant, but I did have a strong feeling that I was crossing a new road, and I wasn't sure who I would be when I arrived on the other side.

At first we may feel only fear. Many of us worry that cancer is a death sentence. Others of us dread the side effects of treatment. How much is it going to hurt? How will I look without my hair? We may resist being part of the "cancer club," where people go around in scarves and wigs.

"Too often the only thing the public sees about cancer comes from a medical standpoint," says Lynn Lane, prostate cancer survivor. "Things like hospitals, doctors, people with no hair, children in a St. Jude commercial, and older people. But cancer affects all kinds of people. If you looked at me at any point prior to and after my diagnosis, for example, you'd never have known I had cancer."

If there's anything good to be said about the disease, it's that it humbles us. Through the struggle, fear, pain, and emotional stress, we come to not only see, but *feel* that we're all fundamentally the same. We are human beings. We're fragile, and we're strong, though not necessarily at the same time. Ultimately, we deserve to receive gentle and tender care—most of all, from ourselves.

Make no mistake: Cancer will change you. When I came to the end of the journey, I looked back on the person I was when I first received my diagnosis and realized I was not the same.

Your hair may fall out, your skin may become dry, and you may (or may not) experience other physical changes in your nails, eyes, lips, mouth, feet, and hands. You may find your memory doing strange things and be unable to multitask as well as you used to. Most likely your emotions will run the gamut from joyous bliss to dull depression, even deep despair. And you may come to question many of the beliefs you've always held.

The one thing you can remember is that no matter what, *you are not alone.*

"No one should ever feel she's the only kid in town with cancer, or he's the only young guy with cancer," says Jonny Imerman, founder of Imerman's Angels. "When you're the only person in your world who has the cancer you have, you start to believe everyone else must have died. It's a false deduction, but that's just what you think, and it's an unhealthy place to be. There certainly are people who have survived—you just don't know them."

Throughout this book, I'm going to help you deal with many of the changes cancer creates, one at a time. I'm going to encourage you at every step to be gentle, and to remember to stop, take a deep breath, and be present in the moment, rather than getting caught up in worries about the future. I'm going to ask you to take the time you need to truly take care of yourself, even if that means reorganizing your priorities. Meanwhile, as we tackle each of these issues, consider this: Cancer will bring about a change, but the nature of that change is up to you.

"You have a role in how this turns out," says five-time cancer survivor Donald Wilhelm. "You're never going to be the same person you were before. It's such an emotional climb, you can't see back to where you came from. But you can choose who you are, today. And you can choose who you will become, tomorrow."

So take a deep breath, and let's talk about the changes that might be taking place in your body.

Who is This "New" Person in the Mirror?

"She told me I would require chemotherapy and that I would lose my hair. I cried and cried and cried. My hair is everything to me."

—Vel, two-time thyroid and ovarian cancer survivor

Many of us have had the experience of changing our appearance somehow, with alterations like haircuts and color, plastic surgery, tattoos, piercings, weight gain and/or loss, makeup, and clothing, and we realize that no matter how the outside changes, the person inside—that indefinable "I"—stays constant.

We know that someday the body will die, but most of us believe the soul will live on, in some form. Even those who believe the soul dies with the body have a sense of separation between the two. "We" are not our bodies.

So why, then, are we so attached to them?

The answer seems obvious. The body is with us every moment of every day and night. We express ourselves through it, experience the world through it, and use it to do everything we want to do.

Our culture, as well, has a way of overemphasizing the body. We learn as children that "presenting ourselves in a good light" is key to success in this world. I was certainly taught early on to use skincare, stay out of the sun (because of aging), wear tasteful makeup, and dress well—all to show the world the best image possible. I believed that I would be judged if I didn't look a certain way.

"I was raised to believe that looks are important," says two-time cancer survivor Vel. "I had to look good and put my best foot forward, so to speak. If I didn't, I was told people would judge me."

No matter how we might like it to be otherwise, people do form opinions of us based on how we look. At least initially. So we learn to present ourselves in the way we want to be seen. As we mature, we (hopefully) become more comfortable with ourselves, and with the face we see in the mirror.

Then cancer comes along and changes all that.

"I ended up with extremely dry skin," says thyroid- and breast-cancer survivor Karen. "I lost my hair. My nails cracked and broke. I had dry mouth. I felt like I lost myself. I was like, I don't even know who this is. Who are you?"

The biggest adjustment for me was losing my hair. It became my mission to do anything and everything to look as if I still had it. You may feel the same, or it might be the loss of your eyebrows and eyelashes that will really bother you. Your skin may become dry and your nails darken. You may lose—or gain—weight, and break out in rashes.

As treatments go on, one day you may look in the mirror and no longer recognize the person who's looking back. She looks different. She looks old. He looks weak. He looks decrepit. She looks *sick*.

We don't want to be "cancer patients." We want to be who we are; but how difficult that can seem when we look in the mirror and see—let's face it—a person who's ill.

That's why it's important, no matter where you are on the cancer journey, to make time for tender self-care. Not only is your body going through the fight of its life, but so are *you*—the soul who lives inside.

"When you're diagnosed with cancer," says Hodgkin's lymphoma survivor Jarrod, "your job becomes getting through it and getting better." The key to dealing with the changes you're seeing, and regaining your confidence and sense of self, lies in relearning the art of self-care.

Looking Good Can Help You Heal

"We splurged on my wig—I think it was the best thing for me because I'm young and I'm pretty social. I was a bridesmaid three different times during chemo, so I wanted to feel like myself. People don't even know I have a wig. I recommend that to everyone. It made me feel better."

—Jamie, non-Hodgkin's lymphoma survivor

Most of us care about how we look. I remember one of my father's most devastating side effects was an acne-rash from the drug Erbitux. I was surprised at how much it affected him. I mean, here was this strong, determined man, concerned about the image that looked back at him in the mirror. That's when I realized that none of us are immune to the changes cancer creates.

"Losing my hair was more traumatic than having cancer," says breast cancer survivor Laurie. "The cancer, I knew we would take care of. But what was I going to wear on my head?"

According to researchers, "Although we are admonished 'don't judge a book by its cover,' we repeatedly defy that warning as we go about our daily lives responding to people on the basis of their facial appearance. The impact of faces is shown in our impressions of people as well as in our behavior towards them, such as whom we help, whom we hire, or whom we ask for a date."[1]

Let's accept that most of us care about how we look and that there's nothing wrong with that. In fact, many studies show that when we feel good about our appearance, it boosts our confidence, energy, and ability to heal—and when we don't, it can have serious health consequences.

"Chemotherapy treatment for cancer can have a profound impact on appearance," says H. Frith and colleagues, "and [this] is often experienced as distressing."[2] Avis et al. also found that body image was related to numerous areas of quality of life in women with breast cancer.[3]

Feeling good about one's appearance can go a long way to boosting well-being. "The clinical and theoretical literature have emphasized the importance of self-esteem to the psychosocial response to cancer," says Katz, et. al.[4] In other words, when you feel good about yourself, you're more likely to reach out to those who can support you.

But the process is not as simple as trying to look like you did before. Instead, the key is to be willing to transform yourself into something that's still you, but fits where you find yourself on this new journey. Only *you* can make it through, despite the challenges, so how can you use the very essence of who you are to climb this mountain and become who you're meant to be?

"Findings suggest," says J.S. Carpenter and colleagues, "that self-transformation may be a factor in the self-esteem and well-being of breast cancer survivors."[5]

Laurie went through such a transformation herself, using colorful turbans and matching earrings and outfits to establish her new look. "I felt that not only did I feel good and look good, but it was cheering up the people around me. It energized me. I mean, when someone gives you a compliment, it energizes you."

Why Does Appearance Matter to You?

How we look—and how cancer changes that—can have a big impact on our self-esteem. I think, however, that to regain our confidence and achieve that transformation so important to healing, we need to examine *why*. Why do we care about our appearance? The answer can determine whether this care becomes self-nurturing or self-sabotaging.

Let's imagine two scenarios. We have cancer patient A—let's call her Sally—and cancer patient B, whom we'll call Barb. Let's say Sally was raised by parents who were overly critical, and as an adult she still considers herself to be unattractive. To compensate, she dyes her hair at least once a month, has had plastic surgery, and uses many products to try to change what she feels is a flawed appearance.

During Barb's formative years, however, her parents complimented her on her intelligence and gentle heart as often as they did her slim figure. Barb grew up to take pride in her appearance. She likes to dress nicely and cares for her skin with a little moisturizer, but she feels good about herself even on days when she can't apply makeup, especially when she's able to help one of her children solve a difficult problem.

How do you think cancer is going to affect each of these women? Obviously, both are going to face emotional challenges when it comes to the changes in their bodies. Barb may want to invest in a nice wig so she feels confident when going out, and she will definitely want a solution for her blackened nails. She will look for ways to care for herself through her difficult journey and will rely on the other parts of her wonderful personality—her gentle heart and her intelligence—to get her through.

Sally, on the other hand, could suffer more difficult consequences. She could become so concerned about her appearance that she piles on more and more products, trying to hide the changes cancer makes to her body. Since her skin may have become more sensitive due to treatments, those additional products may irritate her skin and cause uncomfortable reactions. In addition, she could be contributing more to her own self-consciousness by failing to remember the other valuable facets of her personality.

I urge you to think about this for a moment. Why do you like to look good? What is it that drives you? When you don't look good, how do you feel?

Let's see where your appearance meter stands. Answer the following questions, choosing the answer that sounds most like you. Be as honest as you can. No one is going to see this but you!

My Appearance Meter Quiz

1. I like to look good because:
   a. I'm afraid if I don't, others will look down on me
   b. It makes me feel confident and energetic

2. When I don't feel like I look good, I:
   a. Feel badly about myself all day
   b. Give myself a break—I know it's an "off" day

3. Most of my life, I have received the most compliments on:
   a. How I look
   b. My personality and/or achievements

4. My parents believed that:
    a. If I didn't look good, no one would respect me
    b. Looking good was important, but so were other things like working hard and nurturing my talents

5. I use:
    a. More than 10 products a day to try to look good
    b. A few key products that nurture my body

Now, add up your A answers and your B answers.

_____ A answers   _____ B answers

If you have more Bs than As, you probably have a pretty positive outlook on your appearance. You like to look good, but it's not the end of the world if you don't. You may still experience emotional difficulties with the changes cancer may create in your body, and I'll help you through those, but you've got a good start on learning to be beautiful from the inside out and on using self-care as a nurturing activity, rather than as something to help you cope with an underlying feeling of inadequacy.

If you had more As than Bs, you may be putting too much weight on your appearance, and thus may have more difficulty dealing with the changes cancer will create. Don't despair! There are many of us   in today's world especially—who end up wrapping our self-esteem a little too tightly into our appearance. Again, I'll help you learn to care for yourself in a way that nurtures your soul as well as your skin, and your heart as well as your hair. At the end of this journey, you may just find many other things that you like about yourself, so much so that hair or no hair makes little difference!

In the end, the question becomes: How can I learn to take tender care of myself and my changing body while nurturing my self-confidence and self-image? We're going to talk about that as we go along, but first, let's look at why cancer treatments cause difficult side effects.

What Cancer Treatments Do to the Body

If you have breast cancer and have to get a mastectomy, that's a radical body change that may require exercise and physical therapy to regain posture and movement. Colon cancer may require adjustments in your diet. Prostate cancer may cause changes in your sex life that require your doctor's assistance.

I'm not a medical doctor, so I won't pretend to be able to solve the health issues that may arise as a result of the disease itself. Please check with your doctor, and always trust yourself and your experiences—you know your body best.

What I can do, however, is help you cope with the side effects that inevitably come with cancer treatments like radiation and chemotherapy. Doctors are excellent at saving our lives, but when it comes to dealing with skin rashes, aching feet, or lost eyebrows, they are often at a loss as to what to recommend. After all, dry skin is not their primary focus—getting rid of the cancer is. When my dad and I were going through treatment, we definitely felt like we were on our own.

Your body makeup and previous condition will work as factors in whatever side effects you do or do not experience. The drugs used, the dosage, and the frequency can all make a difference. However, things like mouth sores, hair loss, dry skin, blackened nails, metal taste, skin rashes, and hand and foot pain are typical with many medications. Why do these things happen?

"The chemotherapy works by affecting the fastest-growing cells," says Dr. Stephen Green, breast surgical oncologist, "which are the cancer cells. What other cells are rapidly growing? Those that create hair, nails, and skin. Think of a guy—he's got to shave every day because the hair grows so fast. Chemotherapy also affects the cells on the inside of the mouth. Think of when you bite your gum—it typically heals very quickly. When you have chemo, you're slowing down that healing process."

Radiation acts in much the same way as chemotherapy—it kills off bad cancer cells. Unfortunately, it can do the same to healthy cells and tissues that are in the way of the radiation beam, causing side effects.

Once treatment is over, normal cells usually recover and side effects gradually go away, giving the healthy cells a chance to grow again. The time it takes depends on the type of treatment you had and on your overall physical condition.

Of course, I'm sure most of us would rather deal with a few side effects and live, rather than die of cancer, and many times that is the only choice we have. So let's review your concerns at the moment. Are you most worried about hair loss? Skin changes? Pain in your hands and feet? Sometimes just writing down the problem can help you feel more in control of your situation. We all know how cancer can make us feel *anything* but in control, so we're going to take baby steps to help you regain a sense of steering your own ship. Remember: No matter what changes you experience on this journey, you *do* have control over how you'll respond to those changes.

10 Things I Like About Myself

While we're talking about appearance, please take a moment to write down ten things you like about yourself that are *not* related to how you look. This will remind you of all the wonderful things you have to offer—hair or no hair!

Need some help? How about your talents, how you show love to other people, your skills, or your way with animals? Maybe you're a great cook, or gifted painter? You can even get silly—no one makes a bed like you do! It all counts.

Your turn.

I am:

1. _____
2. _____
3. _____
4. _____
5. _____
6. _____
7. _____
8. _____
9. _____
10. _____

"Most people, when they're given a cancer diagnosis, think: 'I'm going to die.' I want to encourage people to take their power back. Don't let cancer define your life. You define it. Be your own advocate, because it is your fight!"

—Lynn Lane, prostate cancer survivor

My Concerns at This Moment

Right now, the side effect I'm most concerned about is:

_____

This really scares me because:

_____
_____

I'm also worried about:

_____

_____

Can Personal Care Products be Harmful During Treatment?

"Some products on the market now are full of petroleum products, parabens, or other toxins that undermine health. I chose to steer clear from those ingredients when I could. Bodies battling and recovering from cancer don't need the extra burden of chemicals."

—Karen, two-time thyroid cancer survivor

Once you get that cancer diagnosis and find out that you have to go through chemotherapy or radiation, you'll probably assume that you'll have some side effects to deal with. Obviously, you'd like to find ways to cope with them that will not only make you feel more comfortable, but more confident.

My father and I certainly felt this way; but when I went out to the department store to purchase a moisturizer to soothe one of his side effects (dry skin), the product I bought actually burned his skin. As I mentioned in the introduction, this was a huge shock to me, and certainly a big disappointment. I never thought that a reputable brand of moisturizer could create such an adverse reaction! *What could have caused this?* I wondered. *What was in this premium cream that could possibly do such harm?* After all, I'm a skincare specialist and makeup artist. This just didn't make sense to me!

I became obsessed with reading labels. Some of the ingredients I couldn't even pronounce, so I did my research, determined to find out what they were. I was shocked to find out that some of them were harmful chemicals. I also found out that most personal care products have never been tested for safety by any public safety organization. Talk about surprising!

I wanted the best products for my father's skin condition and now I was dealing with products that lacked regulation, and some that had ingredients linked to cancer. As you can imagine, I took this very seriously. It changed my whole outlook. I started being much more careful about how many and what kind of products I was using.

Let's talk about how many products we all use every day just to get clean and look presentable. We've got toothpaste, mouthwash, deodorant, shaving cream, body wash, soap, antibacterial hand cleanser, shampoo, conditioner,

Who Am I Now?

In addition to taking our hair, our eyebrows, and even our breasts or testicles, cancer can make us feel endlessly tired, depressed, and worthless. Having to cut back on work hours, cancel appointments, or ask for help with regular tasks like shopping or cooking can all take a toll on self-confidence.

First, we have to deal with looking different, and then with feeling different. Remember—this isn't forever. Tell yourself you will get better. (Your cells will listen!) In the meantime, you are more than just a professional, just an errand-runner, or just a parent. Even when you're exhausted for weeks, you have something to offer.

Consider these ideas; then add some of your own.

I can still:
1. Make my friends laugh.
2. Write meaningful poetry.
3. Crochet a beautiful blanket.
4. Read and share good books.
5. Share a good movie with someone I love.
6. Tell others what I have learned through my experiences.
7. Help my child recover from a difficult day at school.
8. Brighten someone's day with a phone call.
9. Enjoy a slow walk with my pet.
10. Care about someone else.

Your turn:
1. _____
2. _____
3. _____
4. _____
5. _____

mousse, gel, hairspray, body lotion, moisturizing cream, anti-aging treatments, lip balm, aftershave, perfumes, colognes, a variety of makeup products, sunscreens, powders, and masks. According to the Environmental Working Group (EWG), most of us use at least ten personal care products every day, and my guess is that's a conservative estimate.[6]

Meanwhile, you may be surprised to know that many of these products can contain harsh and potentially carcinogenic ingredients. In a letter to

Congress, for example, the Cancer Prevention Coalition wrote that non-Hodgkin's lymphoma is increasing by 76 percent, due mostly to phenoxy herbicides and phenylenediamine hair dyes; that ovarian cancer (mortality) for women over the age of sixty-five has increased by 47 percent in African American women and 13 percent in Caucasian women, due to genital use of talc powder; and that breast cancer has increased by 17 percent due to a variety of factors, including estrogen replacement therapy and toxic hormonal ingredients in cosmetics and personal-care products.[7]

"Cosmetic products contain toxic chemicals that have been linked to cancer, endocrine (hormone) disruption, allergies, asthma, birth defects, and other health problems," says Dawn Mellowship, author of *Toxic Beauty: How Hidden Chemicals in Cosmetics Harm You*.[8] "Women, in particular, have a skin-care regime that exposes them to around 500 chemicals every day, and that doesn't include other chemical exposures from furniture, environmental pollution, household products, and more."

The EWG further reports that nearly 90 percent of the 10,500 ingredients used in personal care products have *not* been tested for safety by the Food and Drug Administration (FDA) or the Cosmetic Industry Review. In fact, the Cancer Prevention Coalition states, "It is now beyond dispute in the independent scientific community…that environmental and occupational exposures to carcinogens are the primary cause of non-smoking-related cancers." They go on to list certain hair dyes, pesticides, hormonal ingredients in cosmetics and personal care products, and talc powder as some of those potential carcinogens.

I was shocked to find out all this information. It was at this point I knew I had to do something! The good news is that we can reduce our exposure to these toxic chemicals and care for our bodies in ways that nurture us, rather than tear us down. Before we talk about doing that, however, let's take a look at your personal chemical burden.

My Personal Chemical Exposure

Read the following questions and write or choose the answer that best fits you.

1. I use _____ personal-care products a day, including things like toothpaste, deodorant, soap, shampoo, and makeup.

2. In the past, I've had reactions to various personal care products; for instance, my skin turned red, started to sting, or I broke out in pimples or a rash. **(Yes or No?)**

3. I often have unexplained sinus issues, like headaches, infections, difficulty breathing, or just a stuffy nose, and I'm not sure why—I'm guessing it's allergies. **(Yes or No?)**

4. I use regular household cleaning products—and I don't like the fumes. **(Yes or No?)**

5. When I bring my dry cleaning home, I notice the chemical smell in my room for several days. **(Yes or No?)**

6. I buy **(regular or organic?)** produce.

7. I often eat fast food, processed foods, and microwaved meals. **(Yes or No?)**

8. I find my underarms often itch as a result of using my antiperspirant. **(Yes or No?)**

9. I use nail polish regularly. **(Yes or No?)**

10. I'm always trying the newest beauty/personal-care products. I have a bunch of old bottles and jars in my cupboards and drawers. **(Yes or No?)**

This short quiz should help you begin to realize how many products you may be surrounding yourself with every day—and therefore, how many chemicals inside those products you may be exposing yourself to. Of course, small amounts of suspect ingredients usually won't hurt you, but when you use eight to ten products every day for decades, the exposure builds up. As you're going through treatment, it becomes extremely important to be very conscious about what you're using on your body on a daily basis. You may want to start using fewer products, for example, with fewer chemical ingredients.

In fact, I think it's so important to look at the potential harm certain ingredients in your personal care products can do to your body that I've dedicated the next chapter to this subject. As you learn to choose more nurturing and safe options, I think you'll find yourself feeling better. In fact, my hope is you may adopt new self-care habits you'll want to hold onto, long after cancer treatments are over!

Let's Review

- Cancer will change you, but who you become through the course of your journey is up to you.

- When you receive a cancer diagnosis, taking care of yourself becomes your new full-time job.

- Looking good can help you heal by boosting your confidence and making it easier to reach out to others for connection and support.

- Discovering *why* you like to look good can help you nurture your self-esteem in a healthy way.

- Cancer treatments like chemotherapy and radiation kill off fast-growing cells, resulting in side effects that need to be managed with tender care.

- Writing down your concerns about treatment and side effects can help you feel more in control and capable of dealing with them.

- By reviewing your regular personal care regimen, you can begin to see how your products may not be as safe as you thought.

Personal Affirmations

Choose the affirmations that resonate with you and speak them daily in front of a mirror, three times in the morning and three times at night!

I love my body. I love my life.

I attract everyone and everything in my life to help me heal.

I welcome change. I embrace change.

2

Your Skin is Fragile:
Be Careful with the Products You Use

"You don't want to have toxic chemicals absorbed into your body if you can avoid it. At least we can use some gentler products. It's one of the things we can take advantage of."

—Deb, breast cancer survivor

REMEMBER WHEN YOU WERE A KID, HOW YOU STUCK YOUR fingers into everything? Back then, it didn't matter if it was mud, glue, paint, clay, ink, frosting, or makeup—everything was open for touch exploration. Even if the material was a little unsavory (if you've seen a child poking his fingers in dog doo-doo, you know what I mean), no harm done—it would wash off well enough.

As we grow older we tend to be a little more careful about what we touch, but most of us still think our skin will protect us from just about everything. Beyond the occasional lasting ink stain, we feel that whatever goes on our skin either washes away, or at most—like in the case of moisturizer—penetrates a tiny sliver of the outer layer, leaving our insides untouched.

If you still believe this is generally true, I have news for you. Your skin is less like a wall and more like a screen door when it comes to allowing things in and out of your body. Cancer treatments like chemotherapy and radiation kill fast-growing cells on the surface of the skin, further reducing its ability to hold onto moisture and shield the body from bacteria and other substances.

Think of it this way. During treatment, your body is already working harder than it ever has to process all the toxins flowing through your system from chemotherapy drugs and radiation. The last thing you want to do is use eight or ten personal care products on a daily basis that can potentially add *more* toxic chemicals to your body's load.

I'm serious. That innocent-looking moisturizer on your nightstand could contain additional chemicals that a) could further irritate your skin now that it's so fragile, and b) could contain ingredients known to be potentially harmful to your health. Ingredients that sometimes are even *linked to cancer*.

Want to have some fun? Take the following quiz, and find out just how much you know about skin's ability to protect you.

What Do You Know About Skin?

1. Skin is the largest organ in the body.
   a. True
   b. False

2. One of skin's jobs is to regulate body temperature.
   a. True
   b. False

3. Skin "breathes."
   a. True
   b. False

4. Substances regularly applied to skin have been found inside the body, according to scientific studies.
   a. True
   b. False

5. Treatments that weaken the immune system have no effect on skin's ability to keep out bacteria and other harmful elements.
   a. True
   b. False

All right, short quiz, and you probably already know where I'm going with this, but let's look at the answers.

1. True. Skin is considered an organ, and it's the body's largest one. It weighs about seven to nine pounds, and removed, would stretch about twenty square feet.

2. True. In addition to covering the body, skin has a lot of jobs. It acts as a shield for your inner organs, regulates cold and heat via the sweat glands, relays messages of pain and pleasure to the brain, fights off disease with bacteria antibodies, rids the body of some waste products, and manufactures vitamin D.

3. False. This is kind of a tricky question. Our skin doesn't "breathe" in oxygen or exhale carbon dioxide like our lungs do. The circulatory system provides the skin with oxygen, but the skin itself doesn't "breathe" it in. As to the myth that if you're covered in paint you would die, you might, but it wouldn't be because of asphyxiation. Since skin regulates body temperature through the pores, and paint clogs pores, you could die of heatstroke.

All myths aside, skin may not breathe oxygen, but it does allow certain things to pass through it. Hormone and nicotine patches are evidence of that fact!

4. True. Yes, dangerous substances found in personal care products have been found—intact—inside the body. More on this in a bit!

5. False. Treatments that weaken the body's immune system (like chemotherapy and radiation) also weaken the skin's natural ability to protect you from bacteria and toxic chemicals.

Apply it to Your Skin—
And It Could End Up Inside You

"My skin was so thin it was translucent. No matter what I put on my hands it was never enough to keep them moist."

—Chris, non-Hodgkin's lymphoma survivor

Did you know that decades ago, scientists believed the skin acted primarily as a barrier—a closed door to anything we put on it? After all, we can take a swim without bloating up with water, so surely skin keeps everything outside us *out*, right?

Today's scientists understand it's not so clear cut. Sometimes skin acts as a barrier—by not allowing water to get inside our bodies when we're taking a shower, for instance. But other times—as during a long bath when our fingers shrivel up like prunes—things *can* get past this barrier and be absorbed by the body.

"A lot of what is put on skin is absorbed," says Alan Dattner, M.D., holistic dermatologist. "If you look back on history, one of the first occupational cancers was when chimney sweeps would get skin cancer from the coal tar and soot. You add moisture and humidity and you're going to enhance the absorption of anything, and then if you break down the skin's barrier because of detergents or medications or treatments, you can absorb things even more."

In fact, according to the *Chemical Hazards Handbook* from the London Hazards Centre Trust, "Although the skin acts as a protective barrier against many micro-organisms and chemicals, some chemicals can penetrate the skin and enter the bloodstream….Chemicals are also more easily absorbed if skin is moist or damaged."[1]

"Some of what you are applying topically is getting inside you," says Dr. Dattner. "We didn't used to think about that, but now we're more aware."

Now that you know your skin—and body—is susceptible to harm from what you apply to your skin, particularly when skin is fragile and compromised due to cancer treatments, let's look at what's in the products most of us use every day.

Traces of Makeup In Your Blood?

"I used to wear makeup, but during treatment, it really irritated me."

—Dee, breast cancer survivor

How would you feel if after a routine blood test, your doctor told you that he found traces of makeup ingredients in your bloodstream?

It's happened—and more than once. A recent survey by the Environmental Working Group (EWG) tested a small group of teenage girls and found chemicals in every vial of blood. Even more interesting is the fact that the chemicals were the same as those often found in everyday personal care products—like parabens, phthalates, triclosan, and musks (fragrances).[2]

Let's take a quick look at these four ingredients. (Don't worry—I won't make you take a chemistry quiz!) Parabens, for example, are preservatives widely used in personal care products. Simply put, they extend the shelf life of the product, keeping out microbes and bacteria that could sour the formula over time.

Look at the ingredient list on the back of your shampoos, conditioners, moisturizers, body lotions, and more, and you're likely to see words like "methyl," "propyl," "butyl," and "ethyl" parabens.

Go ahead. Take a look. I'll wait....

Found them? Okay. Want to know something a little scary? A 2006 study took urine samples from 100 adults and found two of these parabens (methyl and n-propyl) in over 90 percent of them, with other parabens showing up in over half the samples.[3] A 2010 study took urine and blood samples from sixty healthy men, and again found methyl and n-butyl parabens in 98 percent of the urine samples, with ethyl and n-butyl appearing in over 80 percent.[4] Methyl and n-propyl parabens were also found in the majority of the blood samples.

"Parabens are used as anti-microbial preservatives in a range of consumer products," wrote researchers, "especially in cosmetics. In vitro and animal studies have shown weak estrogenic and other endocrine disrupting effects of parabens, including reduced testosterone levels in exposed male rats."

In fact, a later study did link butyl paraben to DNA damage in men's sperm.[5]

Have I got your attention?

Next, let's look at phthalates, the second chemical found in the teens' blood samples. These are used as solvents in cosmetic products like nail polishes, perfumes, and hairsprays. (They help the product cling to the nail, hair, or skin.) They're also produced from the oil used to make plastics. An easy way to think of phthalates is to imagine them as the "product-changing" chemical. They can make hard plastics flexible (for products like shower curtains), make some products cling to other surfaces, and make fragrances last longer.

Unfortunately, these useful chemicals have been found to be potentially dangerous. One of the most common, called DEHP, has been classified as a "probable human carcinogen" by the Environmental Protection Agency. Animal studies have found phthalates to be associated with liver cancer and damage to the kidneys, heart, and lungs, as well as to adverse effects on reproduction.

In vitro (lab) studies have found phthalates disrupt hormones, causing potential developmental problems.[6] Yet according to studies by the Centers for Disease Control (CDC), phthalates were found to be present in the general human population—in a way the group described as "widespread."[7] In other words, virtually all of those studied had some level of phthalate byproducts in their urine.

7 Quick Tips to Lower Your Toxic Exposure

Want to start ridding your body of toxic chemicals from personal care products and the environment? Here are some quick tips:

1. Don't smoke (or quit smoking).

2. Clean up any mold around the house.

3. Buy organic produce.

4. Limit dry cleaning, and/or air out the clothes before bringing them indoors. (Hang it in the garage for a day or two.)

5. Choose your hairsprays, deodorants, and other personal care products more carefully: Read labels and look for natural ingredients you can actually pronounce.

6. Look for greener household cleaning products.

7. Choose nontoxic bug repellants.

How are these chemicals getting inside our bodies? According to researchers, through ingestion, inhalation, and by skin contact with products that contain phthalates. Further proof: Sathyanarayana et al. collected urine samples from wet diapers and found evidence of at least one type of phthalate in all of the samples. Over 80 percent of the infants had at least seven types. Where were they coming from? According to the researchers, the most likely candidates were baby lotion, baby shampoo, and baby powder.[8]

Did you know that the European Union has banned the use of phthalates in toys made for children under the age of three, as have Mexico, Japan, and Argentina? Cosmetics that contain parabens have been banned in Japan and Sweden as well. Yet these ingredients are still allowed in the U.S.

What's happening to our health as a result of this exposure? So far, science doesn't know. In other words, no one can say that this exposure *isn't* doing us harm, and preliminary studies show that odds are, it's not good for us. Of course, using a shampoo that contains phthalates a total of two or three times probably won't hurt you, as the concentration of phthalates is so low. However, as I've mentioned, when we use ten to twenty products daily for thirty to forty years or more, it adds up. Why put yourself at risk? Especially now that your body needs all the strength you can muster?

Your Current Routine—How Dangerous?

"When I see all these cancers in people who shouldn't have cancer—they have no family history, no genetic markers, nothing—it has to be our environment."

—Laurie, breast cancer survivor

I'll talk about the other two ingredients found in the blood samples—triclosan and fragrance materials—later in the book. For now, I'd like you to take a closer look at your own daily exposure to potentially dangerous chemicals like these we've been talking about.

Let's do a fun experiment. Gather all the personal care products you use frequently and spread them out nearby, like on a table, on a towel on the floor, or anywhere you can reach them easily. Include things like hairspray, toothpaste, body lotion, aftershave, nail polish, nail polish remover, body sprays, deodorants, sunscreens, anti-aging creams, masks, perfumes—anything you use on a daily or weekly basis as part of your grooming routine.

Now, let's look at how many times you're exposing yourself to ingredients that could be harmful to your health. Take a look at each container, and mark down how many times you see the following ingredients. Just make a mark for now—we'll count them up in a minute. For ingredients like parabens, make a mark for every one. For example, if a product has both methyl-paraben and ethyl-paraben, mark it twice.

If you see ingredients not on the list below, don't worry about it. We're not going to get an exact count here of all the ingredients that could be potentially dangerous. And don't worry   you won't have to learn or memorize all these difficult names! We just want to get the general idea of the chemicals surrounding you on a daily basis.

Ready? Go ahead.

My Daily Chemical Count

1. Aluminum:

2. Acetone:

3. Oxybenzone (or benzophenone-3, octyl methoxycinnamate, PABA, dioxybenzone, p-aminobenzoic acid, octyl salicylate, and other chemical sunscreens):

4. Sodium myreth sulfate (or any other "sulfates"):

5. PEG:

6. Oxynol:

7. Ceteareth:

8. Oleth:

9. Polyethylene:

10. Ethyl acetate:

11. Formaldehyde:

12. Fragrance (unless from natural sources like essential oils):

13. Hydroquinone:

14. Parabens (all types):

15. Mineral oil:

16. Toluene:

17. Petroleum oil:

18. Propylene glycol:

19. Dimethicone (or dimethicone copolyol, cyclomethicone):

20. Stearalkonium chloride:

21. Dyes (like FD&C yellow no. 5):

22. TEA, DEA, & MEA:

23. Urea:

24. Phthalates (like DBP or di-n-butyl phthalate, DEP, DEHP, BzBP, or DMP):

Now, total each line and take a look at the numbers. I'm willing to bet you had at least ten, and probably a lot more. If you were exposed to these only once a month or so, you may not have much to worry about, but remember—you're putting these products on your body *every day*, and usually two or more times a day. Let's say you had a minimum of ten of these chemicals, times 365 days a year, times thirty years—that's nearly 110,000 times that you've been exposed to these chemicals by the time you hit middle age.

You may be asking yourself—why are you bringing this up *now*, when I'm dealing with cancer? Is it really that important?

I think it is. Cancer tears down all your defenses. Not only inside your body, but outside it, too—and that means your skin. You may have absorbed some of these chemicals before your diagnosis, but now that you're going through treatment, you're likely to absorb even more, due to your skin's compromised barrier.

Truly, getting a cancer diagnosis makes you re-evaluate how you've lived your life, and I think that's a good thing. It made me look at my daily habits, diet, and stress levels. It was like getting a wake-up call to start over and make changes that would be best for my overall health.

This is the time you need to be building the body *up*, right? Not further tearing it down, or adding extra toxins it has to process through your liver, kidneys, and intestines. Your body is fighting a disease *and* dealing with treatments. It pays to be extra cautious! Besides, if you make changes to guard your health now, these changes will carry over for the rest of your life, helping you feel better than you may have ever felt before.

Alert: 3 Healthy Things to Think About

Before we finish talking about potentially harmful products and ingredients, I want to bring three more things to your attention. You're probably starting to get the idea that when you go through cancer treatment, your defenses take a hit, making you more susceptible to harm from whatever you may come into contact with. As you're learning to change your habits and take more care in what you put in and on your body, be particularly cautious of the following.

Antioxidants

I know you've heard about them. Maybe you've even studied them extensively. They're molecules capable of slowing or preventing what's called the "oxidation" of other molecules. You can think of them as cell protectors, for that's what they typically do in the body—protect cells from damage, including damage that can lead to cancer.

Antioxidants come in many different forms. Some of the most well-known are the vitamins C, E, and A, all of which are now proven antioxidants. Others are naturally present in foods like fruits and vegetables, and come in the form of "phytonutrients"—things like resveratrol, beta-carotene, and lycopene. Still others are present in minerals like selenium, which has antioxidant enzymes.

I mention antioxidants here because at the time of the printing of this book, most doctors want you to stay away from antioxidant supplements during treatment. That means no vitamins A, C, or E, and no supplemental lycopene, resveratrol, quercetin, etc. You may also want to check the ingredient lists on your skin care products for antioxidants, as skin can absorb them, particularly those used in moisturizers. (You can, however, eat all the antioxidant-rich foods you like.) The fear is that supplemental antioxidants will protect your cancer cells as vigorously as they do your healthy cells, making your treatment less effective. This is a very serious concern, and I advise you to always listen to your doctor.

As to whether or not this concern is valid is still up for scientific debate. Many studies, for example, have found different types of antioxidants to actually be helpful during treatment. Women in China who took vitamin E and C during the first six months after they were diagnosed with breast cancer, for example, had a reduced risk of death and recurrence of their cancer.[9] Another recent study found that antioxidant drugs, such as those used to treat malaria and diabetes, could help treat cancer, with researchers suggesting that we reconsider using antioxidants as anti-cancer agents.[10] And there are many more studies like these, showing that antioxidants can help kill tumors and reduce side effects during treatment.

Other studies, however, have found that cancer cells seem to soak up antioxidants like vitamin C, leading researchers to question whether the cancer cells might then use the vitamin to shield themselves against radiation and chemotherapy.[11] One animal study found that mice receiving antioxidant-depleted diets experienced reduction in their brain tumors, compared to mice receiving extra vitamins E and A.[12] Clinical trials in humans, however, are limited.

So far, we just don't have enough studies to draw strong conclusions. The whole thing is pretty complex, and it will probably be a while before science can give us any definite answers. Meanwhile, the best advice is to eat a healthy diet, and if you're considering taking antioxidant supplements, always check with your doctor beforehand to be sure you won't be affecting your treatment.

Essential Oils

Typically, essential oils are wonderful things that can enhance our health and well-being. We use them in aromatherapy to help relieve stress and clear our heads, and they're also often included in nurturing skin care formulas because of their protective and moisturizing benefits.

When you're going through cancer treatments, however, your skin and body are much more sensitive than usual. Things that never bothered you before may now make you nauseated or irritate your skin. In addition, some oils have the potential to act as hormone disruptors in the body. Following are some oils that you may want to avoid during treatment. These are not all-inclusive lists, so be sure to check with your doctor or naturopath if you have questions.

Potential skin irritants:

• Bergamot
• Lemongrass
• Melissa
• Peppermint
• Thyme
• Verbena

Some essential oils have what are known as "phytoestrogens," which have the potential to mimic hormonal function in the body. If you have an estrogen-positive cancer like breast, endometrial, uterine, or prostate, you may want to avoid these essential oils altogether during treatment:

• Jasmine
• Geranium
• Peppermint
• Rosemary
• Thyme
• Lavender
• Clary sage
• Tea tree oil
• Aniseed
• Citronella
• Eucalyptus
• Fennel
• Verbena

Soy

Soy, though naturally good for you, contains an abundance of phytoestrogens—natural plant compounds that can behave as weak estrogens in

Pink Ribbon Products May Be Too Harsh

You've probably seen the array of pink products that hit the market every October, which is breast cancer awareness month. You'd think that these products would be safe for cancer patients, right?

Not necessarily. According to the watchdog organization "Think Before You Pink," there have been several instances where either a product used to raise money for breast cancer contained ingredients linked with breast cancer (what's called "pinkwashing"), or where a company marketed pink-ribbon sales, but ended up giving little actual proceeds to the fight against cancer.

To protect yourself, ask a few more questions. How much of your money will actually go to breast cancer? Does the company have a cap on the amount they will donate? In other words, do they quietly say that after they've donated $10,000, they won't donate anymore, but may still sell the pink ribbon product?

Finally, read the label of the product you're purchasing, especially if it's one you're going to apply to your skin. Choose only those that do not include potentially harmful ingredients.

humans. Currently, there is a similar scientific debate going on with soy and cancer as with antioxidants and cancer. Some studies show that women can reduce their risk of recurrence with a higher intake of soy, but others have shown that phytoestrogens may increase risk of tumors. The type of soy we're talking about can also come into play, with soy in its natural form (as in soybeans or edamame) considered safer than processed soy, such as that found in soy milk.

Again, the current recommendation is that if you're suffering from an estrogen-driven cancer, you avoid soy products. I think you can probably still enjoy a few soybeans now and then, but you probably want to stay away from heavy intake of soy milk, soy sauce, miso, tempeh, and tofu. Watch out for your skin care products as well, as some include soy or soybean oil for its moisturizing and protective benefits.

Speaking of skin, let's talk briefly about how chemotherapy can break it down—another reason you want to be cautious with the products you use.

Where to Find Safer Products

In choosing the products you'll use during treatment, you're most likely to find natural, organic, and chemical-free formulas in Whole Foods stores, health food stores, and online websites like Saffronrouge.com, Beautorium.com, and Spiritbeautylounge.com. (Look at Appendix VII at the end of this book for more shopping locations.) Always read labels. Even if it says "organic" or "natural," refer to the "Ingredients to Avoid" list at the back of the book (or the abbreviated version in Chapter 2).

Chemo Skin is Fragile Skin

"Chemotherapy has a direct effect on the skin. You shed skin cells every day. The chemo slows down the reproduction of those cells, so that as they shed, nothing comes back. The skin gets progressively thinner and more sensitive."

—Dr. Stephen Green, M.D., FACS, board-certified surgeon

Chemotherapy causes dry, fragile skin. My father's skin, for example, was extremely thin during his treatments, and it took forever to heal. Plus it could no longer tolerate alcohols, synthetic fragrances, and harsh preservatives in conventional skin care products.

The drugs used in chemotherapy treatments kill off the fast-growing cells that usually renew skin's appearance, reducing the skin's ability to hold onto hydration. Lipids (or fats) between the skin layers are reduced, opening up spaces between them—sometimes big enough to let bacteria through. The fact that your skin is extra dry shows you that the barrier, which usually keeps water inside the cells, is malfunctioning, or breaking down. Side effects can include redness, itching, irritation, flaking, and dryness.

"Healthy skin cells are turning over fast enough," says Dr. Dattner, "that there is complete regrowth of skin from the basal layer up every 28 days or so. If you throw poison in the form of chemotherapy drugs into those cells, you're going to interrupt that cell division process, slowing the normal turnover and reducing normal thickness. The cells can no longer respond or generate as fast."

Dry skin, one of the most common side effects of cancer treatments, can create cracks, opening the door for products applied to the skin to get inside the bloodstream. "Cancer patients undergoing chemotherapy frequently

10 Tips for Gentle Skin Care

While going through chemotherapy or radiation, your skin is dry, fragile, and inflamed. Changing your daily habits can make you more comfortable and help your skin and body heal and repair.

1. Use only mild, fragrance-free soaps and hair-care products.

2. When using a towel, pat the area dry rather than rubbing.

3. Use a safe sunscreen (like zinc oxide) whenever going outside, on all exposed areas of skin. Cover tender areas with clothes and hats.

4. Avoid perfumes and alcohols.

5. Use lukewarm water instead of hot to wash with—hot water can increase itching and irritation.

6. Use an electric razor rather than a blade to shave when you need to. (Electric razors are less likely to result in cuts that can lead to infection.)

7. Wear loose-fitting, cotton clothing that feels good on your skin.

8. Apply a nontoxic moisturizer while skin is still damp to seal in the moisture.

9. If the air is dry where you live, use a humidifier in your room.

10. Add baking soda or ground-up oatmeal to the tub to soothe irritated skin.

experience skin problems such as xerosis," say researchers in a 2007 study.[13] (Xerosis is the scientific name for dry skin.)

Patients receiving radiation also experience fragile, "thin" skin, typically because of redness, burns, and even wounds and sores. On top of that, cancer treatments increase skin's sensitivity to the sun, making sunburns and itchy rashes more likely with exposure.

All of this adds up to one important thing you must do while going through cancer: Be much more tender and careful with your skin. This means you may need to adopt some new habits. Before you put something on your face or body, imagine if that something were *inside* you. Would you be okay with that? Of course, your skin is still going to protect you to a certain extent, but much less than it did before treatment.

So the first step is to choose your products carefully, which we'll talk about in the next chapter. The second step is to change your regular routine. Your skin can no longer hold up under fierce scrubbing, strong exfoliants, or extreme temperatures.

You'll find a few tips on how to be gentler with your skin in the sidebar, "Tips for Gentle Skin Care." Meanwhile, we've been talking about all these chemicals in our personal care products. Some of you may be wondering: Aren't there government agencies out there protecting us? Surely the Food and Drug Administration (FDA) wouldn't allow us to be exposed to dangerous ingredients, would they?

Well, let's look at just what the FDA does—and doesn't—do in the area of personal care products.

Look Now—the FDA is Not Watching

On the whole, our government does a pretty good job of protecting us. Take our food supply, for example. We have experienced a few salmonella outbreaks, but on the whole, we can purchase food in most places around the country and rest assured it's not going to make us sick.

I used to think it was the same with personal care products. If they were on the shelf, I figured they must be safe for my body. But according to the law, not necessarily. Cosmetic products, on the whole, are *not* subject to FDA pre-market approval. Here's a quote from the FDA website on the subject:

"The Federal Food, Drug, and Cosmetic Act (FD&C Act) does not authorize FDA to approve cosmetic ingredients, with the exception of color additives that are not coal-tar hair dyes. In general, cosmetic manufacturers may use any ingredient they choose, except for a few ingredients that are prohibited by regulation."[14]

Yep. You read that right. *Any* ingredient they choose. Of course, most manufacturers have voluntarily agreed to stay away from a few things that cause severe reactions, and from items that have been classified as poisonous. However, regarding the common preservatives and solvents and softeners and other chemicals I've told you about, there are no similar restrictions.

So who's responsible for the safety of our cosmetics? Ready for this one? The companies themselves.

Here's more from the FDA's website: "Cosmetic firms are responsible for substantiating the safety of their products and ingredients before marketing."[15]

That makes you feel safe, right? All you have to do is trust the people who are making money from these products to do everything possible to make sure they're harmless!

You may ask, "Why would companies put potentially harmful chemicals in these products in the first place?" First, they're cheap to use, so they help companies maintain their profits. Second, manufacturers have been using the same chemicals for decades and no one has required them to do anything different, so they continue as they always have, often ignoring studies calling attention to the potentially harmful effects of these chemicals and neglecting innovation that may provide safer options. After all, it's much easier to just keep doing business as usual, especially if no one seems to care.

There are many smaller companies out there that are more conscientious about what they're using and that work hard to create items that won't harm our health. As more people have become aware of the issue and have started buying from these companies, they have started to grow. However, even for these companies, there are some gray areas. Many of the chemicals we've been talking about—like phthalates and parabens—are under research right now because preliminary studies have shown them to be harmful, but no one (including the FDA) has come right out and said that companies have to stop using them...*yet*.

"The FDA doesn't have the authority to regulate the industry," says Stacy Malkan, co-founder of the Campaign for Safe Cosmetics and author of the book *Not Just a Pretty Face: The Ugly Side of the Beauty Industry*. "We're operating in an environment where companies, for the past 60 years, have been allowed to put millions of tons of synthetic chemicals into our environment and into the products in our homes, with no public safety testing required. Decades later, as the science catches up, we're starting to realize that the old way of thinking about chemicals doesn't work anymore."

Unfortunately, *proving* beyond a shadow of a doubt that these ingredients cause health problems is difficult, and expensive. You need the money to support the research, carefully controlled studies that come up with clear results, and methods to isolate subjects so you can determine what is causing the issue. Even then, there are so many variables involved in disease, particularly cancer, that isolating one particular cause is near impossible.

"You can't isolate a person for years," says Stacy, "exposing them only to carcinogens in baby shampoo to see if they develop cancer. Even if you could, that wouldn't be considered absolute proof. So we have to move away from this idea that you have to be able to prove something that isn't provable before taking action. When the weight of the scientific evidence suggests a chemical is harmful, we must find a safer alternative."

Meanwhile, some organizations—like the CDC, the American Academy of Pediatrics, the National Toxicology Program, and others—continue to work on research that will help determine the potential harm in many chemicals used in our daily products, but the results may not be complete until far into the future.

What we know now is this: Many of the ingredients used in our daily personal care products have been found to be potentially dangerous to our health in human, animal, and lab studies. The FDA has limited jurisdiction over what cosmetic manufacturers can and cannot do. That means it comes down to the individual to make the decision: What kinds of products will you use? Will you grab whatever is on the shelf and just "wait and see" if it causes any damage, or will you be more conscientious in your choices? I say, why take chances? Why not go with a precautionary approach and use clean, honest, and safe products?

In the next chapter, I'm going to show you how to become a more savvy shopper, so you're bringing home only those products that will truly nourish you—not add to your already staggering burden.

Let's Review

- Skin is less of a wall and more of a screen door when it comes to allowing things in and out of your body.

- One of skin's jobs is to protect you from potentially dangerous chemicals and bacteria, but during cancer treatments, the outer skin barrier breaks down, making this protective function less efficient.

- Science has found evidence that most of us are carrying chemicals around inside our bodies that, in many cases, may have come from personal care products.

- Your current daily routine could be exposing you to many potentially harmful chemicals.

- While you're going through chemotherapy or radiation, your skin is more fragile than ever and must be treated extremely gently.

- The FDA and other governmental regulation agencies allow cosmetic manufacturers to use most any ingredient they want in their formulas, except for a few restricted ingredients.

- Companies and manufacturers continue to use chemicals because they're cheap and because they haven't been required to come up with alternatives.

Personal Affirmations

I love and respect my body. I choose to use safe,
healthy products on my skin.

I lovingly protect myself and my body.

3

Enough Already!
Five Ways to Lighten Your Toxic Load

"The radiologist suggested a cream that had three different parabens in it. I asked the nurse about it—'I'm not doing this,' I said. She told me there were only small amounts in the cream, but I said, 'They found these in tumors!' And I got a paraben-free cream instead."

—Joanna, breast cancer survivor

AS A CANCER FIGHTER OR SURVIVOR, MOST LIKELY YOU'VE already been exposed to an overload of chemicals through chemotherapy or radiation. Surgery and drugs may have further assaulted your body with all sorts of toxins that your liver and kidneys and intestines and the rest of your organs have had to do their best to get rid of.

On top of that, you've been exposed to chemicals your entire life, probably at a much higher rate than your parents or grandparents were, simply because of the increase in chemicals present in today's environment. How much damage these chemicals have done is yet to be determined, but is it just coincidence that the incidence of breast cancer rates, for example, has increased by more than 40 percent between 1973 and 1998?

"A substantial body of scientific evidence indicates that exposure to common chemicals and radiation, alone and in combination, are contributing to the increase in breast cancer incidence observed over the past several decades," say researchers.[1]

The Centers for Disease Control and Prevention (CDC) have long been studying the chemical "body burden" of Americans, conducting a series of ongoing assessments of the U.S. population's exposure to environmental chemicals by measuring those found in a person's blood or urine. Their findings? Here are some of the highlights.

Polybrominated diphenyl ethers (PBDEs)— chemicals used to make certain materials fire resistant—accumulate in the environment and in human fatty tissue. One type of PBDE was found in nearly *all* participants.[2] Bisphenol A (BPA)—used to manufacture plastics and found in some beverage containers (like water bottles), plastic dinnerware, in the linings of food cans, and in children's toys—was found in nearly all the people tested.

Perfluorinated chemicals (PFCs)—used to make products that resist heat, oil, stains, grease, and water—were found in most participants. Mercury—which many of us ingest by eating seafood—was also found in most participants, as was acrylamide, which is a chemical formed when starchy foods are cooked, and is also present in tobacco smoke.

These are just the highlights. Over the years the studies have examined more than 200 chemicals. As mentioned in Chapter Two, the report indicates that phthalate exposure is also widespread in the U.S. population, and that triclosan—present in many antibacterial products—was found in nearly three-quarters of the people tested.

Why talk about all these findings? I want to get you thinking about toxins in *all* areas of your life—not only in personal care products, but in your food, your cleaning products, your gardening products, and in the environment around you. I'm hoping you'll begin to take seriously your exposure to chemicals that could be harming your health.

"When I plugged all the products I had used as a teenager into the Skin Deep Database," says Stacy Malkan, co-founder of the Campaign for Safe Cosmetics, "I found out I had been exposed to about 230 chemicals every morning. That included 17 classified as carcinogens, more than two-dozen hormone disruptors, lots of things toxic to the skin and/or immune system, and a whole bunch of fragrances. I did some research and realized that there are other choices—there are some really good products on the market that work wonderfully and aren't toxic." (Determine your own exposure at Skin Deep Database, www.cosmeticsdatabase.com.)

Stay Away from Synthetic Fragrance

Look on the label of any of your personal care products, and most likely you'll see the innocent looking word "fragrance."

That single word could stand for as many as 200 chemicals combined to create the scent. Manufacturers aren't required to list those chemicals because they're "trade secret," so you don't know what you're putting on your skin.

Science reports that 99 percent of chemicals used in fragrances are synthetic compounds derived from petroleum, including benzene derivatives, aldehydes, and other known toxic ingredients capable of causing cancer, birth defects, nervous system disorders, and allergic reactions like sneezing, itchy, watery eyes, wheezing, and headaches. Few of these chemicals have been tested for safety—particularly in combination with one another.

Give your tender skin a break and choose safe, fragrance-free personal care products, or those with natural source fragrances like fruit extracts. Some essential oils could still be irritating for your fragile skin, so it is best to stay away from them until after treatment.

After my father and I had both had cancer, we had a few "aha" moments as we realized some of the stresses we had unwittingly put on our bodies. I hope that as a cancer fighter, survivor, or caregiver, you'll realize your body needs your help to regain health and vitality. One thing you can do right away is to cut down on the amount of toxins it has to process.

The good news? Changing your daily habits to clear out the chemicals isn't that hard. Here are the basic steps:

1. Read labels on your personal care products.

2. Avoid certain ingredients.

3. Buy organic produce.

4. Safeguard your home.

5. Clean carefully.

That's it. You don't have to be a chemist, and you don't have to study for hours. It's really very simple and straightforward, and could give you the edge you need to heal from cancer and regain your energy and vitality afterwards.

Let's go over each step in more detail.

Step One: Read Labels on Personal Care Products

"I've gone to aluminum-free deodorant, and I use it only when I'm going out. I've gone to fluoride-free toothpaste. We have filtered water on the fridge. I've gone to a line of hand soap and hair products that don't use sulfates."

—Dee, breast cancer fighter

Our country is facing an obesity epidemic, and all around us we're hearing messages telling us how to change our habits to achieve a healthy weight. Many of these messages revolve around reading labels. Avoid trans fats, they tell us, which are now listed in the Nutrition Facts on the labels of most foods. Avoid excess sugar—you can see the number of grams listed right on the label. Many of us also need to watch our sodium intake, which we can find listed as a percentage of a set daily recommendation. (Go to Appendix VI to check out other ingredients to avoid in food.)

Isn't it wonderful that we have these clear labels to help us avoid foods that could sabotage our goals? Unfortunately, the personal care industry doesn't make it so easy for us. There are no "chemical exposure facts," for instance, like food "nutrition facts." Maybe one day our government organizations will require such a thing. Wouldn't that be helpful? I imagine change would happen a lot more quickly if shampoo bottles were labeled with daily exposure facts like: 21 percent phthalates, 15 percent parabens!

In the meantime, you can at least find out if a potentially dangerous ingredient is in a product by reading the ingredient list at the back or bottom of the container. You may have already learned to avoid "high fructose corn syrup" listed on food ingredient labels. You can just as easily learn to avoid "sulfates" listed on the ingredient lists of personal care products.

"But wait," you may say, "can't I just look for the words 'natural' and 'organic' and let it go at that?"

Well, yes and no. Organic products are a good place to start, but you still need to read labels. Just because a manufacturer stamps the word "organic" on a product doesn't mean it doesn't contain potentially harmful chemicals—or that it's safe for tender, sensitive skin.

"Organic" and "Natural" Don't Always Mean "Safe"

Personal care companies that want to make organic products are often on the right track. In other words, when seeking out safer products, organic brands are a good place to start. These are the companies that are, on the whole, formulating with fewer synthetic ingredients and chemicals.

Typically, if you turn over a bottle from an organic brand, you're more likely to read things like "aloe, orange extract, olive juice extract, and patchouli essential oil" instead of "bis-diglyceryl caprylate, ceteareth-12, methylparaben, and sodium laureth sulfate."

However, be sure you *do* read the ingredient list, as some organic brands still use potentially dangerous chemical ingredients that may be irritating to sensitive skin. The personal care product industry conforms to only limited regulation, so companies can put a lot of things on their labels without having to be held accountable.

The food industry has standards that a product must follow to be able to claim that it's organic, but there are currently no such restrictions on personal care products. The FDA does not check up on the word "organic" as it applies to makeup, body care, or personal hygiene items. That means that any manufacturer can apply the term to their labels—or other words, like "natural" or "pure"—even if the product itself contains few organic or natural ingredients.

Some organic products will carry a certified-organic seal on their labels (e.g. USDA, Soil Association, or Ecocert). These products adhere to a certain set of standards, but since there are no overarching organic regulations, or even an agreement on standards for personal care products, there are a myriad of different seals that any product may carry. The seal may signify a truly organic product, but it's difficult to be sure what percentage of the ingredients are organic (unless it's stated on the packaging), or what standards the ingredients had to meet to qualify as organic.

Remember, too, that "organic" doesn't necessarily mean "safe." Organic standards are not safety standards, as regulation committees are not toxicologists. Those who set organic standards are usually more interested in environmental sustainability than they are in safety for compromised skin.

When you go through cancer treatments, your skin changes. It becomes drier, thinner, and more sensitive than ever before, so even some ingredients that may be acceptable to normal skin may irritate yours. In addition, some ingredients that stayed on the surface layers of your skin before may now seep into your bloodstream because of the skin's reduced barrier ability.

That's why it's important to watch out for ingredients that can be harsh and drying, as well as those that have been linked to cancer, hormone disruption, and reproductive abnormalities. Unfortunately, even some products labeled "organic" could carry such ingredients.

The only solution is to read labels and avoid ingredients that could be harmful to you during treatment.

Step Two: Avoid Certain Ingredients

"I was always trying to put something on my face, but the creams felt like they were burning. I'd never had that before. I became blotchy in a way. So I went to this clinic and the lady there said to find something very natural, without a lot of chemicals."

—Chris, non-Hodgkin's lymphoma survivor

Now you know you can't rely on product manufacturers to tell you which products contain fewer chemicals. You're going to have to read ingredient lists. But every time you try, your eyes glaze over. After all, who can decipher all that mumbo jumbo?

I'm looking at a label right now. (On a product I would never use, by the way!) Let's see, we have water, cetyl alcohol, quaternium-18, stearamidopropyl dimethylamine, hydroxyethylcelluluse, dimethicone, fragrance, glyceryl stearate, citric acid, propylene glycol, DMDM hydantoin, PVP, disodium Peg-12 dimethicone sulfosuccinate, limonene, disodium EDTA, F239 di–boythisstuffistoohardtoread. (Just checking to see if you're still with me.)

No wonder most people give up! Who can ever be expected to decipher all that?

Don't worry! You don't have to understand all of it to protect your health. All you have to do is avoid certain ingredients that, so far, have been linked to harmful health effects. I've given you a list of those ingredients, and you can take it with you whenever you go shopping. (See sidebar, "Ingredients to Avoid List.") This abbreviated version works perfectly as you're getting started. Then, when you're ready to learn more, you'll find the complete list at the back of the book in Appendix V.

Easy enough, right? Anyone can do it. And it's a great way to get started on buying products that are better for you.

How did I choose these particular ingredients? Let's look at a couple of them.

I've already mentioned parabens, and that researchers found them in almost all urine samples studied. Let me tell you a little more about these preservatives. Not only do they have the ability to penetrate skin and accumulate in the body, they've been found to disrupt normal hormone function. Animal studies have shown that parabens have weak estrogenic activity, which means in the body, they can act like estrogens, interfering with the natural estrogen function.[3] Since some estrogens are known to drive the growth of tumors, you can see why we wouldn't want additional estrogen-like materials inside us.

Cosmetic manufacturers would point out that the amount of parabens in any one product is small, and they'd be right. But they're not taking into account the many products we're using on a daily basis that contain parabens and how our exposure accumulates over the years of our lives, to a point that could be potentially damaging to our health.

Another ingredient on my list is 1,4-dioxane. The Environmental Protection Agency considers it a probable human carcinogen.[4] Animal studies conducted by the National Cancer Institute have found that rats and mice

Ingredients to Avoid List

Copy this list and take it with you for reference at the supermarket, drugstore, or cosmetic counter. You may also go to www.cincovidas.com for a convenient print-out card.

1,4-Dioxane: known carcinogen; easily penetrates skin; watch out for "sulfates," "PEG," "oxynol," "ceteareth," "oleth," and "polyethylene."

Aluminum: found in mastectomy breast tissue; acts like estrogen in the body.

Hydroquinone: has mutagenic properties; hastens aging.

Parabens: potentially carcinogenic preservatives.

Petrochemicals (PEG): may cause premature skin aging; a.k.a. mineral oil.

Phthalates (DBP, DEP): linked to birth defects and organ damage.

Propylene Glycol: causes allergic reactions, hives, eczema; drying to the skin.

Sulfates (sodium lauryl sulfate): penetrate to the heart and lungs, promote allergies.

Synthetic Dyes (FD&C, D&C): most come from coal tar; carcinogenic.

Synthetic Fragrance: may contain hundreds of hidden harmful chemicals.

TEA/MEA/DEA: toxic ammonia compounds, unclassified carcinogens.

Toluene: in some nail polishes; linked to reproductive abnormalities.

Triclosan: can be contaminated with dioxins; endocrine disruptor; may lead to "super bugs."

Ureas (DMDM hydantoin): linked to dermatitis; release formaldehyde.

exposed to 1,4-dioxane in their drinking water had increased incidences of liver cancer.[5] And research by the Environmental Working Group has found that 1,4-dioxane readily penetrates skin.[6] Yet this ingredient is found in many of our personal care products, particularly in bath products used for children.[7]

You won't find this one on the label, because it's typically a by-product of manufacturing. In other words, companies don't put it in the formula on purpose, but it's created when other ingredients are processed.

For example, a common manufacturing process called "ethoxylation" adds ethylene oxide to other ingredients to "soften" them or make them "less harsh"—producing 1,4-dioxane as part of the outcome. Isn't it interesting to note that certain organic standards don't allow ethoxylation at all? The solution is to use less harsh ingredients in the first place!

"Companies should absolutely not be using ethoxylated chemicals that produce 1,4-dioxane," Stacy Malkan says. "Ethoxylation requires the use of ethylene oxide, a known breast carcinogen, in the processing of chemicals. Any company saying they're a friend to women with cancer should not be using them."

Dioxins Could Be Present in Your Tampons

Over the past few years, there has been concern about "dioxins" in feminine hygiene products. Dioxin is a by-product of the chlorine bleaching process and other manufacturing processes used to produce paper and rayon products. Tampons, for example, are usually made of cotton and rayon—rayon being a synthetic fiber made from wood pulp. During that process, dioxin is created.

The Environmental Protection Agency (EPA) has reported that dioxins are known to cause cancer in animals and probably in people. Because dioxins are widely distributed throughout the environment, most people have detectable levels in their tissues, and "this background exposure is likely to result in an increased risk of cancer," the EPA says. Research on monkeys has linked dioxin exposure with increased risk of endometriosis.

New bleaching methods have reduced the dioxin in these products, but it's still detected in tampons—even those made with 100% cotton. Even trace amounts are cause for concern because tampons come into contact with some of the most absorbent tissue in the body. The effects of dioxin are cumulative—it hangs around inside us for years.

Since current studies show little difference between brands of tampons and sanitary pads, you may want to look for all-cotton tampons that are unbleached, or switch to pads, since they have less contact with sensitive tissues.

You won't find 1,4-dioxane on the label, but you can avoid the other ingredients that may be contaminated with it, like sodium laureth sulfate (also on my list) and chemicals that include "xynol," "ceteareth," and "oleth" in their names.

We'll continue to talk about dangerous chemicals in our personal care products throughout the book, so for now, let's continue with the other steps in your new shopping routine.

Step Three: Buy Organic Produce

"I eat organic. I'll use natural products to color my hair. I get organic shampoo. I will not buy produce unless it's organic—same with meats. I shop at the health food store. I don't want to do anything chemical."

—Laurie, breast cancer survivor

Though important for everyone, it's critical for cancer patients and survivors to buy organic produce for one simple reason: It contains fewer pesticides, and the link between pesticides and cancer is quite strong. A National Cancer Institute (NCI) study, for example, found that applying pesticides (particularly for farmers) doubles the risk of developing MGUS, an abnormal blood condition that can lead to cancer of plasma cells in the bone marrow.[8]

Another study found that pesticides used on cotton, peanut, and soybean crops increased risk of colon cancer. They also found a link between pesticides used on food crops, pasture land, and lawns and increased risk of rectal cancer.[9] Other studies have found links between pesticide use and prostate cancer.[10]

Organic produce isn't necessarily pesticide free, but studies have shown that on the whole, organic fruits and vegetables have fewer pesticides than

Pesticides and Childhood Cancer

A study by researchers at Georgetown's Lombardi Comprehensive Cancer Center found a higher level of common household pesticides in the urine samples of children with acute lymphoblastic leukemia (ALL).

Researchers are quick to add that so far there's no proof that the pesticides caused these cancers. Still, according to another study published in *Environmental Health Perspectives*, children who live in homes where parents use pesticides are more likely to develop brain cancer.

non-organic.[11] So buy organic produce and thoroughly wash your produce before eating it. These simple steps can go a long way in reducing your exposure to dangerous pesticides.

Step Four: Safeguard Your Home

"I switched all the plastic containers to glass. I still use plastic wrap, but only if it's not going to touch the food. I put leftovers in canning jars instead of wrapping them up in plastic."

—Karen, two-time thyroid cancer survivor

Let's say you're reading labels, avoiding certain potentially dangerous ingredients, and buying organic foods. If so, you've already made great strides in taking better care of yourself and your family—congratulations! There are other areas, however, where chemicals can be present and make their way into your system. The biggest risk? Your home!

It's true. Many of the toxins that pose dangers to our health are present where we live. The bad part about that is they're close to us, which increases our risk of health problems. The good thing is, our homes are under our control, so we can make them safer.

Again, this doesn't have to be overly difficult. There are a few things you will want to be on the lookout for, and many of these you may have already taken care of. Let's take a look at them one by one.

1. Antifreeze. It's great for your car, but be careful where you store it. It's highly flammable, and if you breathe it in, you could end up with headaches, nausea, dizziness, and shortness of breath. If your dog laps up any spills, he could suffer kidney failure and death. Check for any leaks when you pull out of the garage (mop them up with disposable materials if you find them), and store any unused portions in a container out of reach of animals and young children.

2. Asbestos. Asbestos contains toxic fibers that can cause mild to severe lung irritation and/or long-term respiratory problems—and with long-term exposure, lung cancer. To get your own test kit, check out the Pro-Lab Asbestos Test Kit in your local Ace Hardware, Lowe's, Home Depot, or other home store, and take note: Houses built between 1930 and 1950 may have asbestos insulation.

Even if your home has asbestos, usually it will not cause health problems if it's in good shape. However, tears, abrasions, or water damage can release the asbestos from the fibers. Take the time to look over your home and stay free of asbestos contamination.

3. Asbestos floor tile. Some floor tiles, vinyl floors, and adhesives used for installing floor tile can also contain asbestos. Have a trained professional install or remove your tile, or make sure you're aware of what's in your materials if you're doing it yourself.

4. Asphalt/roofing tar. According to the Occupational Safety and Health Administration (OSHA), exposure to asphalt fumes can cause serious injury and permanent damage.[12] Some people worry they may be exposed in their homes during roofing projects. The Department of Environmental Health and Safety (DEHS) says that typically, exposure to roofing tar during projects is too low to be of concern, but recommends you keep windows that are downwind of roofing tar closed during the project, set the air conditioner (if there is one) to recirculate inside (not outside) air, or simply vacate the premises until the project is completed.[13]

5. Batteries. Household batteries are perfectly safe unless they explode, releasing toxic substances like lead, nickel, mercury, and lithium. Never throw batteries in a fire, and don't put regular batteries into a rechargeable battery station. (Attempting to recharge a disposable battery can lead to an explosion.)

Replace batteries all at the same time. Mixing old and new can increase risk of leakage. Finally, don't store batteries in your pocket or purse, as they could leak or rupture if they become overheated.

Wet cell batteries used in cars, trucks, tractors, and other motor vehicles contain lead and sulfuric acid, which can cause blindness, severe skin burns, and nerve damage. Never break the seal of these batteries, and be especially cautious when charging them—they can explode.

6. Arsenic. Some types of wood are treated with arsenic to prevent rotting. However, exposure to arsenic can cause cancer, dizziness, numbness, rash, headaches, and possible liver damage. To safeguard your family, ask about raw materials before purchasing them. Some alternatives include wood treated with non-arsenic preservatives and wood that doesn't require pressure treatment.

Dangers in Plastics

A lot of plastics contain bisphenol-A, or BPA—a chemical used to make plastics, but which has been suspected of being hazardous to humans for decades. More recently, it's been linked to breast and prostate cancer.

The National Institutes of Health also found evidence that BPA may have adverse effects on childhood development, saying, "…there is some concern for neural and behavioral effects in fetuses, infants, and children at current human exposures."

Found in the resin used to line food cans, BPA has been detected in the bodies of 93 percent of Americans tested by the Centers for Disease Control.

How do you avoid BPA?

- Limit your exposure to foods in cans or plastic containers.
- Buy frozen, fresh, or glass-stored foods instead.
- Seek out manufacturers that use BPA-free containers.
- If microwaving, use glass or ceramic containers, or plastics marked with a #1, 2, 4, or 5, which don't contain BPA. Don't cover food with plastic wrap—use a paper towel instead.
- Choose stainless water bottles, glass, or BPA-free plastic baby bottles.

For existing structures that may contain arsenic (like decks or picnic tables), apply a sealant to the wood at least once a year, and wash your hands after coming in contact with it. If you saw or sand existing wood, be sure to properly clean up and discard the wood chips and dust.

7. Shoes: Where did you walk today? What did you step in? Take a moment to think about all the places you've been, and then imagine all those places coming inside your home, for that's what happens when you wear your shoes inside. Recent studies have found heavy concentrations of coal tar (a known carcinogen) in family driveways,[14] and we all know how particles and debris can get trapped in carpets; so to protect yourself and your family—especially if you have small children crawling on the floor—leave your shoes at the door.

8. Water: City water or well water can be contaminated with small amounts of toxins. To protect yourself, use a water filter on your faucet or invest in a household drinking water purification system, which often includes reverse osmosis to trap chemicals. Beware of bottled water, as it is often no more purified than tap water and can contain harmful chemicals that have leached into the water from the plastic container.

9. Air Fresheners: A survey evaluated fourteen air fresheners and found phthalates in twelve of them, including those labeled as "all-natural." The report says, "The fresh scent of air fresheners may mask a health threat— chemicals called phthalates that can cause hormonal abnormalities, birth defects, and reproductive problems."[15]

According to the Global Campaign for the Recognition of Multiple Chemical Sensitivity (MCS), "Indoor air quality experts recommend *against* using chemical air fresheners and/or chemical room deodorizers of any kind."[16]

What if you want to clear the air in your house? Don't rely on candles, unless you choose safe alternatives. (See sidebar, "Candles Can Be Toxic.") Instead, try these steps:

- Use baking soda, which is nontoxic.
- Find and remove sources of bad odors.
- Keep windows open when possible.
- Add drops of organic essential oils to cotton balls and place around the house or use in a diffuser.
- Simmer desirable spices like cinnamon and cloves in a little water on the stovetop.
- Invest in an air purifier with carbon filtration.

Step Five: Clean Carefully

"I try to use cleaning products that are natural and don't have chemicals for disinfecting, the laundry, and for cleaning the bathtub. I use a lot of vinegar and baking soda. It's hard if you've done it a certain way your whole life, but I want to be around to see my granddaughter's children grow up. What am I going to do to get there? When you look at the things you need to change it's not really that hard. If I continue to do the things that contributed to weakening my immune system in the first place, I'm not going to get to my goal. For me, it's worth it.

—Karen, two-time thyroid cancer survivor

When I was growing up, my German mother was (and still is) a clean fanatic. She thought that a clean house was a healthy house. When I had cancer, she would change my sheets every second day and clean my bathroom

Candles Can Be Toxic

Researchers found that paraffin-based candles give off potentially toxic chemicals like astoluene and benzene (labeled as probable carcinogens by the EPA). Some candles have metal-core wicks, which can release lead and other harmful toxins, and some imported and older candles can contain lead-core wicks. Oils used in scented candles are often petroleum-based synthetics.

You can get around all these dangers with a few simple steps:
- Avoid paraffin-based candles. Purchase those made of natural waxes like vegetable, soybean, or beeswax.
- Keep wicks trimmed to one-quarter inch.
- Avoid candles in jars, as they don't get enough oxygen and can cause toxic black soot.
- Avoid synthetic-scented varieties and use candles scented with essential oils only.

daily. She did the same for my father. Towels were changed every second day as well. Watching her, I quickly learned to equate dirt with disease.

Though it *is* important to keep things clean when you're going through cancer treatments—particularly if your white blood cell count is down—we must be more careful of what we're using to do that cleaning. Just like long-term exposure to personal care products carries a risk of health damage, the chemicals we use to clean can do the same. After all, most of us clean our clothes, dishes, kitchens, and bathrooms on a regular basis.

I have made the switch to nontoxic cleaning products (and so has my mom!), especially with the new information linking some household cleaners to cancer. (See sidebar, "Household Cleaners Double Risk for Breast Cancer?) Again, all it takes is a few easy changes in your shopping habits.

1. Dishwashing soaps (hand). The Environmental Protection Agency has listed chloroform as a probable human carcinogen—capable of causing cancer. Did you know that if your dishwashing soap contains triclosan, that triclosan could react with chlorine in your water to create chloroform?

Many regions use chlorine to clean the water supply, so even if you don't add the chlorine yourself, it could still be there. Avoid dishwashing soaps with triclosan.

Household Cleaners
Double Risk for Breast Cancer?

A new study suggests that our everyday household cleaners and air fresheners could contribute to cancer risk.

The study involved more than 1,500 women. Researchers found that overall, those who used a combination of cleaning products were up to 110 percent more likely to develop breast cancer than those who rarely used them. The biggest culprits? Solid air fresheners and mold-and-mildew-control products—particularly when the air fresheners were regularly replaced, and the mold-and-mildew cleaners used more than once a week, which seemed to *double* cancer risk.

Researchers caution that though the study is worrisome, there could be other explanations for the connection. However, they write, "Because exposure to chemicals from household cleaning products is a biologically plausible cause of breast cancer and avoidable, associations reported here should be further examined prospectively."

2. Dishwashing detergents (automatic). Each time you put your dishes through the dishwasher, some residue is left that can later mix with your food. These detergents can contain chlorine-based sanitizing ingredients, as well as phosphates capable of choking off life in our rivers and streams. For a natural alternative, mix equal parts of borax and baking soda and store in a tightly sealed container. Use two tablespoons per load. If you have hard water, double the amount of baking soda.

3. Bleach. Bleach can irritate or burn the skin, eyes, and respiratory tract. Combined with acidic toilet bowl cleansers or ammonia, it creates toxic fumes. Furthermore, the chlorine in bleach can bind with organic material in the marine environment to create toxic compounds dangerous to fish. Use a bleach alternative, or try adding a cup of lemon juice to the wash cycle for whitening.

4. All purpose cleanser. All purpose cleansers can contain a synthetic solvent and grease cutter called butyl cellosolve, a hazardous petroleum-based chemical that can irritate skin and eyes, and over time, cause liver and kidney damage. Search for green alternatives.

5. Carpet cleaner. Some carpet cleaners can contain an ingredient called "2-butoxyethanol," which if inhaled or absorbed through the skin can cause blood disorders, liver damage, and kidney damage—even reproductive damage if exposure is long-term. In addition, they can contain perchloroethylene, a known carcinogen, as well as 1,4-dioxane, ammonia, and unknown fragrances.

If you clean the carpet in an entire room, your exposure could be high. Look for nontoxic alternatives.

6. Laundry detergents. We clean our clothes every week, sometimes more often. The clean clothes then carry traces of detergent in their fibers, including surfactants, brighteners, and fragrances—all of which can harbor suspected toxins. Since clothes come into contact with our skin for hours every day, skin can absorb those chemicals, to say nothing of the airborne particles that enter the sinuses.

To clean, most detergents use either anionic or nonionic surfactants, used to lower the surface tension of water. These present low-level toxins to the environment and can cause skin irritation. One common surfactant used in laundry detergents is nonylphenol ethoxylate, which in studies has been found to stimulate the growth of certain types of cancer cells.[17]

Fortunately, there are two easy solutions. First, you can purchase organic or natural laundry detergents that are fragrance-free and don't contain these chemicals. Second, you can make your own detergent, using ingredients like borax and washing soda.

7. Dry cleaning. Most dry-cleaning shops use a chemical called "perchloroethylene" (perc) as the primary cleaning solvent. The International Agency for Research on Cancer classifies perc as a probable carcinogen, with occupational exposure resulting in elevated rates of kidney cancer.[18-19]

What about organic dry cleaners? There's no regulation on the word "organic" in dry cleaning, so a company claiming to be organic may still use perc. Ask your dry cleaner what they use to clean. Right now, wet-cleaning (a system that uses biodegradable soap and water, computer-controlled dryers, and stretching machines) seems to be the least toxic option out there.

If you can't find a cleaner in your area offering this option, air your dry cleaning outside or in your garage for at least a day before wearing, buy clothes that don't need to be dry cleaned, and choose spot cleaning and a press when you can.

Goals

Three things I'm willing to do today to start shopping with my health and safety in mind:

1. _____

_____

2. _____

_____

3. _____

_____

Three things I'm willing to do this month to improve what's in my cupboards.

1. _____

_____

2. _____

_____

3. _____

_____

Let's Review

- To reduce your body's "chemical burden" and increase its natural defenses, all you have to do is make five changes in your regular shopping habits.
- **Change #1:** Read labels on personal care products. Organic and natural products are a good place to start, but be sure to always read the ingredient labels.
- **Change #2:** Avoid certain ingredients that are potentially dangerous to your health and/or have been linked with cancer. Take my "Ingredients to Avoid" list with you when you go shopping.

- **Change #3:** Buy organic produce whenever possible to limit pesticide exposure. Thoroughly wash fruits and vegetables.

- **Change #4:** Safeguard your home by becoming more aware of the toxins around you. Properly store potentially dangerous items, and keep the air in your home fresh and clean through open windows and essential oils rather than synthetic air fresheners and candles. Take shoes off at the door to avoid tracking in outside toxins.

- **Change #5:** Clean carefully, using homemade and nontoxic cleaning products and laundry detergents.

Personal Affirmations

I am teachable. I can learn. I am willing to change.

I am doing the best I can. Each day gets easier.

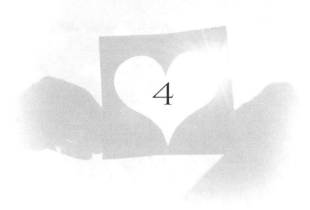

Emotional Coping:
What Are You Thinking About?

"If you meditate, if you exercise, if you play video games, whatever it might be, that's going to help your overall struggle. It's common sense to me that if you're mentally positive, you have something to balance out the negative, physical things you have to deal with."

—Jarrod, Hodgkin's lymphoma survivor

YOU MAY HAVE HEARD SOMETHING ABOUT THE IDEA THAT a positive attitude may help you in your journey with cancer.

You may have well-meaning people around you encouraging you to keep your spirits up, look on the bright side, and banish any negative thoughts as soon as they arise.

You may have seen or heard about other cancer patients fighting the good fight with big smiles on their faces and ribbons on their shirts and endless courage in their hearts.

These ideas may have left you feeling that you have to put on a fake smile even when all you want to do is cry. That you have to find the "gift" in this disease while your hair's falling out and your skin is flaking off. That you have to show others how strong you are when you can barely crawl out of bed, and that by will and optimism alone, you will come out healthier, more attractive, and a better person overall when it's all said and done—if only you have the right attitude.

Cancer isn't a test you have to pass. You don't have to put on your game face and proclaim to the world that you're a winner, and you don't have to "be positive" all the time. What you do need to do, however, is realize that, just as harsh chemicals can harm your fragile body, negative thoughts and emotions can overtax your fragile emotional state.

Cancer is as powerful an emotional struggle as it is a physical one. And science has proven that negative emotions weaken the immune system, while positive emotions help fortify the body's defenses. So there's no doubt that a positive attitude *can* make a big difference as you go through treatment and recovery. But I'm not talking about pretending to feel strong, or pretending you feel better than you do. I'm talking about processing those negative feelings that naturally come up and encouraging the positive ones every chance you get.

During my father's eight-year battle with cancer, he seemed to handle it so well that the running joke among his colleagues was that for him, the disease was like an allergy and all he had to do was take an antihistamine to go into remission. Of course this wasn't true.

My father had his share of difficult times throughout his journey, but his secret was he knew how to deal with them, and he knew how to keep himself on top of the fight. His colleagues didn't see the low moments that we did. They only saw how he continued to bounce back.

I always felt that I, too, recovered quickly because all I wanted to do as a sixteen-year-old was get better and get back to my life. I think my naïveté about the whole thing actually helped. But I also had my father's example to follow, and he was constantly saying that we make our own fate—that we can't give away our power to anything, including a disease.

Cancer can make us feel some of the most negative feelings we may have ever felt in our lives. The first time my dad's cancer returned (it had spread to his lungs), he told my family he needed some time. Then he went into a sort of cocoon, and I don't really know what he did there. I know he slept. I think he cried. Who knows how any one of us, in our most personal moments, deals with bad news?

But after the time was over, whatever time he had allotted himself, he would read, and read, and read, every encouraging book he could get his hands on. And then he would emerge, ready to fight again.

"When you're sad and stressed," says Colleen, a breast cancer survivor,

Guilt Has No Room in Your Survival Plan

Many of us, when we get cancer, hear this negative little voice in our heads whispering, "It's your fault. You could have avoided this!"

Then we get to thinking—was it because I didn't handle stress well enough? Maybe I ate too many hamburgers or drank too many sodas? I didn't exercise every day—was that it?

Stop! Guilt does nothing but tear down your immune system, stir up the release of harmful hormones, and leave your body more susceptible to cancer's harmful effects. There's no way you can know what caused your cancer. Doctors and scientists have been researching for years and even they can't be sure what triggers it.

What we do know is that a healthy diet, regular exercise, a productive approach to stress, and lower toxic exposure can help us not only reduce our risk of cancer or cancer recurrence, but can boost our body's natural ability to keep us healthy and strong.

I encourage you to do what you can to win this fight and survive. But don't waste a moment on guilt. It's a confidence-sapping, immune-busting emotion that has no room in your survival plan.

"and when you get bad news, you need to try not to sidestep the despair. You need to walk into it, breathe it, and live it, and then you will walk out the other side. When they told me I might have cancer in the other breast, I parked the car and screamed as loud as I could; then I cried and cried for an hour until I thought I was going to throw up. After that, I went home, feeling like it was done. If you really allow yourself to go down, the only way left is up."

I'm not denying that cancer sucks. It does. None of us would ever wish the disease on ourselves or anyone we love. Obviously we're going to feel angry about having it. We're going to feel frustrated dealing with the side effects of treatment. We're going to feel despair after six months of chemotherapy if the doctor tells us it's not all gone. And we're going to feel cheated if after a long fight, we end up losing.

I don't know how you've managed emotions so far in your life. Many of us aren't very good at it, as we were never taught how to process the more difficult feelings we often have. What I do know is that now is not the time to play the strong and silent type. Stuffing your feelings under a rug has been shown in studies to be toxic to your health, to say nothing of creating constant anxiety and uneasiness in your mind

Look at your emotions the same way you look at the drugs that are pumped into you—as things you have to process. Imagine them like a dam blocking the flow of a river: Until those emotions are processed and removed, we're stuck. The river doesn't flow because of the blockages, and we suffer because of it.

Taking an active role in dealing with the emotional side of cancer, however, brings you into the "eye of the storm," if you will, that place where your heart and spirit still reside, even while so many other things about your life seem to be blowing out of control.

"This project," says non-Hodgkin's lymphoma survivor Jarrod, speaking of a charcoal drawing, "kept me going through the most difficult of times and proved to be a great source of positive energy and purpose. Working on it seemed to offer me an oasis in a desert of despair and fatigue."

Let's explore some of the ways you can process your feelings, find joy in life even during treatment, and discover more about yourself during this difficult journey.

Make an Appointment to Process Your Feelings

"I kept focusing on myself getting better, and being able to have a future with my husband and my children and seeing my grandchildren. I had to think positively. My friends would read passages to me that would make me feel good. I said to myself, 'I'm not going to let this take me. I'm going to fight this with whatever I've got. Whatever I have to do, I will do it."

—Chris, non-Hodgkin's lymphoma survivor

The first step in dealing with cancer is to accept and acknowledge your feelings about it. The last thing you need after you've just found out you have cancer, for example, or just discovered it has come back after you thought it was over with, is to feel pressured into "positive thinking" by well-meaning loved ones. Feel however you feel, and realize that's perfectly okay.

"I believe in authenticity," says Colleen, "living the moment you feel truthfully. If you feel like, 'Oh my God, I'm going to die,' you don't want your friends to say, 'Oh come on, don't be ridiculous.' You need people who will say, 'I'd be afraid, too.' I wanted to be around people who let me talk about that."

What I like about what Colleen says here is her point about how important it is to find people who are willing to really listen to you.

People who dismiss your feelings can actually harm you without realizing it. If you're truly feeling scared about your life, the last thing you want is for someone to say, "Come on, get over it." Instead, you need to give voice to your feelings and be around people who have the strength to listen to your fears.

Science has been looking into the pressure put on cancer patients to "think positively" all the time, because it's become so prevalent a suggestion in the cancer community. One study, for instance, found that cancer patients should definitely not blame themselves.[1] "You may think if cancer were beatable, you should beat it, but you can't control your cancer," researchers said.

So the point is this: You can *relax.* You don't have to put on your game face when you don't feel like it. Cancer will take you through a whirlwind of emotions, and it's okay to feel those emotions. Your mood may change from day to day, and even hour to hour. It's normal, it's to be expected, and it's okay. You may have bad days, but you'll also have good days. Try to remember that the bad times—like the good times—never last forever.

What do you do when those negative feelings come up? Do you stuff them down inside you because you have too much to do at the moment to deal with them? Or because you don't want to scare your loved ones? Or because you have to look strong around your friends?

Many of us do this, including me! To this day, I still miss my dad. Sometimes those emotions will well up in me, but I won't take time to cry. The tears start coming, but I look at the clock and it's midnight and I have to get up at six A.M., so I think to myself, *I just don't have time to deal with this right now. I can't cry right now.*

I choke down the tears and go to sleep. But for several days after that, I don't feel well. I don't feel right until I've really allowed those emotions to come through my body. I've learned over time to allow my feelings to pass like waves. Most of the time, we resist actually *feeling* our painful feelings because we fear we won't be able to handle them. But it's not like that. A feeling simply has to pass through you. You need to acknowledge it, process it, and let go of it; then it's gone. It doesn't hang around anymore. However, if you don't go through these steps, the feeling stays with you. Most of the time, your resistance to the feeling is a lot scarier than the actual feeling itself.

Cancer requires so much of us. We have doctor's appointments to go to, work schedules to manage, families to care for, support groups to attend, and our own bodies to nourish. Where on earth are we going to find the time to process emotions?

I encourage you to make an appointment to do so. It's that important! Schedule it on your calendar. Maybe you'll take a weekend after your diagnosis to get away and process it all. Maybe you'll ask your family to leave you alone for an evening after a difficult setback so you can get through it.

I learned an exercise I'd like to share with you. I do this often, as it allows me to release any anger and to process feelings like sadness and fear. This is just one of your many options when dealing with emotions, and if it works, great. If not, I've got other suggestions coming up.

The Exploring and Emptying Exercise

Find a quiet space. This could be your bed, your couch, a spot under a shady tree, or parked somewhere in your car. Just be sure you won't be interrupted.

You may want to use a timer to give yourself ten minutes. During that ten minutes, scan your body from head to toe. You can start at the top or bottom, but go slowly, inch by inch, through your entire body. How does each part feel? Where do you feel pressure or tension? Where do you feel pain?

As you come to each area of discomfort, ask yourself: What is this discomfort about? Is it a side effect of chemotherapy or radiation? Or is it tied to some emotion?

Can you give the feeling a shape, or a color?

Feelings like anger often show up in our stomachs or in our muscles, as tightness or pain. Sadness can feel dull, like an ache in your shoulders. Anxiety can feel like pins and needles, under your ribs or in the lower part of your belly.

Whatever emotions come up, resist the temptation to stuff them back down. Let them come out however they want to. If you feel like crying, cry. If you feel like screaming, scream. If you want to pound on something, do so. (Make sure you don't hurt yourself.)

Stay in your body for the full ten minutes (or however long you need) until you feel whatever it is that's there. Sometimes it takes longer, particularly if you're used to stuffing your feelings. In that case, take as long as you can, then come back the next day or the next week and do the exercise again. The more you do it, the easier it will be to find those hidden emotions inside you.

When you're finished with the ten minutes, reflect on your experience. If you need more time, take it. If you need to process the feelings further, use one of the techniques we're going to discuss in the next section to do so.

Next, write down five things you discovered through this exercise. Maybe you're not sure the treatments are going to work, or you feel awful after your last chemotherapy treatment, or you're angry at God. Maybe you're worried about who's going to help you take care of your children, or you're embarrassed about how you look. Whatever feelings you're having, don't judge them, just write them down. If you need more space, use another sheet of paper.

I feel _____

_____

I feel _____

_____

I feel _____

_____

I feel _____

_____

I feel _____

_____

If you prefer to get help with this sort of exercise, check with your doctor as he or she may have a recommendation. Many psychologists and therapists are schooled in this sort of exercise. You may also want to try other practitioners who specialize in: a) craniosacral therapy, which focuses on enhancing the body's natural healing capabilities around the central nervous system, b) core energetics, which uses the body as a base for therapeutic work, or c) Bio Energetics Synchronization Technique (B.E.S.T.), a hands-on process that reestablishes the healing potential of the body.

The key is, you must take time to do this. If you keep putting it off, you're allowing those feelings to take up residence in your body. As my friend and spiritual teacher says, "If you don't do it now, you'll have to deal with it later."

The Mind/Body Link: How Emotions Affect Healing

"People were telling me, 'You need to be nice to yourself.' I was always pretty self-aware and I realized that not giving myself time to rest was being self-destructive. I remember thinking, you need to change the way you're thinking or you're not going to get through this."

—Alli, ovarian cancer survivor

Let's imagine a day after a chemotherapy treatment. "Your body goes through this roller coaster," says Dee, breast cancer survivor, "as though you've been hit by a truck." You have aches and pains, you can't get out of bed, your mouth is full of sores, your hair covers your pillow in chunks, and you feel nauseated. "You're on the couch and sick as a dog," Jarrod says.

On a day like this, most likely you're not going to feel positive. You're going to find it hard to smile. You're mind is going to hammer at you with thoughts like, *I'm never going to be the same again. I'm never going to get through this.*

Obviously these thoughts aren't pleasant, and they're going to make you feel worse than you already do. On this, we have scientific proof. For example, one study found that negative thoughts increase pain sensations.[2] Another found that the participants with the highest levels of brain activity in a region linked to negative thoughts had the worst immune reactions to a flu vaccine.[3] (Those with a pattern of brain activity associated with more positive emotions had the best immune response.)

Research has also found that ruminating or catastrophizing about your situation can make everything worse. "Research has shown that the more patients catastrophize, the greater their levels of pain…and frequency and duration of hospital stays."[4]

Negativity is just like the toxins we've been talking about in the environment and in our homes and personal-care products. We have toxins inside us, too, in the form of negative thoughts. "The way a person copes with stress has been suggested to be of importance for both mental and physical health," say researchers. "Negative thoughts may have detrimental effects on health."[5]

The solution is not to stuff the negative thoughts. When you do that, they hang around *longer*. It's like expecting the toxins inside you to naturally disappear without drinking water to flush them out of your system. The idea is to take the time you need to process your feelings—walk through them, so they naturally dissipate. This way, you don't give them power by building on them, nor do you allow them to stay with you by ignoring them.

For example, when you're thinking you might die of this disease or forever be miserable, instead of building on these thoughts, you can say to yourself, "It's okay to feel this way today. But I won't feel this way forever. I will get better."

If that doesn't work and the negative thoughts are still there, you can take a moment to write about them, or call a close friend to talk about your sadness, which will help you let them go.

"I think attitude is a huge player," says Meghan, three-time cancer survivor. "It doesn't mean you have to be happy all the time. It's okay to be sad. But it's not okay to stay in that sadness for days and months and years. It's okay to feel it, but you have to be able to move through it."

Tools to Help Process the Negative

"I think the attitude of concentrating on today and not yesterday or tomorrow has helped me get through it. It's important not to dwell—and it took me a long time to get there—but not to dwell on the negativity. Once you get into the negative mode it's hard to get out."

—Alli, ovarian cancer survivor

While going through cancer—or even just going through life—you're going to experience negative emotions. The key is learning how to deal with them, so they don't get the best of you.

One study found that patients with breast cancer who suppressed emotion felt higher levels of emotional distress both before and after diagnosis.[6] The opposite approach, however—expressing emotions—has been found to benefit physical and psychological health.[7]

Researchers found that breast cancer patients who coped by expressing their emotions surrounding the cancer had fewer medical appointments, enhanced physical health and vigor, and decreased distress.[8] In a study on women with breast cancer who used online support groups, those who expressed both positive and negative emotions experienced psychological benefits.[9]

Fortunately, there are many healthy ways to express and process negative emotions. In addition to the "exploring and emptying" exercise we went through earlier, here are some other options you can try:

- Write about it. Expressing your negative emotions in a journal (or a blog) is a good way to get them out so you can move past them.

- Write a letter. If you're angry at something—at cancer, at chemo-therapy, even at God—try writing a letter. Let all your feelings out—don't hold back. When you're done, burn the letter to signify letting those feelings go.

- Talk. Discuss your feelings with someone you trust, with a thera-pist, or with an online or in-person support group.

- Scream. Get into your car or another private place and just let it all out, as loud as you can for as long as you can.

- Exercise. Walk, jog, swim, punch a pillow—anything to get you moving to get the anger out.

- Forgive. Forgive yourself if you are feeling guilty about something, and work toward forgiving others if you need to. Forgiveness helps you release the anger you feel.

- Put your feelings into art. Paint, draw, crochet, knit, do wood-work—anything to help you express the feelings you're having.

- Try one of the many alternative therapies mentioned later in this chapter, or come up with your own. Music, dance, guided imag-ery, meditation, and more can help you express and let go of bad feelings.

Another thing I like to do is name the negative thought-bringer. You've heard of the old idea of how we all have an angel on one shoulder and a devil on the other. I like to use a little more imagination and create characters out of the doomsayers. Let's call this one Jason, after the character from *Friday the 13th*. (No offense if your name is Jason!)

Next time Jason comes along with all his predictions of doom, you can say to him, "Okay, Jason. I hear you. Thanks for bringing this to my attention. Now go away. I choose to think more positive and nourishing thoughts."

Then, you invite the sunnier thought-bringer into your mind. Let's call him Benji, after that adorable dog. Benji comes in with his sparkling eyes and wiggling body and cuddles up next to you and says, "It's going to be okay. You're going to get through this."

Do you feel the difference inside you? Can you imagine how your body feels when Jason is talking to you, as opposed to when Benji is around?

My Plan to Process the Negative

Within the next week, make an appointment with yourself to process any negative emotions you may be feeling. You can use any of the tools mentioned above, or choose one of your own.

Review the list below, choose the ones you're going to try, and next to each one, write the date you're going to do it. If you want to know more about these methods, keep reading, as we'll talk about them in the next few sections.

____ Exploring and Emptying   ____ Journaling

____ Letter Writing   ____ Talking with a Friend

____ Therapy   ____ Exercising

____ Painting and Drawing   ____ Dancing

____ Forgiving   ____ Guided Imagery

____ Meditation   ____ Music Therapy

____ Other (describe here) _____

Tools To Help Accentuate the Positive

"You have to be positive. You don't want to be looking at the downside. The downside says, 'I'm going to die.' I don't want to die. I have a lot of living to do. It was not my solution to die. My solution was to work at getting better and getting healthier."
         —Chris, non-Hodgkin's lymphoma survivor

Once you've used one of the tools mentioned above to process your negative feelings (don't cheat—you must actually *do* the exercise to get those feelings out!), it's time to encourage positive emotions. Below are several methods you can use, all of which will help you feel things like hope, joy, lightness, humor, and more.

Affirmations

Affirmations were my dad's tool of choice in helping direct his thoughts toward positive outcomes. It worked for him, especially when he did them in front of a mirror, and it works for me on a daily basis.

Affirmations are also great tools to use when your "Jason" (negative doomsayer) starts whispering in you ear. For instance, if Jason says, "You look horrible today, and people are going to notice," I say one of my most cherished affirmations, like "I am beautiful and whole just the way I am."

Remember that what you say to yourself is programmed into your sub-conscious mind, much like you might program a computer. It's a game of odds. You may not always be able to stop the negative thoughts from speaking, but you can consistently replace them with positive thoughts, until it becomes easier and easier to do so. Your daily practice is like learning to type: The more you do it, the easier it gets, until those thoughts become a part of you. Within a few weeks, you'll find you're thinking positively more and more often.

Laughter

Laughter is one of the best coping techniques there is when it comes to making yourself feel better. When I'm laughing, somehow I feel like everything is going to be all right.

"My husband is bald and he has a very good sense of humor," says Rayette. "After I lost my hair and I was bald, too, we got into bed and we both had on stocking caps because it was so cold. I told him, 'If we die in the night, I hope whoever finds us will jerk these hats off so they can tell who's who!'"

Studies have found that laughter increases the presence of health-promoting hormones in the body. For example, Dr. Lee Berk found that the anticipation of "mirthful laughter" increased beta-endorphins (that elevate mood) by 27 percent, and the human growth hormone (which helps optimize immunity) by 87 percent, and that the physiological effects of watching a humorous video last up to twelve to twenty-four hours.[10] Later studies found that the same anticipation reduced the levels of three stress hormones.[11]

"Laughter was the thing that got me through the first two cancers," Meghan says. "When I was thirteen years old I wore a hat. I was with my cousins and my aunt and my mom in the car, and we were driving along, and we pulled up next to this man smoking in his car. I whipped my hat off and said, 'Smoking kills, Buddy!' And we drove off laughing. What else do you have? I tried to make light of a really heavy situation."

"I don't think you have to take it so seriously," Rayette says. "You realize that if you can laugh at something then you're not giving in to it. It's kind of a way to fight. Instead of sitting around thinking this is the worst thing that can happen—and I did think that—but once you find the humor in it,

Music Therapy

Many cancer centers are now using music therapy as a complement to other therapies for their residents. Several studies have found that it's helpful for cancer patients; it increases well-being and relaxation, boosts the immune system, decreases stress hormones, and can even reduce post-operative pain.

Music therapy uses sound and music to treat physical and mental conditions. The methods are wide and varied. You may listen to certain musical recordings, play different instruments, chant, or simply put on your favorite tunes.

If you enjoy music and are sensitive to sound, check around your area for music therapy sessions, find soothing and healing CDs online, and/or incorporate music in your own way to relax and encourage positive emotions. In addition, be more aware of the sounds around you. Try to reduce hard noises like television, traffic, harsh music, and people shouting, and take more time every day for healing, soothing sounds.

as sick as it may sound, there are some things that are funny with cancer. There's some funny stuff! You have to decide it's kind of funny."

What else do fighters do to encourage laughter? "A fun coping thing for me was scheduling a movie with friends," says Jody, breast cancer survivor. "We'd go out to lunch and go to a funny movie. I remember seeing *Something About Mary*. We laughed till we were silly."

Something my family did quite often when my dad wasn't feeling his best was to order pizza and stay in to watch funny movies. Hearing him laugh always made all of us feel better.

Another nice side effect is that laughter increases blood flow to the face, invigorating the skin and brightening skin tone. Laughing people just look more attractive!

To get more laughter into your days, try these options:

- Treat yourself to a funny movie, and invite some friends.

- Try a laughter yoga class. I tried this one once and it's amazing how much I laughed! It was a total high—I loved it!

- Make it a habit to read the comics, or online joke-a-day websites.

- Try exaggerating your troubles to hilarious levels. Boost your self-pity to new heights until you can't help but chuckle at the silliness of it all.

Gratefulness

"I always felt lucky," Jarrod says, "with the kind of cancer I had, that it had a high cure rate. I felt lucky that I had a twin brother who helped me, and that I had a good job with health insurance. I really had that sense a lot."

By the way, Jarrod didn't have it easy. He had surgery and chemotherapy, and after six months of remission the cancer returned, after which he had chemotherapy again, radiation, and a stem-cell transplant.

Whatever your situation, you can find things to be grateful about. For Rayette, it was those precious days between chemotherapy treatments when she would feel more like herself again. "It feels so good to feel good after you feel bad; you'd be amazed how much energy you can have!" she says.

I know that gratitude can shift my mood in minutes. If I turn my attention from what I think I lack to what I have, and focus on all the gifts and blessings in my life, it's as if I'm suddenly looking out a different pair of eyes that see my life as rich and full of miracles. Sometimes when I need to get out of a funk, I'll write a gratefulness journal every morning for a week or so. It helps me every time.

Researcher Robert Emmons has long researched the effects of gratitude on mood and health problems. He found that participants who regularly counted their blessings were more likely to have feelings of well-being and optimism.[12] He has also found that people suffering from disease who wrote in daily gratitude journals got more sleep, felt more refreshed in the morning, and felt more optimistic about the future.[13]

"Every day I'm grateful for what I've got," says Chris. "I'm grateful to see sun shining and birds singing. I'm grateful for my husband, my children, that little compliment from a friend or coworker, and all the little things that make me feel good."

To bring more gratefulness into your life, try some of my favorite activities:

- Keep a daily gratitude journal. Set aside time each day to record at least five things that you're grateful for. On bad days, it may be things as simple as having a pillow under your head, or loved ones around you.

- Use reminders. Sticky notes, e-mails to yourself, or cell phone signals can remind you during the day of those things you have to be grateful for. For example, I have my cell phone programmed to go off every four hours with a message that says, "Take three deep breaths and be grateful for this moment that God has given you." It's amazing how that has turned things around for me on some days!

- Change your own self-talk. When it starts getting negative, switch to counting your blessings. Eliminate "should," "can't," "have to" and "but" from your vocabulary. You don't "have to" do the laundry right now. Instead, decide. Do I want to do the laundry because I like having clean clothes? Or would I rather wait until tomorrow? Choosing gives us freedom.

- Be creative. How else might you work gratefulness into your life?

Let's start now. Below, write five things you're grateful for. To help you, I'll go first.

1. I'm grateful that I woke up. Today is a gift, not to be taken for granted.

2. I'm grateful for the hot shower I get to take every day that helps my muscles and my mind relax.

3. I'm grateful the sunshine came out this afternoon, which reminds me there is always light at the end of the tunnel.

4. I'm grateful that my best friend accepts me exactly as I am.

5. I'm grateful for my father's spirit, who reminds me every day to go after my dreams relentlessly.

Okay, your turn:

1. I'm grateful for_____

_____

2. I'm grateful for_____

_____

3. I'm grateful for_____

_____

4. I'm grateful for_____

_____

5. I'm grateful for_____

_____

Meditation

Meditation has changed my life. It not only helps calm my mind and keep me centered, but it also allows me to better cope with stress. What's even more amazing is that in cancer patients, studies have shown meditation helps improve mood and anxiety and enhance coping and well-being.[14-15]

"You have to find that even, emotional space to live in," says Hillary, melanoma survivor. "Meditation has been an incredible tool that helps me see things for what they are, find more levity in day-to-day living, and not take things so seriously. I find when I meditate for twenty minutes a day on a regular basis, I have a skip in my step."

Meditation helps quiet those negative thoughts so they don't get out of hand. "We talk to ourselves all the time," says Fran Greenfield, author and mind/body healing teacher. "The mind judges, complains, compares, and generally does a running commentary on life at every moment. Unless we find a way to disengage from this morass of undirected, unconscious thought, we run the risk of giving our bodies toxic messages that can literally make us sick."

Meditation can be as simple as taking twenty minutes every day to sit in a quiet room, perhaps with a lit candle, and concentrate on your breath. You can take a walk in the park and focus only on the movement of your body, or try some of the many guided meditation videos and CDs available online or at your local bookstore. I've also listed my favorite meditation CDs in Appendix IV. Whatever you do, the idea is to regain a feeling of calm and bring yourself back into the present moment—because the present moment is really all we've got!

Prayer—Have Faith

"Focusing on God's word brings me calmness," says Joanna, breast cancer survivor.

"I'm a church member and my church family was very supportive," says Chris, non-Hodgkin's lymphoma survivor. "The power of prayer is important to me, too. I had a lot of people praying for me and helping me through it."

No matter what your own personal beliefs, prayer can be a powerful way to process your emotions and encourage healing. Every night, I turn over all my worries and fears to God. I know he can handle them a lot better than I ever could! My faith brings me serenity and peace of mind like nothing else in my life. I talk to God about everything. I bring him to my doctor's appointments, my meetings, and any situation I don't want to deal with. Life is so much smoother when I let him handle all the details.

If you're feeling angry at God, or whatever ultimate power you believe in, don't be afraid to talk to him about it. Express your feelings and ask for answers. Pray for your own acceptance of where you are in life, and ask for signs to show you the purpose in your journey.

Whatever religion or spiritual practice you may have tried before in your life, now is a good time to reconnect, or to seek out a faith that feels right to you. Friends and loved ones can be of enormous support during this time, but you also need something that feels greater than you—a powerful energy in which you can put your trust.

"I think it's a combination of a certain spiritual belief that there is a universe or a God or whatever you want to call it," says Deb, breast cancer survivor. "For me, it's a belief in God, a faith that there's somebody greater than me in charge. If I have faith and choose to live my life in faith and hope and love and gratitude, I will continue to come to a better place."

Prayer can give you strength. It can give you peace. It can help you to step outside yourself and realize that no matter what happens, you're not alone.

Guided Imagery

"Once we wake up and acknowledge that thoughts and beliefs wield power," says Fran Greenfield, "we can create a new relationship with life and with ourselves."

The term "guided imagery" refers to a wide variety of techniques that focus and direct the imagination to help speed healing, relieve pain, and process negative emotions. It may involve visualization, game playing, dream interpretation, drawing, and more. The idea is to use the unconscious to help the conscious mind deal with current life issues.

You can find information and guided imagery techniques online and in bookstores. Fran recommends the following exercise if you're ever feeling "stuck."

- Close your eyes and breathe out three times.

- See yourself in the museum of your life.

- See all the statues and artifacts that fill these rooms and hallways.

- Sense and know how these creations prevent you from living freely and wholly in the present.

- Breathe out one time.

- Walk through this museum and in any way you choose, break apart and destroy these constructions.

- Once you have done this, clear away the debris and get rid of it.

- See what happens and notice how you feel.

- Breathe out, open your eyes, and return.

Journaling

"I wrote in my journal all the time," says Jamie, non-Hodgkin's lymphoma survivor. "I was able to say what was going on and keep track of everything. It helps you to write stuff down. I think it's just because you're able to get your thoughts out. You don't want to be constantly talking about it. I had that place to vent."

A study of students with a history of trauma showed that whether the participants were writing about coping themselves or helping others cope, just the act of writing improved their physical symptoms.[16] Another found that patients with mild to moderately severe asthma or rheumatoid arthritis who wrote about their experiences actually got better.[17]

Even more to the point—another study found that cancer patients who wrote about their feelings prior to treatment said the writing changed their thoughts about the illness, and these changes were associated with improved physical quality of life.[18] After the exercise, patients said things like "Writing helps me stand back and reflect on what has happened" and "I felt a lot calmer and more able to move on after writing about it and being forced to think about it."

This comes back to processing those negative feelings we were talking about earlier. Journaling helps you empty your thoughts on paper, which helps you get out of that negative funk. For me, my blog (www.cincovidas. com) has been an amazing way to get my feelings out, and at the same time help so many people. It's encouraged me to deal with my own journey with cancer as well as to grieve for my father. I know many other survivors, as well, who have started a blog to share their experiences and to keep their friends and family updated on their journey.

"I used to write a lot of times in the middle of the night when I couldn't sleep," says Alli, ovarian cancer survivor. "I didn't overthink how I was typing, I just typed how I felt. It allowed me to release those feelings, let them go, and keep them from building up."

Pet Therapy

For many survivors, pets help them cope with those days when nothing seems to be going right.

"At the time I had my dog," Alli says, "my Golden Retriever who was the love of my life. He would get up on the bed with me and let me cry into his fur."

Researchers examined the effects of animal contact on a group of patients with cancer. Fifteen patients took part in a ten-week study of ninety-minute weekly sessions with visiting dogs. Results showed that those who had contact with the visiting dogs experienced decreased anxiety and despair.

Do you need something to get you up and going? Someone with whom you can share an afternoon walk? A pet is a big investment, but it may be just what you need.

Writing down your experiences can also help you find some meaning in the challenges you overcome. "I'm writing a memoir about my journey," says Meghan Black, three-time cancer survivor. "I've had cancer from my very early teen years to my mid-teens to my later twenties, when I was married and trying to have kids. I've had a full life, and more than half has been dealing with this disease. Part of my book is that I want to try to give someone a nugget, a piece of hope, just as much for other patients as for their friends, husbands, wives, and parents. To help them all understand."

My father always wanted to write a book. He survived so much in his life, including cancer in five different areas of his body (colon, lung, liver, bone, and brain). I think that's why writing this book became so important to me, as I think of it as a book for both of us. In a lot of ways, it's been an extension of the healing I started with the blog.

Try it. Of course, you don't have to write a book or a blog, unless you want to. You can just write whatever you feel in whatever notebook you like. It costs very little to find that special notebook or journaling pad or blogging page where you can pour out all your frustrations, sadness, anger, and despair—as well as your joys, gratitude, prayers, and funny stories. Once it's all on paper, you may find it a lot easier to see the bright side of things.

You may also find writing workshops in your area that are specifically for cancer patients. Check on "Writing Through Cancer" and "Wellspring Writers" to get started.

Reading

I mentioned earlier that when my father was struggling through difficult times, he would read whatever books he could find that would inspire him.

What we put into our minds can make a huge difference in how we feel. For example, how are your emotions after seeing a sad movie or reading a tragic story? Most likely, you feel a little down. You can create the opposite effect by reading books that pump you up, encourage you, and help you feel good about yourself.

I've created a reading list at the back of this book that contains the materials I felt were most helpful while my father and I were going through cancer. Please feel free to peruse that list and read anything that resonates with you, or take a trip to the bookstore and look around.

If you like to read, use it to encourage yourself to feel better. Even a comic book can do the trick!

Art Therapy

You don't have to be an artist to benefit from art therapy. Studies have found it helps cancer patients improve self-esteem and lower anxiety and depression.[19-20]

Many cancer centers now offer art therapy classes. Typically, these involve more than just drawing or painting, though these activities can be helpful as well.

"One thing I did during chemotherapy," says Laurie, breast cancer survivor, "is called 'soul collage.' You take a 5x8 card, make a collage on it with different pictures, and then you tell something about it. I had one that was this big scary fish with big teeth. It was my fear card. It helped me identify my fears, and my courage."

If you like working with your hands, look for art classes at your cancer center or in your area. You may even try learning something new, like painting, ceramics, or woodwork. While you're engaged in the activity, you'll find yourself thinking less about your cancer and more about how you're enjoying yourself.

"Art was a major thing to get me through all of it," Jarrod says. "It was something to do, something to keep me occupied, and it was fun, too."

Forgiveness

You've probably heard about the power of forgiveness. In the realm of health, forgiveness is huge because it helps release built-up negative emotions, allowing the body to let go and relax.

Science has confirmed this. One study showed that when people who felt victimized by others forgave their offenders, they experienced more self-control and less stress in the body. Nursing grudges, on the other hand, prompted more negative emotions and created higher blood pressure and heart rate.[21]

Another larger review of several studies concluded that forgiveness is more important than ever as an issue in healthcare.[22]

There are many times I've gotten help in forgiving someone who has wronged me. I actually went to a therapist for it, as I knew that only by going through the process and truly *feeling* the forgiveness could I ever reap the benefits. Now, I make it a habit in my daily prayers to do a mental scan of my feelings. If I'm holding onto any resentment, I forgive that person, then visualize myself cutting the rope connecting the two of us and setting him or her free. This sets me free as well, and helps me avoid the "heavy burden" I walk around with when I carry resentment.

If you're nursing some old hurts, try the following simple steps. If these don't lead you to a true feeling of forgiveness, care enough about yourself to seek help. By not forgiving others, you're only keeping yourself a prisoner. You need all your energy to heal right now, and you can't afford to be spending it on old grudges.

1. Face what happened to you. Write about it, talk about it, or just go over it in your mind. It happened, and you can't change it now. Realize that your feelings about it are hurting you.

2. Resolve to let go of your angry and bitter feelings.

3. Remember what it was that really hurt you. Write it down if you want to.

4. Recognize that the person may not have realized how his actions would affect you. Even if he did, perhaps he was acting out of an old pain or injury he had experienced. Maybe she didn't know how else to handle her own emotions. Try to find compassion for the person.

5. Imagine what it would feel like to forgive. Imagine how much better you would feel, how much lighter. Feel in your body the airiness that comes with letting go of this hurt.

6. Ask yourself: What purpose is it serving to keep holding on? Am I ready to let go now?

7. If you can let go, feel the release inside you, and experience the peace.

8. If you're not yet ready to let go, ask yourself, "Okay, when will I be ready?" Repeat this exercise again at that time, but realize that you will continue to carry around these negative emotions until then.

Deep Breathing

How do you normally breathe? Are you uptight, breathing mostly from the chest? Did you know that it's healthier and more relaxing to breathe from lower in the body, near the belly?

When you relax and breathe deeply from the diaphragm, it has numerous benefits. It relieves stress, improves circulation, assists proper digestion, helps eliminate toxins, releases anxiety, lowers your blood pressure, and helps release feel-good hormones.

I'm not exaggerating here. Learning to breathe more slowly and deeply can really have all these health benefits. In fact, one study found that patients who performed deep breathing exercises after heart surgery had better heart function afterward.[23]

According to Michelle Maniaci, physical therapist, energy medicine practitioner, and yoga therapist, diaphragmatic breathing increases lymphatic flow, which is rich in immune cells; encourages the release of oxytocin, which is a healing hormone; and helps the nervous system function more efficiently. Current research shows that as you train yourself to better use your diaphragm for breathing deeply, you improve lung and immune function, increase blood flow, improve digestion, and experience better sleep and reduced stress.[24]

"When we breathe using our diaphragm," Michelle says, "we are better able to process and release emotions we may have suppressed and that may have been restricting our ability to feel calm and centered. This helps dissolve tension in the body-mind, allowing healing to occur more efficiently."

You can practice breathing from the diaphragm in just a few simple steps. First, lay down on your back with pillows for support underneath your head and outer thighs. Place the soles of your feet together and your hips away from each other. You can also lay on your left side with pillows in between your legs so your knees and ankles are positioned parallel to one another. (Use other pillows under your head and neck and between your arms so your shoulders and wrists are parallel.)

Deeply relax your mind and body. Place your right hand over your abdomen, and left hand over your chest. Breathe in the deepest and longest inhalation you can through your nose. Notice how the inhalation causes your whole center to expand—abdomen, rib cage, and pelvic floor. Hold the end of your inhalation for a few seconds, then exhale, creating a *shh* sound through your mouth or blowing through pursed lips while activating your corset muscles to push all the air out.

Taking long and slow inhalations followed by long and slow exhalations will ensure the most benefit. Once you're comfortable doing this while lying down, try it during everyday life activities, such as sitting in a chair, driving a car, walking, or climbing stairs. Make sure to keep your head, spine, and pelvis in a neutral position with shoulder blades down and back to inhibit overuse of the upper-chest muscles. According to researchers, six breaths per minute (count to five during inhalation and exhalation) has been shown to induce optimal psychological effects and optimal autonomic nervous system functioning.[25]

The most important thing to remember: Imagine breathing in the fun and pleasure that life brings us in every moment. Don't view this exercise as "work." Nurture, heal, and purify your whole being with your breath.

Volunteer/Service Work

You know how good you feel when you do something for someone else? Giving always makes me feel more positive (especially when I'm in a funk) because it takes my focus off myself, and I realize my problem wasn't so bad after all. It's amazing how, when we get caught up in our own minds, things can seem worse than they are, and how doing some little thing for someone else can give us a more realistic perspective while helping someone else along the way. It's a win-win!

You may think that you can't do anything for anyone else while you're going through cancer treatments. You have so much on your plate already, right? Well, consider it part of your treatment. Maybe you can go to the hospital and talk to other people there who are sick. Maybe you can volunteer in the children's department. Maybe you can crochet a blanket for your sister's new baby, paint a picture for a loved one, or help a child with homework, or simply share your experience, strength, and hope in a support group. What you have to say might be just what someone else needs to hear.

If you play a musical instrument, maybe you can entertain at a senior living center, or play for students at your local elementary school. It doesn't matter what you do, big or small. Giving to someone else helps get you out of your own world—out of that same mode of thinking running over and over in your head.

Try it and see. I think you'll find that the day you give to someone else is just a better day.

Counseling, Support Groups, and Accepting Help

It's so difficult for us to ask for help, isn't it? We think we should be strong enough to handle cancer and continue to do the things we've always done. We think we should be tough enough to deal with all the emotional backlash that comes with treatment. Then, somewhere along the way, we start to crumble.

"It was really hard for me to ask for help," Alli says. "I've always been very independent and have lived on my own for a very long time. It was easier when people said, 'This is what we want to do, is that okay?'"

It was really hard for my father to ask for help, too. He was always very independent and had achieved everything on his own. To ask someone else to help him was foreign to him.

However, cancer is *not* something you should do alone. You need supportive people around you. You may feel like you want to go into your own little hole and never come out, but if you remain alone too much, your symptoms could get worse. In fact, animal studies have shown that social isolation enhanced tumor growth and affected survival of mice with liver cancer.[26-27]

I think my father may have thought it was weak to ask for help. Until the very end, he wanted to do it all himself. But this kind of thinking can put undue pressure on you and actually make it harder for you to heal, and can also put more stress on your friends and loved ones.

People can't read your mind, so communicate as effectively as you can with those who are willing to help you.

"I went to major therapy," Meghan says. "I found a nonprofit organization that deals with the emotional and spiritual side of having cancer. They were my lifesavers. If I hadn't found something like that, I don't know if I'd even be where I'm at now."

Meghan found her help at a nonprofit organization in Vancouver called Callanish. You may want to ask your oncology nurse or doctor about similar programs that may be available in your area.

Another part of reaching out for help is to join a support group. Friends and family will do all they can, but nothing compares with sharing your experience with others who have actually been there. It's when we identify with others that the healing really starts.

"I felt like I was the only one going through this," Alli says. "Once I started meeting other cancer patients, I learned from their experiences. I would chat with someone online at three o'clock in the morning when I couldn't sleep or I would call someone when I was having a total meltdown. I had other friends, but with them it would feel like I was bitching about my life. The people in my support groups could identify with me."

Research on support groups has found them to be very helpful to cancer patients. For example, one study of women in four community breast cancer self-help groups found that women felt the groups were extremely helpful for navigating the short- and long-term impact of breast cancer.[28] They felt it helped to connect with other survivors, to feel understood and share experiences, and to share healing laughter.

"Cancer transforms your life and connects you to other people on a level someone who hasn't experienced it could never understand," Laurie says. "We didn't ask for this, but here we are, and we are connected in this web."

To find support on your journey, try these tips:

- Ask your oncologist or oncology nurse about support groups in your area.

- Sign up for online support groups, like Cancer Compass (www.cancercompass.com), The Cancer Survivors Network (www.acscsn.org), Cancer Forums (www.cancerforums.net), and OncoChat (www.oncochat.org).

- Ask your doctor for a referral to a psychiatrist or psychotherapist who works with cancer patients.

Be Kind to Yourself: This is Where the Healing Starts

"You have to realize things aren't in your control. You have to let go and heal. If you can't find the blessings in everyday life, in every moment you have, it's going to be very tough on you. You have to accept where you're at and look for that pleasure, or that sense of peace, or whatever you need to get you through."

—Joanna, breast cancer survivor

Encouraging positive feelings while processing negative ones all boils down to one thing: Be kind to yourself. The more you accept, express, and process your feelings while showing kindness to yourself, the more relaxed and positive you'll feel.

"Surround yourself with the best books," says Colleen, "and the best flowers, and let people cook for you, and make yourself a milkshake, and lie on the couch and curl up with your daughter and read together. Just surround yourself with loveliness and joy."

Healing for me started when I realized how I was talking to myself. Have you ever stopped to listen to your thoughts? I highly suggest that you become more aware of what you say to yourself on a daily basis. My spiritual teacher calls it the "critical parent." It sounds something like this: "Why would you even think you could do that in the first place?" Or, "Yeah, it's your fault for sure." Or, "You never know how to handle things."

My teacher asks me, "Would you ever speak to a child like that?"

Of course not. I would encourage that little girl to be the best she can be.

This is precisely what we need to do with ourselves, especially during cancer treatments, when we're already feeling so beat up and fragile. We know most of the things we tell ourselves aren't true. We're not failures, nor did we cause this disease.

In a few minutes, I'd like you to make a list of how you might encourage positive emotions and be kinder to yourself in your daily life. To get you started, let me share with you a few ways that I'm kind to myself:

1. I look in a mirror and repeat that I love and approve of myself as I am. There is nothing to fix because I am already whole.

2. Sometimes when I'm feeling sad and vulnerable, I hug myself and tell myself that everything will be all right and that I'm doing my best.

3. I do things I want to do, not because I "should" or "have to," but because I've chosen to for the benefits I will experience.

4. I follow my truth. If I don't feel like doing the laundry today, and I'm craving nature, I will take a walk instead, making sure I don't beat up on myself on the way!

5. If I need to hear something, I will ask a close friend—someone I really trust—to look into my eyes and repeat a few times what I need to hear: "Britta, you are at the right place in your life," or "Britta, trust and let go." It's very powerful to have another person say your name and tell you something like this.

Britta's Balanced Living Philosophy

I have ten things I do daily that keep me balanced, happy, centered, and grounded. When I take care of these things, everything else takes care of itself. They work for me—might they work for you?

1. **Be still/silent.** I meditate for 20 minutes each morning.

2. **Prayer.** I talk to God daily, ask him to guide me, and hand over my worries anxieties to him. I feel connected and lighter after I do this.

3. **Affirmations in the mirror.** My favorite one is, "I love and approve of myself."

4. **Take a few slow deep breaths.** I inhale love and exhale fear.

5. **Do something nice for someone.** For example, I will call someone and just listen or send a loving e-mail or note.

6. **Read** something that inspires me.

7. **Move** my body.

8. **Write** a few sentences in my journal.

9. **Drink** my daily green juice (mix kale, dandelion, parsley, cucumber, spinach, romaine, lemon, and ginger in a juicer; add ½ green apple for a touch of sweetness)—and I try not to overeat.

10. **Stay present** with every task I'm doing.

As you continue through your cancer experience, you may find that the skills you attain—learning how to deal with your emotions and cultivate joy in your life—will be useful to you long after the cancer is in remission.

"I dropped a lot of habits that weren't really effective," Jody says. "Cancer gave me a picture of what can happen if you don't have this opportunity in life. This is an opportunity we have. An opportunity to just be here as much as I can be, to do as much as I can do, to give as much as I can give, and not to waste it."

One of the biggest things cancer taught me is to love me for everything I am—unconditionally. Some days it's easier to feel this than others, but that's why I do my exercises. My daily work helps me to honor my feelings, accept where I'm at, and continue to love myself a little bit each day.

I hope you'll give some of these tools a try. Cancer is as much an emotional fight as it is a physical one. The more weapons you have in your corner, the better. Remember: Be patient. It takes practice. Be gentle with yourself.

Emotional Coping Techniques I'm Going to Try

You did this exercise earlier, for processing negative emotions. Now, circle three or more of the following activities you're going to try for encouraging positive emotions, and/or add a few of your own at the end of the list.

Art Therapy	Meditation	Guided Imagery
Laughter	Gratefulness	Music Therapy
Counseling	Aromatherapy	Support Groups
Pet Therapy	Journaling	Gardening
Quilting	Woodworking	Crafts
Reading	Deep Breathing	Volunteering
Forgiveness	Self Appreciation & Kindness	

Other _____

Other _____

Let's Review

- Cancer taxes your emotions as much or more than it does your body. To foster healing, take an active role in dealing with the emotional component of the disease.

- Unless you specifically make an appointment (with yourself or with a therapist) to deal with your emotions, you're more likely to stuff them. Make time to process negative feelings.

- When negative emotions come up, it's important to accept them, work through them, and then let them go.

- One effective exercise for processing negative emotions is to explore the body, identify uncomfortable areas, and determine what emotion may be speaking to you through that discomfort.

- Science has proven that emotions affect the body. Negative emotions bring down the immune system, while positive emotions help fortify the body's defenses.

- You can control your thoughts. You do not have to listen to negative ones—you can choose to replace them with positive ones.

- You can use many tools to help you process your negative emotions, including journaling, forgiveness, therapy, and more.

- There are also many things you can do to help encourage positive emotions, including affirmations, meditation, guided imagery, group therapy, art therapy, pet therapy, and more.

- Most of the time, encouraging positive emotions is as simple as being nice to yourself. By loving yourself a little bit every day, you pour loving energy into your body and mind.

- Whatever emotional coping skills you learn now will help you through the rest of your life.

Personal Affirmations

I accept whatever feelings come up, and I'm gentle with myself in dealing with them. I know they are just feelings and that they will pass.

Using my daily coping techniques, I find myself experiencing joy and happiness on a regular basis.

I let go. I trust the universe is taking care of all my needs.

Your Face: Acne, Dryness, & Photosensitivity—Be Gentle!

"I've never seen a smiling face that was not beautiful."

—Author Unknown

THE FACE, MORE THAN ANY OTHER FEATURE, IDENTIFIES us to the world. It's no wonder, then, that as side effects start showing up on the face, many of us suffer a blow to the self-esteem.

I remember how badly I felt when my face started puffing up, and when it got dry and dull looking. My first thought was, *How can you do this to me? Stop it!* I felt that somehow my body was not cooperating with me, and not doing its job. I had enough to go through. I didn't need to be dealing with all these changes that made me look different than my old self—the self I liked.

"I could see as I went further into treatment," says Jody, breast cancer survivor, "that everyone gets a pale kind of color. That's to be expected. But I would also get these cystic pimples that wouldn't heal. They're way underneath the skin and they never go away. You don't want to take more medication to alleviate a couple of pimples. It's just a bummer. It feels better if your skin is clear."

My father suffered a similar side effect—pustular acne all over his cheeks and neck—and it was one of the most difficult for him to deal with. While he had it, he would come out every morning and say, "I'm not feeling that well, the chemo's not working, and I have acne." These three things were equally difficult in his mind. He would ask me, "Can you go get me something? I just don't like looking in the mirror."

I tried to tell him it didn't matter. We were trying to keep him alive. "It's just a side thing," I said. "It will go away."

But he didn't want to leave the house. Granted, it was bad acne, all over his face. But he'd fought through years of cancer and cancer treatments, and hardly ever complained. He was a strong man, but the acne was devastating him.

I realized then this wasn't a beauty thing or a woman thing. This was a human thing. My father took pride in how he looked. He could handle the bald head, the lost weight, the flushed skin, the burned hands and feet, even the nerve damage, but not the acne.

After he died, I wondered if maybe this effect had somehow triggered memories from his childhood, when he was an insecure teenager struggling to make his way in the world. Whatever it was, at that point in his life, it became the most important thing to address. Not the cancer. Not the chemo. The acne.

Those of you who are suffering similar side effects—I completely understand what you're going through. It's hard to explain sometimes to our loved ones and friends, but cancer treatments can really affect our confidence in ways we probably weren't prepared for. That's why it's so important to do everything we can to tend to the problem, while encouraging ourselves to keep our heads high.

Sometimes it helps to remember that most of the symptoms you're experiencing are *temporary*. Once your treatment is over, your face will most likely return to how it was before cancer came around. You may have some lingering long-term side effects, and I'll talk about how to deal with those in a later chapter, but for the most part, the redness, the rashes, the acne, the dryness, and the puffiness will eventually fade away.

In this chapter I'm going to talk about caring for things like acne rashes, photosensitivity, and dryness, and about choosing nourishing products. In the next chapter, I'm going to give you some makeup tips to help hide some of those embarrassing side effects like redness, hyperpigmentation, scars, under-eye circles, and more. (Men, this goes for you too—don't think just because I said "makeup" that you're excluded. My father was able to feel more confident going into business meetings with a few of the tips I'm going to share with you.)

I'm not kidding when I say you're probably going to have to completely change your regular routine, all the way down to how you wash your face. That said, let's start there!

Step 1: Adopt a More Tender Routine

"The skin's barrier is made up of layers of cells and various lipids that are put together in a brick-and-mortar type arrangement. If you use harsh detergents and you disturb that function, you can strip the skin, remove some of that barrier, and then you have less protection to keep material from going in or out."

—Dr. Alan Dattner, holistic dermatologist

Most likely, you're familiar with giving a baby a bath. Whether it's your own child, a younger sibling, a niece or nephew, or even when you watch your friends who are moms, you know the care one takes in the task. First, the water has to be just right—not too hot. Then, the cloth must be

My New Facial Care Routine

During cancer treatments, skin becomes dry, flaky, red, irritated, itchy, and extremely fragile. To help you feel more comfortable, adopt these new habits:

- Avoid hot water; it makes itching worse. Use lukewarm instead.
- Pat (don't rub) dry.
- Avoid drying soaps. Use organic, nontoxic cleansers or just plain water. (Read your labels!)
- Apply a nontoxic heavy moisturizing cream when skin is still damp to seal in moisture.
- Use chemical-free sunscreen (zinc oxide is best) every day, and avoid long sun exposure. Wear a hat and sunglasses, and opt for shady areas when you do go outside.
- Avoid synthetic fragrances.
- Use a humidifier in your room.
- Drink at least eight glasses of fluids daily, preferably water.
- Sleep with a satin pillowcase so your skin can move freely over the material without tugging or pulling.

very soft, not too harsh for baby's tender skin. Only the most gentle baby soap and shampoo will do.

When going through cancer treatments, skin is extremely fragile and needs to be treated much like a baby's skin. It's sensitive, reactive, flushed, thin, dry, and vulnerable. Water that's too hot, pressure that's too hard, soap that's too harsh—all these things increase your risk for abrasions, bruising, tearing, more dryness, flaking, irritation, redness, and itching. Want to be more comfortable in your own skin? Think like a mom does when she's caring for her little baby, and treat yourself with a new, gentler touch.

We're so used to rushing through our own routines that it can feel strange, even self-indulgent, to slow down and be tender with ourselves. There are so many other things to do, right? So you run the water hot, scrub hard, use harsh cloths and drying soaps, splash the water again, rub your face with a towel, and out you go. Or maybe you swab over the face with a stinging alcoholic toner first, *then* go.

All that has to stop. Your skin is baby skin now, and you have to treat it that way. If you can slow down and enjoy the process of giving yourself a little extra attention, your skin will most likely respond by becoming less irritated. I've given you some easy tips in the sidebar, "My New Facial Care Routine."

Soothing Solutions from Your Kitchen

The solution to your compromised skin may be right in your kitchen cupboards. Fortunately, these ingredients are safe and don't contain harsh chemicals.

- Massage itchy areas with an ice cube, or cover them with a cool compress.

- Rub the inside of an avocado on your face, leave for 15 minutes, and rinse dry.

- Mash ripe bananas in a bowl, add some honey, and apply to face for 10-15 minutes.

- For very dry skin, try natural oils like olive, almond, or sesame oil.

- For a mild cleanser, try mixing a little yogurt with some honey, lemon juice, a tablespoon of instant mashed potatoes, a bit of finely sliced apple, and a teaspoon of wheat-germ oil.

- To reduce itch and redness, blend natural oatmeal with a little water, spread over skin, wait 10 minutes, and rinse.

Perhaps most important is that you use products that will not irritate your sensitive skin. Instead, you need to choose those items that will help nourish and protect it.

Step 2: Use Safe, Nourishing Products

"Stay away from anything that's going to strip the rest of the health off your skin. Avoid formaldehyde releasers, like imidazolidinyl urea, and harsh solvents, like alcohol, and of course, anything that's a suspected carcinogen."

—Dr. Alan Dattner, holistic dermatologist

On Your "Not" List

While you're looking for options to nurture your skin, make sure you stay away from these, at least during treatment:

- Acids like retinol, salicylic, and glycolic. These exfoliators work when your skin is healthy, but during cancer treatments, they're way too harsh. Be careful—they're found in all kinds of products, even foundations.

- Acne products contain salicylic acid, retinol, benzoyl peroxide, and other ingredients that can dry and irritate fragile skin.

- Alcohol, menthol, and peppermint can further dry, sting, and irritate your skin.

- Anti-wrinkle creams are helpful when your skin is strong, but they're too harsh while you're going through treatment.

- Chemical peels use powerful acids to remove dead skin cells. They could cause burns and permanent scarring on fragile skin.

- Eyebrow and upper lip waxing are much too harsh during treatment and can lead to irritation, redness, and scarring.

- Microdermabrasion is gentler than a peel, but it still assaults the skin with sand-type crystals. You have baby skin—you wouldn't blast sand on a baby's skin, right?

- Synthetic perfumes & fragrances are actually mixtures of many chemicals that can irritate dry and sensitive skin. Choose fragrance-free, or products scented with essential oils and other natural extracts.

- Vitamin C products are great for fine lines and wrinkles, but they're acidic and easily oxidized when exposed to air (which can encourage the formation of free radicals). Wait until after treatments are over.

Chemotherapy affects your skin's natural moisture level. Your glands don't secrete as much oil as before, so even if you're gentle and caring during your regular routine, you may find that your skin needs more nourishment.

Try not to get desperate and use the first heavy cream you can find. Moisturizers aren't designed to rinse off, so many of the ingredients are absorbed into the skin and may make it into the bloodstream. Fragile skin affected by chemotherapy or radiation has fewer defenses and a compromised protective barrier, so you want to choose brands that are safe, clean, and free of potentially harmful chemicals—like hormone-disrupting preservatives.

"The data on hormone disruptors is real," says holistc dermatologist Dr. Alan Dattner, "but the exact effects of these chemicals is not clear to me. However, if I had someone with a hormone-related cancer, I would probably stay away from them. Be on the safe side. Why expose yourself? We don't know what they're going to do, and you don't want to be part of the evaluation."

There is also some evidence to show that skin prefers ingredients it can identify with—those that have not been created in a chemical laboratory. Synthetic chemicals can sometimes cause more harm than good to skin that's too fragile to deal with them. Reactions are more common, as are irritations and dryness. Natural ingredients also undergo some processing to pull them out of the plant they come from, but on the whole, these ingredients arc less damaging to the environment and better for humans.

You don't have to break the bank to go toxin-free in your facial care. Some of the best moisturizers for dry, irritated skin can be found right in your refrigerator and kitchen cabinets. (See sidebar, "Soothing Solutions from Your Kitchen.")

When you do go shopping for safer products, seek out ingredients that are moisturizing, soothing, calming, and nourishing. Here are some great ones to look for:

Aloe: Known to promote healing of damaged and dry skin, aloe is very soothing and moisturizing. This is also a great ingredient for skin burned by radiation.

Chamomile extract: Known for its soothing and softening benefits, chamomile is naturally cleansing, but not harsh or dehydrating.

Calendula: This plant extract is soothing and has natural anti-inflammatory properties, which makes it great for irritated, sensitive skin. Often referred to as a skin "tonic," it also helps heal scars and soothe pain.

Cucumber: A natural source of silica—a trace mineral that contributes to the strength of connective tissue—cucumber helps maintain skin cohesiveness and elasticity. With ascorbic and caffeic acids, it also helps prevent water retention, helping improve the appearance of swollen, puffy eyes and soothing burns and dermatitis.

Honey: This ingredient helps the skin hold onto whatever moisture it has. It also has natural antibacterial properties. You can use it in combination with other ingredients from your kitchen to soothe and moisturize.

Jojoba oil: As with many natural oils, jojoba is moisturizing, without being too heavy, so this ingredient is great for acne-prone skin.

Oat extract: Ground oatmeal has been used for thousands of years to cure itchiness and soothe irritation. It's also known to relieve rashes and ease the pain of insect bites. Combine oatmeal or oatmeal powder with water and apply to your face to help moisturize and comfort your fragile, overtaxed skin.

Olive oil: This ingredient deeply moisturizes, while protecting your skin with its powerful antioxidants. It may be too oily to apply directly to your face, but can be very helpful in a skin-care moisturizing formula.

Omega 3 fatty acids: These are not only great for your diet, but they're good for your skin. Considered "good fats," omega 3s keep your skin moist and help prevent sagging. They also protect against environmental damage that can lead to aging.

Shea butter: This butter is made from the nut of the mangifolia tree in central Africa. It's a great natural hydrator, which helps the skin retain moisture and regain its softness. Shea butter also encourages skin repair.

Reishi mushroom: Long used by the Chinese for beautification of the skin, reishi mushrooms help condition, promote delivery of nutrients, and reduce the appearance of sun damage.

Gentlemen—Go Easy on the Shaving

Okay, guys, I know how tough you are, but if you're going through chemotherapy or radiation, your skin is *not*, which means you need to be a little more careful during your morning shave.

- Your skin is fragile during treatments, making you more vulnerable to nicks and cuts, which can lead to infections and sores.

- Use an electric razor and take your time to avoid pain or bruising.

- When washing, use tepid—not hot—water. Hot water can increase itching.

- Pat, don't rub, your skin dry.

- Since most shaving products are made with harmful chemicals that can be absorbed by the skin, opt for organic, chemical-free formulas that are mild and labeled "sensitive." Always read the labels on your products.

- Steer clear of perfumed and alcohol-based aftershaves. They can be highly irritating and drying.

- Invest in a chemical-free moisturizer with calming ingredients like aloe, chamomile, shea butter, and oat extract.

- Don't forget a good, chemical-free sunblock when you head outside.

- Take a break from shaving now and then (over the weekend?) to let your face rest.

Rose hip oil: This oil has a reputation for treating dry skin and scar tissue. It absorbs quickly, so you can try it alone or in a natural formulation.

Rosemary: Great for purifying the skin, rosemary also has antimicrobial properties.

Turmeric: A soothing and healing ingredient, turmeric encourages wound healing, calms eczema, and has historically been used to treat skin ulcers and scabies. It also smoothes skin and contributes to a healthy glow.

Vegetable glycerin: You may see "glycerin" on the labels of many moisturizing creams, but make sure it's the natural version, not the synthetic. The synthetic one can be very irritating, but vegetable glycerin is a rich lubricant extracted from vegetable oils that can be very helpful for dry skin.

Vitamin E: This vitamin is a powerful antioxidant that will protect your skin from harmful free radicals. It also has natural hydrating properties. (Check with your doctor before using.)

There are many more natural ingredients that are beneficial to your skin. As you start using these more natural ingredients, you'll see and feel the difference. Keep reading labels, and soon you'll grow used to choosing products that nourish and support your skin.

The Doctor Recommended It—Should I Use It?

Many doctors (or nurses) may recommend moisturizing creams or ointments from the drugstore that contain petroleum-based ingredients. These chemicals can cause damage to the immune system and the nervous system after prolonged exposure, and some studies have connected them with cancer.

For example, hairless mice treated with four different brands of moisturizer after UV exposure had an increased rate of tumor formation.[1] Researchers took out a few ingredients they thought were to blame, then ran the experiment again with a new moisturizer. It did not have the same effect.

The culprit ingredients? They included mineral oil, which is a petroleum-based ingredient, and sodium lauryl sulfate. This is just one small animal study, but several have warned of the health dangers linked with petroleum.

Petroleum ingredients appear in many common cosmetic products and cleansers. Look for words like mineral oil, paraffin gel, propylene glycol, or PVP/VA copolymere. Choose organic formulas made with petroleum alternatives like waxes and oils that work just as well.

Keep Your Products Bacteria Free

When you're going through treatment, your immune system is compromised and your defenses are down. That means you're more at risk for infections. Your bathroom, no matter how diligent you may be at cleaning, most likely has airborne microbes that can easily contaminate your skin care or beauty products.

Decrease your chances of bacteria exposure by following these few tips:

- Use only products that come in a tube or with a pump, ideally an airless pump. These products are less exposed to air and thereby less at risk of contamination.

- Keep formulas fresh and effective by storing out of direct sunlight. Place them in a dark, dry place like a closet or dresser drawer. It may seem convenient to leave products on your sink or countertop, but steam from daily showers can lessen ingredient effectiveness, so choose an alternate place.

- Stop using jars whenever possible. Because you have to frequently dip your fingers into them, they become breeding grounds for bacteria.

- Wash your hands before using any product on your skin.

- Always dispose of sponges and cotton swabs after one use. Launder washcloths after one use as well. These things can all breed bacteria, and when your white blood cell count is low, you're more prone to infection.

- Regularly clean your bathroom environment with green, nontoxic cleansers. If you're too tired during treatment, ask for help with this one!

Step 3: Protect from the Sun

Cancer treatments make your skin more sensitive to the sun. Remember— treatments kill off the cells that form the outer layer of skin, exposing the more tender cells underneath, which can be easily damaged by UV rays.

If you're not careful, exposed areas may suffer redness, exaggerated sunburn that lasts for days to weeks, and even itchy rashes.

Fortunately, the solution is easy. Apply sunscreen to your face *every day*, even if it's cloudy outside. Just because you can't see the sun doesn't mean that UV rays aren't coming through the clouds.

A good sunblock will do a lot to protect your skin. However, even the best ones fade after a couple of hours, or become less effective if you get wet or perspire. During treatment, it pays to be extra careful. Avoid direct sunlight, especially during the hours of ten A.M. to three P.M., when the sun's rays are at their most powerful.

When you go out, wear a wide-brimmed hat, long sleeves, long pants, and even light gloves when you're in the middle of treatment. All these precautions will help keep your skin softer and more comfortable.

You get the idea. Sun protection is a must. Let's talk about the *kind* of sunscreen you'll want to use. Unfortunately, many are formulated with all the ingredients I've been telling you about—ingredients that might be harmful for your skin or body. They may have parabens, formaldehyde, fragrances, and other harsh chemicals, so it's important to always read labels.

What About My Lips?

Lips can get just as dry, flaky, and irritated as the rest of your skin during treatment. Dryness can lead to chapping and even cracks, so remember to extend your new tender-care routine to your lips.

- Avoid lip balms with menthol or petroleum jelly. These can actually make the skin dryer.

- Parabens and phthalates are lurking in many lip products. Read labels!

- Look for formulas in tubes rather than jars or pots, which can easily become breeding grounds for bacteria.

- Yes, there are organic lip balms, which often have natural waxes and oils. Seek them out.

- Ingredients like beeswax, propolis, jojoba and sunflower oils, shea butter, vitamin E, herbal extracts, and light essential oils are all good choices.

- Choose lip moisturizers with an SPF of 15 or higher; your lips need sun protection, too.

There's something else about sunscreens, however, that you'll want to pay attention to. They come in two basic types: chemical and physical. For ease of understanding, we can think of the physical sunscreens (or so-called mineral sunscreens, which include titanium dioxide and zinc oxide) as those that reflect or scatter UV radiation before it damages skin. They're reputed to offer broader protection against both UVA and UVB rays, but are sometimes more visible (as a white or colored cream).

Chemical sunscreens, on the other hand, absorb UV rays and chemically alter them to decrease their damaging effects. These include oxybenzone, PABA, octyl methoxycinnamate, salicylates, avobenzone, and menthyl anthranilates. They usually vanish on the skin and have been shown effective against UVB rays, but not so much against UVA rays, though some manufacturers have already started working to change that.

Chemical sunscreens can irritate sensitive skin, as the harsh chemicals in them can cause allergic reactions. The preservatives, particularly, and the synthetic fragrances can cause dermatitis and rashes, which may sometimes not show up until the treated skin is exposed to the sun. People who are more sensitive to the sun—which includes anyone going through cancer treatments—are more at risk.

Which type of sunscreen should you choose? Can you guess? Let me give you a few more clues. Physical (or mineral) sunscreens currently protect against a broader range of UV rays, which is important, as it's the UVA rays that penetrate more deeply into the skin and may be more to blame for skin cancer.

Second, only one chemical sunscreen (avobenzone) is legal in Europe. They've banned the rest. Why? Because chemical sunscreens have three primary defects: 1) they generate free radicals that can damage cells, 2) they can contain estrogenic (hormone-altering) chemicals, and 3) they contain synthetic chemicals that can be harmful.

In fact, one study found that certain sunscreens containing PABA damaged DNA in test-tube experiments.[2] Some researchers believe that the increased use of chemical sunscreens is the primary cause of the skin cancer epidemic.[3] Another study found that benzophenone (BP) UV filters act as endocrine disruptors—mimicking the female hormone estrogen and interfering with the male hormone, testosterone. The effects were detected at levels found in human blood after applying sunscreen.[4]

Finally, one more thing you should know: One study found that sunscreen agents do penetrate the skin, with benzophenone-3 passing through in significant amounts.[5]

By now I'm sure you know which sunscreen I would recommend for your fragile skin. Go for a physical (or mineral) sunscreen like titanium dioxide or zinc oxide, with zinc oxide having the reputation for being the safest option.

Do make sure the product doesn't contain nanotechnology, however. Recent advances in technology have enabled manufacturers to make ingredients in particles so small you could fit tens of thousands of them across a human hair. These tiny ingredients (called "nanoparticles") allow products to feel lightweight on the skin and fill in microscopic crevices; but that also means they may be more likely to penetrate the skin and enter the bloodstream.

Many organizations, including the Natural Resources Defense Council (NRDC), have expressed concern over the lack of safety testing on nanotechnology.[6] Because of their tiny size, nanoparticles are more readily taken up by the body and can cross membranes to access cells, tissues, and organs that larger particles cannot.

So far, the FDA is not requiring safety testing of these nanoparticles in our sunscreens. Look for brands that aren't using them. Check with organizations like Friends of Earth (www.foe.org—search "nanotechnology" and "sunscreens") and the Consumer's Union (www.consumersunion.org—search "nanoparticles") for lists of companies that are avoiding these particles. The Environmental Working Group (EWG) also has a safe sunscreen guide (www.ewg.org/2010sunscreen).

Step 4: Be Gentle with Your Rash—It's Not Acne!

Chemotherapy drugs can often cause an acne-like side effect. You may want to reach for the harsh acne products that are so popular on today's market. Please read this first!

As I mentioned, my father suffered from this side effect. He asked me to get him the harsh acne medications, but I knew that these would only scar and burn his very fragile skin. He kept on asking, so I got him some, but it burned his skin and did nothing to heal the acne.

Not only are traditional acne products drying and irritating for fragile chemotherapy skin, they're also formulated to treat traditional acne, and usually the side effect that comes about as a result of cancer treatments is *not* regular acne. Instead, it's more like a rash.

What you'll see on the skin is red spots and tiny "pimple-like" blotches. You may also experience severe dryness and redness, like sunburn. It can come and go, so it seems a lot like acne, but it's not acne.

Some people deal with adult pimples before cancer, but the side effect I'm describing can be much worse, as it can be so noticeable. In the next

Flushing and Burn-Like Pain

Sometimes your skin may flush or feel burned (even though it looks fine) as a result of treatment. Skin reactions like these are common, but always check with your doctor.

Flushing is a temporary redness that comes up on your face and neck. Chemotherapy drugs can cause it, although spicy foods, caffeine, stress, and alcohol can also encourage it. Soothing ingredients like calendula, cucumber, aloe, and oatmeal can help calm the skin so the redness fades. Make sure you're avoiding the sun and any harsh products that will further irritate skin.

Sunburn-like pain can be the result of radiation, which we will discuss in a future chapter. However, if you're experiencing pain not related to radiation, check with your doctor, as it could be an allergic reaction. Then try some anti-itch or anti-burn lotions (that include aloe) as well as cool compresses for relief, and protect your skin fiercely from the sun.

chapter I'll show you some ways you can hide the effects with makeup, but for now let's concentrate on how to help your skin heal.

Some of the things we've talked about, like switching to sensitive skin cleansers and moisturizers (natural baby formulas and organics are good options because of their low-to-negligible chemical content), using non-chemical sunscreens, and switching to more moisturizing, toxin-free makeup options will all help your skin deal with the changes it's going through.

Once you have the rash (or acne-like condition), try washing with soothing chamomile and water. Add ground oatmeal to your bath, and apply a mixture of oatmeal and water to your face to cool irritation and redness.

There's some research that supports the idea that omega-3 fatty acids can help reduce rash, so try increasing your daily intake of fatty fish (salmon, sardines), nuts, and flaxseed. Clay pastes can reduce symptoms very well. You can also try almond oil, or another deep moisturizer that you may want to apply a couple of times a day. (Don't be fooled into thinking you need to dry the acne out—your skin is crying for moisture.)

If natural remedies don't work, check with your doctor, who may recommend a cream with hydrocortisone or clindamyacin, or even antibiotics. Continue to moisturize to prevent scarring. This is another reason you want to avoid harsh acne products—they can contribute to scarring, which may hang around on your skin long after the acne is gone.

Step 5: Heal Your Skin and Spirit at the Spa

"As I'm getting new products, I love the natural stuff. When I get a facial, that's what I do. I don't want to do anything chemical."

—Laurie, breast cancer survivor

You may think that a trip to the spa is a luxury you can't afford during treatment, but I'm telling you this is the *best* time to get a gentle facial targeted to sensitive skin. It's a great way to relax and recharge, which you definitely need during this stressful time, and it will help your skin to become more hydrated and energized.

I'm not talking about harsher treatments like chemical peels and microdermabrasion. Choose a place that uses organic, toxin-free products (call ahead of time and visit their website), let the technicians know you have cancer, and tell them you want only gentle, safe products applied to your sensitive skin.

Numerous businesses are proud to advertise themselves as "organic" spas and offer herbal, organic, and natural skin treatments that are gentle and relaxing. Typically you'll receive a gentle cleansing, toning, and a masque that's usually full of fresh fruit pulp and intoxicating herbs. Many times you'll enjoy a complimentary beverage, some quiet time by the fire, or a calming walk around well-manicured grounds.

Did you know that many spas across the nation offer discounts and even free services for cancer patients? If you're too tired to make the arrangements yourself, ask a good friend to accompany you. You really do owe it to yourself to do something that will relieve your stress, nourish your skin, and help you feel refreshed and renewed.

"There are so many benefits of touch," says Vicky Weis, founder of Faye's Light, a nonprofit organization providing free spa services for cancer patients. "It can help relieve pain, get circulation going, and relax pinched muscles. After a few spa treatments you can just see patients open up. Fear and anxiety melt away."

Before you go, check with your oncology nurse for recommendations. Your hospital or area cancer centers may offer free or reduced-cost massages or other spa treatments for cancer patients. If not, look for spas that have certified oncology estheticians on their staff—people who have been trained to work with people living with cancer. Make sure you bypass the more aggressive offerings, like deep tissue massage and cupping, and just go for something that is gentle and will make you feel good.

I encourage you to make a trip to the spa as often as you can during treatments. If you're still unsure where to go, my website, www.cincovidas. com, has a list of certified oncology estheticians and organic spas near you. You'll walk away with much more than a glowing complexion. The power of human touch, combined with the quiet, relaxing atmosphere, is a powerful way to rejuvenate and be kind to yourself.

Let's Review

- Side effects that show up on the face can make you feel self-conscious and insecure. Be kind to yourself, take steps to care for and nourish your skin, and remember these effects will go away after treatment is over.

- **Step 1:** Adopt a more tender routine when washing and caring for your face. Treat your skin as you would a baby's.

- **Step 2:** Use only nourishing products, and avoid harsh, synthetic ingredients. Read labels on the products your doctors or nurses recommend, and choose those with safe ingredients when necessary. Store your products carefully, and dispose of cotton swabs and sponges after one use. Launder washcloths regularly and keep the bathroom clean.

- **Step 3:** Protect your skin from the sun at all times. Use a physical sunscreen like zinc oxide and wear a wide-brimmed hat when you go out. Avoid products with nanoparticles.

- **Step 4:** If you get an acne-like rash during treatment, avoid harsh acne products. Choose gentler treatments instead, and ask your doctor for solutions if the side effect gets worse.

- **Step 5:** Take the time to treat yourself to an organic facial at a spa. You'll emerge refreshed and relaxed, and your skin will feel more hydrated and energized.

Goals

Three things I've done in the past that I now realize may not have been nourishing for my face:

1. _____

_____

2. _____

_____

3. _____

_____

Three things I'm willing to change this month to take better care of my skin.

1. _____

_____

2. _____

_____

3. _____

_____

Personal Affirmations

My complexion is glowing, healthy, and vibrant.

No matter how cancer treatments may be challenging my body,
I know that I am perfectly okay, whole, and complete as I am today.

Makeup: Sallow Skin? Eyelashes Gone? No One Needs to Know!

"I didn't know how to make myself look good without looking like a painted doll. It was nice to have people show me how to apply [makeup] and make it look natural. It was like, okay, I can do this and I don't have to look like a washed-out sheet. I can look good every day, even if I'm not seeing anybody. It was a real confidence booster."

—Chris, non-Hodgkin's lymphoma survivor

WE TALKED IN AN EARLIER CHAPTER ABOUT HOW IMPORTANT it is to keep your spirits up during and after cancer treatment. It boosts your immune system, helps you better cope with the challenge, and improves the quality of your life while you're on this journey.

I know that on some days the last thing you want to do is leave the house, and that's okay. Some days you just need to hole up in your room and rest. But on other days, when you do feel a little better, do you find yourself staying in because of how you look?

My aunt Chris, a non-Hodgkin's lymphoma survivor (you may have noticed her quotes throughout this book so far), had a hard time reaching out for social support during treatment. She felt she just didn't look her best and didn't like the idea of going out when she felt self-conscious about her appearance.

"You're not feeling good, and you're not looking good," she says, "so you don't want to see people. I wouldn't go out and socialize. After receiving some makeup advice, I felt more like seeing people. 'I can do this!' I said to myself. 'I can put on a nice scarf, I can apply makeup to look natural, and I can go out looking good.'"

During cancer treatment, makeup becomes more than just a way to bring out your best features. It can become a tool to help maintain your lines of emotional support to your friends and loved ones, which is so important! With a little makeup (and I'm talking to the guys, here, too!), you can cover up the flaws that cancer creates on your skin, and still feel confident enough to go to work, go out to dinner, or join your friends for a movie.

My father was deeply affected by how he looked, as he had a flushed face, dark circles, acne, and a pale, bald head. However, he was very proactive in doing things to make himself look better. For example, he would use self-tanner so the tone of skin on his head would match his face. Half the time you couldn't even tell he was sick.

He used to tell me, laughing, "I'm still so good-looking without my hair, aren't I?" Of course, I would agree! It's funny, but he was, as by doing things to make himself look better, his strong, confident spirit shone through. He could go off to work and focus on things other than his cancer, which gave him motivation to keep up the fight. Being around people helped him feel purposeful, whereas hiding away at home made him feel defeated.

If you're thinking you just *have* to get out and do something fun, but then you look in the mirror and go, "Ew, that rash looks awful," or "I have no eyebrows—I don't look right," and decide to stay in because of it, you're depriving yourself of a necessary mood-boost, and therefore not making the best decision for your health.

When you feel good about yourself, you can go out and enjoy the company and support of other people, and return reenergized for your fight with cancer. In fact, getting social support is *so* critical that in one study, it was related to quality of life in cancer patients;[1] in another, it assisted patients in coping with cancer;[2] and in a third study of nearly 3,000 breast cancer patients, those who were more socially isolated had an elevated risk of mortality.[3]

To boost your self-confidence, help you get out among friends and family, and encourage you to do more of the things that make you feel good, I'm going to give you some targeted makeup tips in this chapter. We'll talk about how to deal with missing eyebrows, thinning eyelashes, scars, sallow skin, and more. And of course, we'll talk about choosing products that contain fewer chemicals, as now that your skin is more sensitive from the cancer treatments, your typical makeup products will probably be too irritating, harsh, and drying.

Avoid Health Dangers in These Five Cosmetic Products

"I use a little makeup when I go out, but I choose chemical-free brands."

—Joanna, breast cancer survivor

We've looked at a few of the toxic ingredients that can be found in everyday personal care products. Now let's examine those found specifically in makeup products.

1—Micronized Powders

Mineral powders have made a big splash on the market in the last few years, with manufacturers praising the even coverage and natural look they offer. However, if these products contain tiny particles called "nanoparticles," as many of them do, they come with a risk. In these cases, the ingredients are broken down into tiny, tiny particles—much smaller than they used to be, some a thousand times smaller than they were even ten years ago. These "nanoparticles" usually measure about 1 to 100 nanometers in diameter. (A nanometer is one-billionth of a meter. A human hair is tens of thousands of times larger!)

The smaller-size particles in these powders create a more flawless look by filling in microscopic crevices and reflecting light for a natural glow. They help the product feel light on the skin and glide easily over your face. However, they're also more likely to penetrate your skin's outer layer and make their way into your bloodstream. (Studies are under way to uncover health risks.)

Ultrafine particles, when inhaled, can also become embedded in the lungs, where the body has a hard time removing them, thus irritating allergies and asthma, and potentially causing inflammation, irritation, and even lung disease.

To lower your risk of irritation and to increase skin hydration while going through treatments, choose a liquid, cream, or mousse foundation or a tinted moisturizer, as these will be less likely to settle into fine lines, and will be more hydrating. (You can ask for ones that "illuminate" or give you a "glow.")

If you're sold on your mineral powder, work it into the brush by swirling and tapping until you don't really see it anymore, tap off the excess, then apply carefully. Try not to inhale the particles, and be sure you're in a well-ventilated room. Finally, look for mineral powders that aren't made with nano- or micronized particles.

Makeup Counters Harbor Germs

Be particularly cautious at makeup counters. "Testers" often carry the germs of many women who have dipped their fingers into them. One study found bacteria like staphylococcus and streptococcus in lipstick, brushes, lip gloss, and eye shadow from makeup counters. Take your antibacterial wipes, and if you want to try a product, apply it to your hand, then wash your hands immediately after leaving the counter.

2—Mercury in Mascara

Mercury has several adverse health effects, including birth or developmental defects, damage to the brain and nervous system, and organ system toxicity. Fortunately, most mascaras don't contain mercury anymore, but some still do, especially the "cake-type" varieties.

How can you tell? In mascaras and other personal care products, mercury comes from an ingredient called "thimerosal," a compound that's about 49 percent mercury by weight and is used as an antiseptic and antifungal agent. (Look for "thimerosal" or "mercuric" on the label.)

Thimerosal has been linked to allergies and skin irritation. Because it's easily absorbed through the skin, the FDA banned the use of it in all cosmetics thirty years ago...*except* in those products you use around the eyes.

The eyes are more susceptible to infection, so products used anywhere around them need to be free of contaminants. Thimerosal has long been the favorite antimicrobial, but with new alternatives now available, regulation is currently outdated.

Though levels of thimerosol in personal care products are low, it can be found in some eye moisturizers; makeup removers; nose-, eye-, and ear-drops; eye ointments; and some imported skin lighteners and soaps.

Choose mascaras made by health-conscious companies, or research your favorite brand at The Skin Deep Database (www.cosmeticsdatabase.com) to make sure it's free of mercury and other harmful carcinogens.

3—Lipsticks & Lip Glosses

According to recent tests conducted by the Campaign for Safe Cosmetics, a whopping 61 percent of brand-name lipsticks contain detectable levels of lead, which can be toxic if ingested.[4]

Chronic exposure to lead can result in increased blood pressure, decreased fertility, cataracts, nerve disorders, muscle and joint pain, and memory or concentration problems. Guilty brands included many well-known in department stores and drugstores. One-third exceeded the FDA lead limit for candy, and many of these were the more expensive, supposedly "higher-quality" products.

A one-time exposure to these small, trace amounts of lead may not be a problem, but lead builds up in the body over time. If you're using a lead-containing lipstick several times a day, every day, it can add up to significant levels inside you.

Why do manufacturers put lead in lipstick? Colorants used in lipsticks can contain lead, or lead may be introduced as a byproduct from other ingredients, like mineral wax or paraffin, even mineral oil. Companies don't purposely *put* the lead in there, but it can form as a result of how they process and combine other ingredients.

Where does that leave you and your favorite shade? The study did find that 39 percent of the products tested had no detectable levels of lead. (You can find these at www.cosmeticsdatabase.com.) With a little research you can find those brands advertising "lead-free" lipsticks and enjoy luscious lips without the tasteless taint!

4—Sunscreens

I mentioned these in an earlier chapter, but want to remind you here to be sure to use a safe sunscreen on your face. Cancer treatments make your skin more sensitive to UV rays, and unprotected, you can get lasting burns that may actually scar your skin. Many foundations, moisturizers, and lotions have chemical sunscreens in them (like oxyenzone, cinoxate, octocrylene, octyl salicylate, etc.). These sunscreens have been found to disrupt hormones and even encourage sun damage, so seek out sunscreen-free makeup products and then get a separate, physical sunscreen, or find makeup products with chemical-free sunscreens like zinc oxide and titanium dioxide.

5—Sunless Tanners

Self-tanners can be lifesavers for your best look. They were for my father; they evened out the skin tone on his bald head and gave him a fabulous glow. The main ingredient—DHA, or dihydroxyacetone—is a nontoxic type of sugar that reacts with skin proteins to create brown or golden-brown compounds. DHA doesn't penetrate the skin, but remains on the top layer (which is why the tan wears off within a few days, with the sloughing off of dead skin cells).

Other ingredients manufacturers include in tanners are not so safe, however. Many contain parabens (toxic preservatives), 1,4 dioxane (byproduct of manufacturing), and synthetic fragrances. These chemicals have all been linked with cancer, so it's best to avoid them in products that you apply to your skin. While the DHA tanning ingredient may not penetrate below the top layer of the skin, other ingredients might.

Are there better alternatives that don't use these dangerous ingredients? You bet. You can even find some that are good for your skin! Look for brands with green tea, ginkgo biloba, and aloe vera, and that contain no parabens and no synthetic colors or dyes. (Read your labels!) Also, choose formulas that are extra moisturizing, as self-tanners have a tendency to dry the skin.

Best Makeup During Treatment

The most important thing while going through treatment is to choose safe products with few potentially harmful ingredients. However, I can also give you some basic guidelines as to what kinds of makeup products may work best for your dry, sensitive skin. These are general guidelines, and you'll want to pay attention to your own skin to see how it reacts, but these tips may help you make some initial adjustments to your makeup routine.

Cleansing and Moisturizing

First of all, don't forget that your skin needs moisture, and lots of it. If you're used to a lotion, switch to a nontoxic nourishing cream for dry skin and apply it morning and night, or as soon as you feel your skin is tight. (This goes for men, too.) As mentioned in the last chapter, be gentle with your skin, and choose a fragrance-free cleanser that won't further dry it out. Depending on how dry your skin is, you may want to skip cleansing in the morning, since there's no makeup to remove, and wash just once at night. Always follow immediately with moisture.

Foundations

- **Liquids** continue to be my favorites because they're so flexible and natural-looking. Oil-based formulas are best for dry to normal skin, and water-based formulas are better for those with oily skin. But remember, even if you had oily skin before, your skin may be drier during treatment. Oil-free options or matte-finish brands are best for those with oily or acne-prone skin.

- I highly recommend **tinted moisturizers,** which are great for those who don't want a lot of coverage but need something to even out skin tone and relieve dry skin. They also combine two steps in one (moisturizer and foundation). Many come with effective sunscreens and are great for normal to dry skin. When going through cancer treatment, this is a nice option for casual days.

- **Stick foundations** come in solid form, have more of a drying effect, and can look cakey, so they're good for covering scars, tattoos, and flaws, but not the best for everyday use in cancer patients with dry skin.

- **Powder foundations** feel light on the skin and are great for people with normal to oily or combination skin. Like other powders, however, they're typically not the best choice for you while going through treatment. Similar to pressed powder, loose-powder foundations help control shine, but they can be too drying. Use these for touch-ups only.

Concealers

Oh, how I love this product! Even guys learn to love a good concealer for the power it gives them in covering up the redness, rashes, pimple-like outbursts, and under-eye circles. My dad became a believer!

Concealers come in all different forms. For the best results, you'll probably want to have a couple around.

- **Solids** come in wand or stick forms. They're great on the go, provide the best coverage, and are particularly effective on scars, bruises, and acne spots. They are my choice for masking any flaws! However, they can also accentuate dry skin, so use them sparingly. The best way to get targeted coverage is with a concealer brush rather than with your fingers.

- **Liquids** are best for those with dry skin and work perfectly for all-around coverage. They're a good choice for under-eye circles, since they're easy to blend on tender skin. Liquids provide sheer coverage and a light finish, and can help make red veins on the cheeks and nose less visible. They can also fade faster, however, requiring more touch-ups.

- **Creams** usually come in tubes or potlike containers. (Choose the tubes to lower your risk of infection.) Coverage is not as heavy as stick concealers, but they will cover better than liquids and are great for all skin types. I love creams, particularly for eye circles. Too much can look cakey, though, so apply carefully.

- **Powders** have a lightweight feel, but they are not the best choice for skin going through chemotherapy. Powder settles into the fine lines and flaws you're trying to cover. It also doesn't cover blemishes very well. Save these for use after treatments are over.

When looking for the right shade, consider your skin tone, and go just a half-shade lighter.

- For pale skin, use a light beige with yellow undertones.
- Cool skin tones do well with peach or apricot colors.
- Warm skin appears more flawless in yellow tones.
- Olive skin should go for medium beige with pink undertones.
- Darker skin should choose a medium-to-dark shade with peach undertones.

A test: If your concealer is too light or too pink, it will emphasize the dark area rather than concealing it. Or, try your concealer over your foundation. If you can't see it, you've got the right shade.

Eyeshadows, Liners, and Mascaras

As in other makeup products, you want to choose more hydrating formulas, so go for cream eyeshadows as opposed to powders for your eyes. Your skin is extra sensitive on and around the eyes anyway, and during treatment will be even more so, which will make the powder more likely to flake.

For mascara, choose a mercury-free brand that's free of chemicals so it won't irritate your already-sensitive eyes. Avoid waterproof and longwearing types, as they're hard to remove. You have to rub, which can cause you to lose your eyelashes.

For eyeliner, you don't necessarily have to buy a separate product. Just use eye shadow and apply with a wet eyeliner brush. Easy, looks natural, and will accentuate your lash line to make for fuller lashes (since they may have thinned out). If you feel comfortable using a liner, however, go ahead; just be careful!

Blushes and Bronzers

- **Powders**. For bronzers, powders are the easiest to use. They easily enhance skin tone and give you a healthy, rosy glow. Just make sure your shade is not too "orange." Apply with a brush for a smooth and even look. For blush, pink and peachy hues are great colors for all skin types. Apply to the apples of the cheeks. Make sure you go back and blend the blush with a brush for a more natural look.

- **Creams**. Anyone can use creams, but they're especially good for dry skin. (If you're going through chemotherapy and radiation and haven't used creams before, you may want to try one.) They're bit easier to blend, and give you more control as to where you put them. They're also great if you're not using foundation underneath, but just want to brighten your complexion. If you have dry skin, however, and don't blend properly, they can make your skin look muddy. You can try mixing some with your moisturizer and then applying. I recommend using a liquid foundation and then a powder bronzer to give it a glow. For blush, I love creams—they last longer and are great for dry skin. Apply after your foundation on the apples of the cheeks and blend with clean fingers.

- **Shimmers.** Use shimmering bronzers sparingly, particularly if you have mature skin. Too much can make the skin look "too made up" and can settle into wrinkles and fine lines. Choose a bronzer with a slight luminescence for a radiant glow.

Lip Color

First of all, make sure lips are hydrated. Find a beeswax or other non-petroleum-based lip balm and keep it with you at all times. Sun protection is important for lips as well, so choose a formula with a sunscreen in it.

Lip color is a great pick-me-up for those days when you're feeling your worst. Cream formulas with moisturizing ingredients like jojoba, avocado, and vitamin E help keep your lips moist while adding color. Shimmer brands add a little shine without attracting UV rays as much as glosses do. Avoid longwearing and matte formulas, as these are more drying. Be cautious with lip liner—it can prevent bleeding, especially when you're using creamy lipsticks, but it can also be drying and may illuminate dryness around your lips. You may want to use it only on special occasions.

Best Brushes to Choose

As you're perusing your drawer of products, you may want to consider your makeup brushes. Where did you get them? What kind are they?

Natural bristles are made with animal hair that comes from goats, ponies, badgers, or squirrels. (If you're allergic to animal hair, choose synthetic brushes.) They may shed, but they hold and distribute powder better than synthetic bristles, which is why professionals often prefer them.

Synthetic brushes are made using manmade materials and can also range from rough-feeling to silky soft. You can tell they're synthetic by their shinier appearance. The biggest advantage is they typically don't shed and glide easily over your face, which can be better for dry, flaky skin.

High-quality synthetic brushes can be just as nice as natural ones, so if you're concerned about animal rights and want to avoid natural hair, you can still find quality brushes. However, watch out for low-quality synthetic brushes, as they can stiffen with use.

Look for trustworthy brands that make tools for sensitive skin. Taklon makeup brushes (a synthetic material) are best for applying cream or liquid makeup, as they hold onto the product and distribute it evenly. Some Taklon brushes have antibacterial benefits, which can be helpful while you're going through treatment. (Natural bristles can trap powders and chemicals in makeup.)

You may want to buy individual brushes as opposed to those in a set, so that you can test each for quality and get only what you need. To test, run the brush over the back of your hand. If the bristles get out of shape or fall out, pass it by. If you're not sure where to look, check out Appendix IV for some great sites that carry quality brushes. You may also find some at your local spa, department store, or health food store.

When to Toss, What to Keep, and When to Clean

Most makeup items don't have expiration dates. Nevertheless, they do expire over time, which can make them more irritating on your skin because of bacteria growth or ingredients that have gone rancid.

Store your makeup in a cool, dry place (away from the bathroom if possible), and always close products securely to limit exposure to contaminants. Here are a few basic guidelines. Throw away:

- Any damaged products (broken containers, cracked seals)
- Mascara over three months old
- Liquid foundations and concealers over three months old
- Lipstick, lip pencils, and eye pencils over six months old
- Powders, eye shadows, and blushes over a year old
- Any product that changes color or texture, or begins to smell funny
- Brushes that are old and shedding, have hairs separated from the wand, or are stiff and hard

Keep disinfectant on your makeup counter, dip your brush into it after *every* use, then swirl into a tissue. Clean your brushes at least once a week, particularly while you're going through treatment. Use warm water and a little toxin-free shampoo, swirl in a cup, use your fingers to clean the hairs gently in the direction of the hair, then run under clean water until the water runs clear.

Air dry on a paper towel with the brush hanging over the sink overnight. Do not dry the brushes upright (with the hair pointing upward), as moisture and particles can collect into the base of the brush and cause the hair to eventually fan out or shed, or even loosen the handle.

Avoid Infection: Create Your Own Tool Set

During cancer treatments, applying your makeup can be risky business. One slip with a pair of dirty tweezers could set you up for a serious infection. One tug with the eyelash curler could leave you with no eyelashes at all. Suddenly that set of styling tools has gone from a harmless batch of brushes to a dangerous stash of weapons!

You have to be a little more careful while your immune system is waging the fight of its life. Here are a few tips for choosing the safest makeup tools to use on your fragile skin.

- **Brushes.** Your fingers may have worked in the past, but fingernails trap bacteria, so if you haven't already done so, get yourself a set of brushes—at the very least a blush brush, eye shadow brush, eyebrow powder brush, face powder brush, and a lip brush. If you're going to use your fingers, be sure to wash your hands thoroughly first.

- **Cotton Balls.** Choose the jumbo-sized, whispy-soft real cotton balls. They absorb better than synthetic and are softer on your skin.

- **Tweezers.** Besides the eyelash curler, this is one of the most dangerous makeup tools while you're going through chemo or radiation. To lower your risk of cuts or other wounds, set aside your pointed-nose tweezers and choose something that won't cut your skin. Try tapered, flat, and round tips, and those that have a soft foam cushion grip.

- **Sponges.** I'd recommend those made of natural materials. Be sure to dispose of them after every use to reduce risk of bacteria buildup.

- **Eyelash Curler.** If you're losing your hair due to treatment, you could lose your eyelashes too. An eyelash curler during this time can be Enemy #1 to your lashes! Use a rounded-rubber curler gently and only when you need to, or try warming a spoon in hot water, dry it, and push the curved part of the spoon against the lashes to curl.

My New Tender-Care Makeup Bag

Now that you know the basics, take a look at the products you currently have. If any of them are old or damaged, throw them out. If you have drying powders or foundations with chemical sunscreens, put those in a bag. (You can decide what to do with them later.) If you have products with petroleum ingredients, harsh chemicals, fragrances, parabens, or lead, in the bag they go!

Below, make a list of the new products you need. To help you, I've listed the basics. Check those you already have, and make note of those you need.

Once you have your new products ready, we'll talk about camouflaging the various flaws you may encounter during treatment.

____ Foundation (hydrating, without chemical sunscreen)

____ Concealer (liquid or cream for under eyes; stick for target areas)

____ Eye shadow (cream is best for dry, sensitive eyes; powder for eyeliner)

____ Blush (creams for dry skin and for long-lasting color; powders for easier application)

____ Bronzer (liquid is best for dry skin; powder for light touch-ups)

____ Highlighter (powder or liquid)

____ Mascara (mercury-free formulas; avoid waterproof)

____ Lip balm (free of petroleum products and filled with natural nourishing hydrators)

____ Lip color (moisturizing, nourishing creams)

____ Sunscreen (no chemical types; zinc oxide or titanium dioxide only)

Troubleshooting and Application Tips

Cancer treatments cause certain flaws to appear on your face that you wouldn't normally have to deal with. This is where makeup can make a huge difference in how your skin looks. I strongly encourage men as well as women to give these tips a try, especially for covering scars and pimples. No one will ever know, but it will make you feel (and look) much better! To help camouflage these drug-related effects, try the following tips.

Facial Swelling
Steroid use during treatment can make your face, fingers, and neck look puffy. These side effects can become more pronounced the longer you're on the drugs.

You can lessen the appearance of the effect by using color to create a little contouring on your face. Try these steps:

- Nose: Use a foundation just a tad darker than your regular skin tone (or a bronzer) and blend it in on either side of your nose. Use a slightly lighter color on the bridge, applying it down the center for a nice highlight.

- Cheeks: Use a soft blush on the apples of your cheeks back to your hairline. If you're in the mood for a little more glow, apply a shimmery lighter color on top of your cheekbones. Blend everything.

- Face: Extra bronzer along your jawline can help further slim the look of your face. Blend down toward your neck.

- Eyes: As the face swells, the eyes appear smaller. Be sure you're moisturizing around the eyes, and apply slices of cold cucumber or potato on the eyes to reduce swelling. Apply concealer around the eye area (near the brow bone and on the lash line too). Then apply liner to the upper lash line to kind of "lift" the eye. Use a lighter color to the inner rim of the lower lash line, and finally, brush a little blush under the eyes to reduce the appearance of bags.

- Lips: If your lips look swollen, stay away from shimmers and glosses. Use a deep shade of moisturizing lip color.

Covering Scars

You may be dealing with an acne-like rash, which can leave scars on your fragile face. As long as there is no open wound, you can use concealer to neutralize the color of the scar.

- Start by using a small concealer brush (your finger is not as effective for such a small area) and covering all areas needed by using a yellow or golden concealer (to hide the redness). Then apply your foundation or powder. Continue with your regular makeup, and then, if the scar is still showing, dab a bit more on top and blend.

- MEN: You may just want to use a powder that matches your skin to set the concealer without making you look like you have makeup on. An easy application of powder will do.

Covering Pimples

A yellow-based concealer in a color close to your foundation is best for hiding breakouts. Apply sparingly, work from the center out, and blend well at the edges with a makeup wedge. For a more natural look, apply concealer after foundation. Use a dab of powder to set, but not too much or you'll have a noticeable light spot.

MEN: Just use the brush and the concealer—no foundation needed.

Under-Eye Circles

The skin under the eyes is particularly thin, so tiny blood vessels can show through, creating a darker look.

- To brighten your eyes, use a concealer with a warm (pink) undertone to counteract the blueness of the dark circles.

- Pat some moisturizing eye cream under the eye first; then apply concealer. I use the ring finger for application, but while going through treatment, you're at a higher risk of infection, so be sure to wash well, or choose a soft, flat concealer brush. (Make sure you wash your brushes often and disinfect daily.)

- Dab concealer, almost tapping the skin, on the inner corner of the eye (always dab, never rub or streak) and underneath the lashes to the outer corner. Apply about an inch below the eye and keep dabbing until blended.

Loss of Lashes

Most of us know that we may lose our hair during chemotherapy. What you may not be prepared for is losing hair in other places—like on the eyebrows and eyelashes!

Chemo drugs can cause you to lose your hair just about anywhere, but eyelashes may arguably be the most difficult to deal with. The good news is that eyelashes usually *do* grow back, so the change is temporary.

To help prevent lash loss, refrain from rubbing your eyes too vigorously. Use a natural, creamy eye makeup remover to gently clean your eyes. Heavy mascara—particularly waterproof brands—can also be too harsh on delicate lashes, so you may want to go with a more natural look for a while.

If your lashes do fall out (or if you lose more than half of them), you may want to use false eyelashes. However, I strongly recommend that you don't. You could have an allergic reaction to the glue, the chemicals may irritate you skin, and there's also a risk of increased infection. You can end up pulling out any lashes you may have left when you remove the false lashes.

A better option is to use makeup to recreate the look of full, healthy lashes. Just line the upper lash line, smudge it, then apply mascara (if you have lashes left). It's okay to use an eyelash curler on occasion, but overuse can cause breakage and eyelash loss, so be careful.

There may be a time, however, when you feel like you *really* need false lashes. If you feel it may be too difficult to do, get a makeup artist at a local makeup store, department store, or salon to help you. Let her know you have cancer and that it is imperative to use fresh, clean tools because of your susceptibility to infection. (Better yet, take your own tool set and some antibacterial wipes.)

- When putting on the lashes, measure them against your eyelid and trim with a pair of sharp scissors so they fit just right. They should fall just short of the inner corner of your eye.

- If you have lashes of your own, there's no need to apply mascara to them first, as it can look messy and clumpy.

- It is best to line the upper lid first, however. A liquid liner is preferable, as it lasts longer and will help create a smooth line.

- Hold the lashes with a pair of tweezers (make sure they're not sharp ones); then use a toothpick to apply a thin coat of eyelash glue to the base of the fake lashes. Wait a minute to allow the glue to become sticky. (Be sure to get clear glue, not black.)

- Position the lashes as close to your own as you can and gently press down, starting with the inner corner and working outward. Hold the lash on your lid for 20-30 seconds. (Smooth as necessary.)

- When you're ready to remove the false lashes, gently pull them, then use eye makeup remover to take off the glue and liner.

Loss of Eyebrows

Unless you're an eyebrow fanatic like me, you may not have thought much about your eyebrows before cancer treatment. Maybe you tweezed them now and then, or shaped them with a little color, but when they start disappearing during chemotherapy, you suddenly realize how important they are. Eyebrows frame your face and make your look complete. They can also help hide your illness.

If you haven't completely lost your eyebrows but are finding them sparse lately, choose a shadow color a tad lighter than your natural hair color (unless your hair is light blond or silver, and then go for a slightly darker shade). Use a brow brush (love the ones from Anastasia). Feather the color into the area where your eyebrow usually is. Then brush through the hairs to create a more natural look.

If your eyebrows are completely gone, you need to determine the eyebrow shape that's right for your face.

- **Determine a shape**. Women with round faces, for example, should choose a more angular brow shape. Rounded brows are great for those with large eyes or a wide forehead. The standard arch shape is flattering to most women, as it helps open the eyes, and the low arch helps give the illusion of length to those with small foreheads.

- **Choose a stencil to guide the desired shape**. The stencil will guide the application of makeup, sort of like a cutout eyebrow. You can find many stencils online, even some made particularly for cancer patients that fit on your face, leaving both hands free to apply makeup.

- **Choose your eyebrow makeup.** Go for shades that most closely match your natural hair color. Use nontoxic formulas to protect yourself from dangerous chemicals, and follow these easy steps:

- Use a pencil to dot along the brow line, creating the line of your eyebrow.

- Take your brow brush and apply the shadow or brow color over the pencil line and throughout the brow area.

- Brush through both pencil and color to blend.

It may be easiest to find an eyebrow kit. Most come with two shades of powder to help you get a realistic look, plus a highlighting pencil to mark the beginning and end of your brows, perhaps one to use as a base before you apply color, the stencil to establish the shape, and powder to set the makeup when you're done.

Remember that not everyone's brows are perfectly even. Most people have one higher than the other, or one with a more pronounced arch or fuller hairs. You don't have to be perfect to create this natural illusion. (Don't forget to check Appendix VII for websites that have great eyebrow makeup and kits.)

Dry Lips

Cancer treatments can dry your skin, and your lips are no exception. The mouth is a very sensitive part of the body and becomes even more so during chemotherapy or radiation treatments. Dryness can lead to chapping and even cracks in the lips, so it's important to keep them lubricated.

- Drink lots of water, and gently exfoliate at night by carefully rubbing a washcloth over your lips. (Be extra careful if lips are tender.)

- Apply a moisturizing lip balm often. Remember to avoid those made with synthetic chemicals like parabens, phthalates, and petroleum (which can further dry your lips over time). Try natural and organic brands that can be purchased at your local health food store or Whole Foods Market. Purchase tubes instead of jars or pots.

- Nourishing lipsticks can help keep lips moisturized while preventing chapping and flaking. Choose creamy, moisturizing options as opposed to matte long-lasting formulas, which can accentuate dryness. Be sure to use a lead-free formula. If your lips are cracked or in poor condition, avoid lipstick until the lips are healed.

- Lip liner can prevent bleeding, which is more likely to happen with creamy lipsticks. (It may be drying, however, so test it out first.)

Pale, Ashy Skin

As you're going through treatment, you may notice paleness on your face, or even on your head if your hair is gone. Bronzers and highlighters are a great way to bring back that healthy glow.

MEN, listen up: A bronzer can really transform your complexion. This is not makeup, per se, but a way to bring back a healthy hue to your face, neck, and scalp (if needed). There are bronzers marketed especially to men, so don't even think twice.

Shade

- If you're just staring out with bronzers, choose suntan browns and golden shades, as these are most universally flattering. If the product looks too orange in the package, it probably will on your skin as well. With bronzers it is best to test them on the skin rather than buying without trying them on. Think this: You want to "warm" the skin, not color it. Try to remember how you looked after your last natural tan.

- Those with cool, pinkish complexions should look for bronzers with touches of pink.

- Warmer olive tones may do better with deeper shades with amber or honey undertones.

- Yellow or golden skin does best with gold, tan, or brown bronzer.

- Brown skin is best with tawny and brown bronzers.

- Women of color who may experience "ashy" skin during treatment may want to choose bronzers with burgundy or copper undertones.

- As a basic rule: Look for something that most closely matches your natural skin tone, similar to the way you would shop for a foundation, only this time you're looking for something just a shade darker.

Application

- When applying on your face, apply foundation and concealer first. Start on the perimeter and move in, applying bronzer where the sun would usually create a tan: upper cheeks, forehead, and nose. If you're wearing your hair back, dust the tips of your ears and your neck. If you end up with too much, use a dry cotton pad to wipe some off, or dust your face with some loose powder.

- For powders, use a brush slightly larger than your regular blush brush, and make sure the hairs are fluffy, not too tightly woven. If you're using a liquid or gel bronzer, squirt a dab on a sponge and apply in circular motions. Use a small amount; you can always add more later.

- Finally, add a bit of blush on the cheeks to keep the bronzer from looking flat.

- You can use a sunless tanner to help bring some color back into your face (and even your head if you like). Just be sure to choose a safe brand that has nourishing ingredients, and go for a slight change in color rather than one that leaves you too orange. Look for formulas just slightly darker than your normal shade of skin.

- MEN: After concealing, if you choose to, dust powder bronzer all over your face, concentrating on areas where the sun would naturally hit: cheeks, nose, and forehead. Make sure you blend in well. Start with an easy application and build up if you need to. Don't forget your ears and scalp if you have no hair. If you end up with too much, use a dry cotton pad to wipe some off.

Dull Appearance—Time to Highlight

During treatment you may find that your complexion looks dull and lifeless. Highlighters subtly enhance the shape of your face, helping to bring out certain features over others (your cheekbones, for example) and creating a new radiance and glow.

During treatment you can use either powders or creams, depending on the effect you're going for. Powders are the easiest to work with. If you want just a subtle highlight, apply foundation first and let it set. Then, using your powder brush, lightly apply powder highlighter just above your cheekbones to make them appear more prominent and to give your face a bit more shape and liveliness.

You can also apply powder highlighter down the center of your nose, which has a slimming effect. Highlighting the tip of the chin brings it out a bit more. Finish by using a blending brush to blend everything in.

The technique is basically the same for cream highlighters, except that you usually apply it before foundation and go back for a touch-up if needed. You can also mix it with your moisturizer or foundation for an all-over luminosity.

Makeup Tips for Emotional Days

If you're having a particularly emotional day and are planning to go out, you may want to prepare for a few tears. No one likes mascara running down her cheeks! Apply your mascara and eyeliner to the upper lash only—leave the lower lash bare. Use water-resistant mascara (avoid waterproof types), and choose a pencil eyeliner instead of shadow for these days, as it tends to stay on longer. Avoid powder eye shadows, as usual, and go for cream. Keep a little concealer, blush, and lip color with you to refresh.

Let's Review

- Feeling good about your appearance can help you feel more confident and more likely to reach out for important social support.

- While going through treatment, your skin is more sensitive than ever before, and requires tender, nourishing care and products.

- Like other personal care products, makeup can contain potentially toxic ingredients like parabens, lead, mercury, nanoparticles, and synthetic fragrances. Be choosy about your products, read labels, and use brands reputed for using safer ingredients.

- No matter what products you used before treatment, your skin has changed, so you may need to throw away or set aside your old products and change to more hydrating and gentle ones until you recover.

- Since you're more at risk of infection during treatment, disinfect your makeup brushes daily, wash them weekly, and throw out cotton balls and sponges after each use. Be careful with your makeup products as well, and throw out old and expired formulas.

- The tools you use for makeup application can make a big difference in how natural you look. Choose very soft brushes and sponges that will feel good on your tender skin.

- If you have trouble areas like under-eye circles, sallow skin, or scars, you can effectively conceal them with careful makeup application, helping you to feel more confident when going to work or out to play.

- Don't forget to check Appendix VII for great sites that offer safe products!

Goals

After reading this chapter, you may want to make some changes in your makeup products and routine. Here are some examples for you. Circle the ones that apply to you, and add some of your own.

- Switch from mineral or powder foundation to liquid, which is better for dry skin and will give it a dewy look.
- Buy a couple of concealers to help camouflage scars, pimples, and dark spots.
- If you don't have makeup tools, get a set of brushes so you can avoid using your fingers on your face.
- Wash your brushes more often.
- Invest in a bronzer that looks good with your skin and use it regularly.
- Change your mascaras from waterproof types to those that are easier to remove.
- Switch your pointed tweezers to a more safe, rounded type.

Other ideas you may have:

1. _____

2. _____

3. _____

Personal Affirmations

I release the need to criticize myself. I love myself.

I am more than my appearance.
I am beautiful/handsome in mind and body.

7

Solutions for a Body Under Stress

"I always stay positive—remind myself every day to keep a good mind, body, and spirit, and to never give up. I just don't want to give up."

—Justin, brain cancer survivor

IS THERE A QUESTION IN ANYONE'S MIND THAT CANCER treatments majorly stress out the body? We're talking about treatments that actually *kill* the cells inside of us. It's great when those cells are cancer cells, but we all know that so far, most of the treatments available can't differentiate between cancer cells and healthy cells.

"All these chemo agents," says breast cancer oncology surgeon Stephen Green, "attack the fastest growing cells in the body. They attack the cancer cells and kill them, but what other cells are rapidly growing? Hair, nails, and skin."

That's not all. According to Dr. Green, fast-growing cells also exist in the mouth, digestive system, and immune system. "Eat something and bite your gum, and it heals very quickly," he says. "If you have chemo, you slow down the healing process. The chemo prevents the immune system from working efficiently."

Radiation, as well, kills cancer cells, but also damages skin on the way. "Radiation has a direct toxic effect on the skin," says Dr. Green. "It's the same as sunlight, creating burns. Most of the energy goes to the tumor, but you get some effect on the skin."

This attack on our cells shows up in symptoms that range from uncomfortable to just plain miserable. I'm talking mouth sores, wounds that won't heal, nausea, burns, bruising and bleeding, fatigue, flaky skin, and more.

For many people, these symptoms can be the scariest part of the experience. "When I first started chemo, I was scared," says Donald Wilhelm, five-time cancer survivor. "I didn't know what to expect, and chemo kicked my butt. I would be sick before I even got to the hospital."

"When they changed my chemo to different drugs it really put me over the edge," says Alli, ovarian cancer survivor. "I would go in for treatment on Friday afternoons and spend my weekend at home. I would go back to work on Monday. It wasn't uncommon for me to be running to the bathroom and throwing up, but I needed my benefits and needed the work."

Most of us have experienced not feeling well at one point or another in our lives. We know what it's like to have the flu, or perhaps to spend a few days in the hospital. We have dealt with pain in the past, but may be completely unprepared for the discomfort of cancer. Still—never doubt that you have what it takes. You can get through it! What you need now is more love for yourself than you may have ever mustered before.

"I remember being really scared about it," says Deb, breast cancer survivor. "Then I remember thinking it wasn't as bad as I thought it was going to be."

Did you know that your mental outlook can affect the pain you feel from cancer and cancer treatments? According to researchers, cancer patients with more optimistic outlooks were better able to manage their cancer pain, and those patients with a strong sense of control over their environment experienced less severe fatigue as well.[1]

Researchers recommend that cancer patients and their loved ones encourage optimistic emotions by watching comedies, laughing, hanging out and talking with positive people; and using prayer, meditation, and counseling to help increase control.

"If you have a negative attitude," says Dr. Green, "you're going to feel terrible, and the chemotherapy is going to make you feel worse. If you're someone who says, 'I want to get better, and I'm going to get better,' you're going to manage very well. It's a matter of how you look at things, and how you handle it."

Of course, it's easier said than done. On those days when you're throwing up or having difficulty eating, an optimistic attitude may be the furthest thing from your mind. I was lucky, as my father was a great example of someone who understood that he needed time to deal with his emotions. He would take a few days on his own, sort of a personal retreat, and then he would get back into the fight. He knew that a positive outlook was critical for his healing. When he was diagnosed a second time, he actually said to the doctor, "You do the medical thing, I'll do the mental thing." Watching him, I realized that I had to be kind to myself, but I also had to be careful not to let negative feelings or thoughts run away with me.

On those days when you're feeling really low, it's more important than ever to take the time you need to pour self-love back into your mind, body, and soul. In this chapter, I'm going to talk about how to deal with some of the side effects treatment can create in your body. Through it all, I hope you'll remember one thing: Love yourself, and love your body. You may feel sometimes that it's betraying you, but it's going through a lot and it needs your support and your good emotions to heal.

Your Body Needs Your Loving Energy

"You have to come to the concept that you're either going to fight it and live longer or you're going to give up. Surround yourself with people who want to help you and be there for you. It makes it so much easier."

—Teresa, colon cancer survivor

When your body starts feeling uncomfortable as a result of cancer or cancer treatments, you may experience a myriad of emotions, ranging from anger and frustration to discouragement and despair. Wouldn't it be nice to just have a button to push to make it all feel better?

According to Dr. Eva Selhub, author of *The Love Response*, we have such a button. It's called love.

"From the very beginning, right after we're born," Dr. Eva says, "the very first thing we learn is love. When we cry, someone holds us. When we're hungry, someone gives us food. These things create receptors that allow us to take in love, which regulates our whole body/mind physiology, turns off the stress response, and teaches us to trust."

The opposite of love, Dr. Eva says, is *fear*. Going through cancer, all of us experience fear, which can leave us defenseless in fighting the disease. Fear breaks down the immune system and further stresses the rest of the body. To turn this destructive emotion around, we must remember what it felt like to be loved.

Am I Loving Myself?

How do you know if you're acting in a loving way toward yourself? Find a piece of paper and answer the following questions. Don't hesitate, and don't hold back because you think you're being "selfish." Job #1 right now is to take care of yourself. It's very eye-opening to become aware of how we usually fall short in this area!

"If I loved myself…"

- What would I do for me?

- Would I be around this person?

- Would I eat this food?

- Would I use products that are full of chemicals and may be harmful to my health?

- Would I put these expectations on myself?

- What would I ask for right now?

- How would I schedule my day?

- What would I tell myself first thing in the morning?

- How would I make this easier?

- Would I ask for help so I can focus on my recovery?

Dr. Eva calls it the "love response"—a place where the mind and body feel loved, cared for, safe, and whole. When we're in this place, the body responds with physical changes that support the immune system, clear the mind, and fuel strength to handle any situation.

"In the love response," she says, "we're turning off stress chemicals, opening up brain centers that allow us to think more clearly, turning off the cortisol that's suppressing the immune system, and relaxing into the experience of love."

The experience of fear can often come about because we don't believe we have the resources to deal with our situation. We fear the cancer is stronger than us and will get the best of us, or that we won't be able to deal with the side effects. These feelings are perfectly natural to experience, but it's important that we learn how to alleviate them and feel better again, because staying in that negative place cripples the body.

"Feeling bad just means something needs to be fixed or adapted," Dr. Eva says. "If your physiology stays in a negative place for too long, the entire system breaks down on many levels."

The solution is surprisingly simple. If you're in a place of feeling bad, whether it be stress, fear, discomfort, or discouragement, the solution is to go to a place of love. "You turn on hormones related to love and the mind will clear, the body will feel better, and you will be more capable of handling your situation."

What exactly is a "place of love?" It involves those emotions that go with love—relaxation, warmth, joy, and strength. "We must change the belief systems that say 'I don't have enough' or 'I'm not enough,'" says Dr. Eva. "We change it to 'I am enough, and I have enough resources to handle this. The situation is here. I have cancer. What are my resources? How can I make myself as resilient as possible to handle this?'"

Dr. Eva recommends a daily practice that takes you into a more loving place in your mind. First, however, you must accept and allow your negative feelings (as mentioned in Chapter 4). "The first thing is, you're allowed to be scared. Screw the 'gotta be strong' thing. Let yourself be scared and realize that you have a support system to hold you up and help you. Tell yourself, 'I'm supported. I'm loved. I don't have to be anything, or do anything.' You don't have to be superhuman. Open up to receiving love and support around you."

How can you practice going into a place of love? Some of it has to do with what we've been talking about—caring about the products you put on your skin, the food you put in your mouth, and the way you take care of yourself. Part of it is being tender and caring toward your own body.

According to Dr. Eva, you can also take certain specific steps to encourage a loving state of mind. She suggests a visualization she calls "SHIELD." When you're feeling badly, perform this visualization and see if you can calm yourself and feel better.

1. **S—slow** down. Take a moment to be quiet with yourself. Imagine a warm, golden light shining upon you, wrapping you up in love.

2. **H—honor** how you feel right now. Don't judge it. Just become aware of it.

3. **I—inhale.**

4. **E**—don't forget to **exhale**.

5. **L—listen** to your needs. What's missing? Do you need love, sleep, comfort?

6. **D—decide**. Shift into the love response and be loving to yourself. Take action to get what you need, and say several times over, "The

support I need is here. I am loved and I am valued." Imagine your best idea of love—someone holding you, arms from above cradling you, the shield protecting you, whatever feels loving to you.

Now that you're in the loving mode, let's talk about how you can be kind and loving to your body—through gentle remedies for various side effects.

A New Approach to Bathing and Showering

Cancer and cancer treatments change your body, skin, hair, and nails, and that means you need to alter your daily habits. If you're like me, you probably love long, hot, luxurious soaks in the tub. They may have felt good before, but now—since your skin is probably dry, irritated, fragile, and delicate—they're likely to make things worse. Hot water robs the skin of its own moisture, breaking down the natural oils and increasing dryness.

That doesn't mean you can't enjoy a little luxury. If bathing is your thing, make sure the tub is clean before you step in. You're more prone to infection, so take the extra time to disinfect, and use toxin-free, eco-friendly cleaners.

Organic Towels & Silk Sheets

One thing you can do to be gentler with yourself and your skin is to invest in a few items that will feel good. Start with your towels. Many store-bought towels are cheaply made with synthetic materials and then processed with harsh chemicals. Choose instead natural fibers, such as fine cotton and silk. (Be cautious with wool and linen; depending on how they're processed, they may feel too rough.)

Be careful, too, about the detergents you use. You can have the softest, most natural towel there is, but if you use harsh detergent, remnants of bleach, brighteners, and surfactants can cling to the fibers and make their way onto your skin.

Silk sheets may be more expensive, but they'll make treatment easier for you. You tend to move with more ease on silk, so you won't get wrapped up in the sheets, and your hair is less likely to break or fall out. If you have radiation burns or other skin wounds, you'll be less likely to catch or hurt the painful area. If you're having trouble sleeping, silk sheets may really help you, as they're known to just put the body in a happier place. They typically last longer than regular sheets as well, which can make the cost worth it in the long run.

Remember to change both your sheets and towels regularly. You can never be too careful while your immune system is compromised.

Tone down the temperature to lukewarm and add about a cup of ground oatmeal, which will soothe skin and relieve itching. (You may also want to try Dead Sea salt or natural bath teas.) Enjoy the moisturizing effects of almond or jojoba oils—even pure honey and evaporated milk.

Light a few naturally scented candles or release homemade scents by placing rose, mint, or lavender leaves in a fabric bag and hanging it under the faucet. Play some soothing music, drink a cup of chamomile tea, and as you relax your tired body and calm your senses, you may find you don't miss the steam at all.

"Baking soda and Epsom salts help draw toxins out of your body," says three-time survivor Meghan. "It helps your skin feel a lot better."

For everyday showering, short, tepid sprays are better than long, hot ones—again, to keep your skin from drying out. If you use soap, which is too drying, switch to a moisturizing, SLS-free (sodium-laureth sulfate or sodium lauryl sulfate) shower gel. (Read the label to steer clear of harmful chemicals.) Avoid aggressive shower puffs and gently wash with your hands instead.

Whether you take a shower or a bath, use a soft towel afterward and go easy on your skin. Make sure your towels are washed with toxin-free, mild, and unscented detergents to reduce allergies and irritation. Pat, don't rub or tug, yourself dry; leave your skin a little damp and apply a natural, chemical-free moisturizer to retain moisture.

On your more tired days, standing in the shower or sitting up in the bath may be too much. I remember when showering was such a difficult chore for my father. It just took more energy than he had on some days to scrub, lift his hands over his head, or twist, turn, and bend as we usually do when washing. I wish I had known then about a handy gizmo called a "shower chair"—which you can also use in the bath. These come in many styles, and you can find them in medical supply stores or online sites that cater to people living with medical challenges. Choose the one that's right for you and take a load off while rinsing.

If there comes a day you just can't get out of bed, you can still enjoy the comfort of a clean head of hair by enlisting the help of a friend or loved one and employing a shampoo basin, which allows you to have your hair washed without having to toss off the blankets.

However you bathe, if you're going through treatment, care for yourself enough to alter your habits for a while. When it's over you can go back to the steam if you like—and with your new, healthier products, it will probably feel better than ever!

What About Shaving?

"I use natural skin-care products—100% pure products. Nothing that can harm you or harm your skin. I feel much better without those products."

—Justin, brain cancer survivor

We talked about how men need to take a few precautions when shaving during treatment in Chapter Five, but what about women and shaving?

Some chemotherapy drugs cause us to lose the hair on our legs as well as our heads, which can create smooth, hairless legs. This was definitely a plus for me during treatment! However, if you do still have hair on your legs, be careful. You're at a higher risk of infection, and razors are notorious for causing nicks and cuts. Use an electric shaver instead of standard blades whenever possible.

If you're sold on razors, make sure they're properly sanitized and sterilized—best to use them and then discard them. Look for chemical-free shaving creams and gels, and try to find those that have soothing ingredients like aloe and green tea.

Waxing and plucking can increase skin sensitivity and may be especially uncomfortable during treatment. I suggest staying away from waxing if your skin has become very thin and fragile or if radiation has left it red and inflamed. If you do decide to go for it, avoid salons or spas that may put you at risk for additional germs. (Think double dipping in waxing pots!) You may just want to go for at-home solutions, where you can use all your own tools and products. Always moisturize afterwards with toxin-free products and protect exposed skin with a chemical-free sunscreen.

The Most Common Side Effect: Nausea

"I did have a lot of nausea. Sometimes I could eat a few crackers with peanut butter and be fine. But then it would change and I didn't want to eat anything. I remember not wanting to drink plain water. It was totally unappealing."

—Deb, breast cancer survivor

Why is it that cancer treatments so commonly cause stomach upset? Chemotherapy-induced nausea and vomiting usually occur because the drugs stimulate a part of the brain that controls the vomiting response. Damage to the intestines from chemo can also stimulate that same response in the brain and also in the stomach. Other causes of nausea unique to cancer include: radiation-induced nausea (when part of the gastrointestinal tract is involved, including the esophagus), intestinal obstruction (due to scar tissue or a tumor), pressure or swelling on the brain, and uncontrolled pain.

Which medication your doctor may recommend typically depends on the cause of the upset. Those used specifically in cases of chemotherapy-induced nausea and vomiting include anti-nausea medications that target receptors in the brain and gut to block the vomiting response. For other types of nausea caused by the cancer itself, or by a combination of causes, doctors may prescribe anti-nausea medications, or "motility" agents, which help get things moving in the intestine.

Medications aren't the only option, however. Many non-medical approaches can be effective at calming the stomach. For instance, when my father drank ginger tea, it helped him a great deal with nausea, especially if he drank it thirty minutes before a meal. In fact, ginger, has been shown in studies to be more effective than a placebo when taken before treatments.[2] (Try about 500 mg a day.)

Researchers have also found that acupuncture prevented post-operative breast-surgery nausea more effectively than a leading medication.[3] Two hours after surgery, 77 percent of subjects who received the acupuncture experienced no nausea or vomiting, compared to 64 percent taking a drug. According to another analysis of eleven studies, acupuncture seemed to reduce the vomiting that can occur shortly after a chemotherapy treatment.[4]

Other solutions that have helped survivors: two pinches of cardamom and a ½-teaspoon of honey mixed into a ½-cup of plain yogurt; or a pinch of nutmeg and a pinch of cardamom into a ½-cup of warm milk. If you like tea, steep a teaspoon of cumin seeds and a pinch of ground nutmeg in one cup of boiling water for ten minutes, strain to remove the seeds, and drink.

You can also try boiling a cup of water and mixing in a teaspoon of cinnamon or one cinnamon stick, a tablespoon of honey, and drinking slowly. Peppermint is also commonly recommended to control stomach upset. Try a drop or two of peppermint oil on the tongue, or take some peppermint candy with you on treatment days.

And remember—just because many people experience nausea and vomiting as a result of treatment doesn't mean you will. Expecting a side effect may help to bring it on. "If you say to yourself, 'I'm going to feel sick, and I'm going to have these side effects,'" says Dr. Green, "you will get the side effect. The suggestion is sometimes harmful."

Dry, Itchy Skin—Nutrition Tips to Boost Hydration

"My face was so dry. My cheeks—everything felt like snake's skin. Not itchy, just complete dryness. It's like having a sunburn all the time."

—Donald, five-time cancer survivor

We've talked a lot about how dry, flaky skin is an uncomfortable side effect of many cancer treatments. Radiation damages skin at the treatment site, while chemotherapy can get you itching everywhere. You apply moisturizer and apply moisturizer, but are there any other natural remedies?

Dry skin seems to occur on the surface, but actually the problem goes deeper than that, down to the oil-producing glands in the lower layers. A healthy diet filled with vitamins, minerals, and omega fatty acids that support healthy gland function can help your skin battle the problem. Fortunately, the foods that are good for your skin are good for the rest of your body, too, so while you're eating for moisturization, you'll reap the benefit of increased immunity and strength.

Water: Believe me, I know how hard it is to drink liquids during treatment. You just don't feel like drinking anything! I would hand my father a glass and encourage him to take a sip. He would do it to make me happy and put it back down, so I'd ask him to take another. Drinking water is so important to your body at any time, but especially so when you're fighting an illness. Take a water bottle with you everywhere, and drink frequently. If you can't drink, just sip, one small sip after another. Your body is always losing water through perspiration, evaporation, and regular organ functioning, to say nothing of cancer treatments that dehydrate you, so please don't neglect this step.

Watery Foods: Goodies like cantaloupe, grapes, oranges, celery, cucumbers, and tomatoes are all bursting with liquids that will moisturize from the inside out.

Nutrients: Foods high in vitamins A, B, C, E, and natural antioxidants to support skin renewal and repair. *Note: I'm recommending nutrient-rich foods, here, not supplements. If you want to try supplements, be sure to check with your doctor first, especially if you're still undergoing treatment.*

- Vitamin A helps maintain and heal epithelial (skin) tissues. Sources include egg yolks, oysters, and nonfat milk, plus beta-carotene-rich

Estrogen In Your Moisturizer?

Researchers have long speculated that estrogen—a hormone necessary for normal development and growth of the breasts and organs important for childbearing— may have something to do with cancer.

Most of us know that hormone-replacement therapy (HRT) after menopause has been linked with an increased risk of breast cancer. However, we don't expect to have to worry about estrogen exposure from food, plastic containers, or skin care products. Unfortunately, that is our present-day reality.

Now environmental estrogens—synthetic chemicals—can act like human estrogen. Research has found that these estrogens can increase cell division and potentially contribute to breast cancer risk. These types of estrogens are found in pesticides, food preservatives like BHT and BHA, compounds used in plastics like bisphenol A and phthalates, food dye Red #3, and formaldehyde (used in making carpets, plywood, and some nail polishes).

Estrogens like phthalates, parabens, and other hormone-altering chemicals are also showing up in our personal care products. Rejuvenating skin creams often contain estrogen itself. Epidermal growth factor (EGF), used in some anti-aging creams to stimulate new cell growth, can also mimic the effects of estrogen on some cells.

To lower your exposure, avoid the ingredients we've listed in Chapter 2 and in the Appendix V. Stay away from products that contain parabens, phthalates, chemical sunscreens, and the like. Since estrogens aren't always listed on the label, buy from reputable companies producing organic and natural products. Check your favorite products against the Environmental Working Group's Skin Deep Database for safety.

gems like carrots, sweet potatoes, papaya, broccoli, eggs, and spinach. (The body converts beta-carotene to vitamin A.)

- B vitamins are involved in healthy functioning of oil-producing glands, so pile on the whole grains, cantaloupe, sweet peppers, green peas, fish, and citrus fruits.

- Vitamin C supports the formation of collagen, which helps your skin hang on to moisture. Sources include orange juice, broccoli, tomato, mango, peppers, and kiwi fruit.

- Vitamin E is great at slowing skin aging and is found in almonds, leafy vegetables, and olive and sesame oils.

- Antioxidants are strong warriors and fight off damaging free radicals caused by sun exposure, pollution, and malnutrition (which can occur during cancer treatments). Try blueberries and strawberries, squash, kale, spinach, kidney and pinto beans, cranberries, artichoke hearts, apples, and potatoes. (Check with your doctor before consuming any supplements.)

- You may also want to beef up your intake of omega-3-rich foods. Fatty acids are essential to the epithelial structures that retain moisture. Foods high in omega-3 fatty acids include salmon, herring, anchovies, sardines, flaxseed oil, soybeans, canola, and walnuts.

Finally, avoid those foods that rob your body of water. These include alcohol, anything with caffeine, salty foods, and high-sugar foods and soft drinks, which can all act as diuretics on your system. Stay away from fried foods as well, as they carry free radicals that damage skin structure.

Remember that cancer and chemotherapy rob your body of critical nutrients that you can replace by eating good foods. Though vitamins and minerals aren't a quick cure-all for dry skin, getting enough of powerhouse nutrients *can* arm your body with the tools it needs to lighten the effects of treatment. Of course, continue with your nontoxic moisturizer as often as needed.

Ouch! Soothing Radiated Skin

"While I was going through radiation, I could only use a certain type of deodorant because the aluminum would interfere. They were suggesting gentle, mild things to use. People don't know that there are so many things in products that you shouldn't have, and they don't know what to buy, because there isn't a lot of information on it. At least I have control of what I'm putting on me and in me. It gave me some sense of control over that."

—Karen, thyroid cancer survivor

Although I was fortunate not to have to go through radiation, my father did get a few treatments. The process can leave the skin red, irritated, and burned around the treatment site, much like a sunburn, although it can vary in severity. Skin conditions that may develop include the following:

- Erythema—skin reddening due to inflammation. Usually occurs seven to fourteen days after the start of treatment.

- Dry desquamation—dry, flaky skin that is usually itchy. Occurs further into treatment as a result of the loss of epidermal cells that are sloughed off.

- Moist desquamation—painful, thin, weeping skin that develops cracks and fissures that drain fluid. May occur after several doses of radiation or in the final weeks of treatment as a result of the breakdown of the skin's outer barrier.

- Radiation dermatitis—inflammation in the skin caused by radiation exposure. Can include any of the above conditions.

- Radiation recall dermatitis—renewed radiation dermatitis that occurs after radiation treatment is over and usually in response to additional treatment like chemotherapy, or even much later as a result of taking other medications or certain herbal remedies. Skin becomes inflamed again at the original site of treatment.

Your doctor may recommend helpful emollients or creams for you to apply to the treated area, particularly if you develop open wounds. Some of those products, however, may contain mineral oil or petrochemicals.

Fortunately, there are natural remedies for burns. Here are several you can try, most of which I used on my dad.

- Use cool compresses on the area for short periods of time. (Be sure they're clean to prevent bacteria.) Be careful, however, not to expose the treated area to extreme hot or cold. Do not use heating pads, hot water bottles, or ice packs.

- Try pure aloe gel that's been cooled in the refrigerator. If you have access to the plant itself, cut off a piece and place the fleshy side directly on the burn. The soothing effects of this plant are amazing.

- Some cancer survivors I spoke to recommend emu oil and tamanu oil for their soothing and moisturizing properties.

- Other creams and ointments that may be soothing include those with calendula for its ability to calm burns, and vitamin E for its healing moisture.

- Manuka honey—made from bees that feed on the Manuka bush, a close relative of the tea tree plant—is considered a better choice than regular honey for treating sensitive skin. It contains antibacterial, antioxidant, and anti-inflammatory benefits, and can help the skin fight off infection while soothing the burn. It has been clinically proven to help with burns and is now used in many hospitals.

- Soothing hydrogel sheets and packs are available from medical and home health suppliers. They're sterile and hydrating and are easy to work with.

Deodorant Linked with Breast Cancer?

No study has been absolutely conclusive yet, but one study reported that, after testing seventeen tissue samples collected from breast cancer patients, "the aluminum content was higher in the outer regions of the breast, in close proximity to the area where there would be the highest density of antiperspirant."

Another study linked underarm shaving and deodorant use to an increased risk of cancer. Subsequent studies, so far, have not duplicated the results.

Aluminum hangs around in the body after it's absorbed and is capable of causing DNA damage. Worse, since it plugs up the natural sweat glands in the underarms, toxins tend to build up in that area, where the lymph nodes are.

Spray-on deodorants often contain parabens, as well. Why take chances with your health? Try natural alternatives like crystal deodorant stones, herbal roll-ons, and aluminum-free varieties. You may need to do a little experimenting, but a little time spent on your own self-care is well worth the effort.

- If your skin is too tender to touch, try sunburn-cooling sprays from reputable manufacturers that use safe, natural ingredients. (Look for those made for babies and children, but don't forget to read labels!)

- Whatever moisturizing product you use, continue with it even after treatment is over to help your skin recover fully. Most physicians recommend extra moisturizing for at least a month after your final treatment.

You may also want to try storing your skin care products in the refrigerator for extra cooling. However, be sure to ask your oncology radiologist about applying any creams. Most will instruct you not to apply anything to the skin on the day of treatment, as lotions and creams can interfere with the radiation and can lead to a more serious skin burn.

"I used calendula on my skin when I had radiation," says Karen, two-time thyroid cancer survivor. "I had to clean it off before the next treatment, but it helped soothe the tissue a lot. I still got really red because that's what radiation does to you, but I didn't have any blistering."

Studies have found some other interesting things that may help with radiation burns. Researchers wondered if the antioxidants in red wine might help. Out of about 350 women, those who drank wine on treatment days had lower rates of skin toxicity than those who didn't. In fact, the toxicity

Homeopathy Relieves
Radiation-Induced Dermatitis?

Homeopathy may help relieve several side effects of chemo, including dermatitis. Based on the principle of "like cures like," a substance that would cause symptoms in a healthy person is used to cure those same symptoms in illness. One remedy used for a person suffering from insomnia, for example, is coffee.

Considered a "gentler" way of healing, homeopathy has been around for thousands of years and typically uses plant, mineral, and animal-based medicines, diluted to form a "tincture." The solution is then agitated (shaken) before being used in treatment.

In a review of several scientific trials, scientists found that skin irritation caused by radiation was less in patients using calendula ointment (a homeopathic remedy) than trolamine (a topical agent). More studies need to be done, but early evidence looks promising on some homeopathic remedies.

Homeopathy can be practiced by all kinds of healthcare professionals, from medical doctors to nurse practitioners to physician's assistants. The important thing is that the person is certified in homeopathy and that he or she has experience dealing with cancer side effects. The National Center for Homeopathy provides a listing of homeopaths. The Society of Homeopaths also offers a handy search engine.

effects were reduced up to 75 percent.[5] Patients drank just one glass—and the wine didn't reduce the effectiveness of the radiation therapy.

Other studies found that red wine makes cancer cells more susceptible to radiation therapy, and normal cells more resistant. For instance, when pancreatic cancer cells—typically highly resistant to chemotherapy—were pretreated with resveratrol (a powerful antioxidant in red wine), then irradiated, the combination induced a particular kind of cell death that is usually the goal of cancer treatment.[6]

If you'd like to try red wine on your treatment days, ask your doctor. Another option might be to consume unsweetened red or purple grape juice, which also contains antioxidants from grapes (including resveratrol). You may also consider resveratrol supplements, preferably in liquid or juice form, since the antioxidant is best absorbed by the lining of the mouth.

Another interesting finding: The natural properties found in the spice "curry" (known as curcumin) seem to help reduce the likelihood of burning after radiation.[7] Mice that were given doses of curcumin prior to radiation had minimal skin damage. The findings have only occurred in animal studies so far, but researchers believe that there is a positive connection between the ingestion of anti-inflammatory foods (like curcumin) during radiation treatment and the lowered likelihood of extreme burning.

To further reduce your own internal inflammation—which may also help reduce the severity of burns—eat a diet rich in anti-inflammatory foods, like whole grains, colorful produce, lean proteins (white meats instead of red), and plenty of healthy fats, like organic fish and nuts. Avoid foods that can increase inflammation, like fried foods, preservatives, white flours, refined sugars, and saturated fats (found in full-fat dairy products, butters, or fatty meats like bacon).

Where Did All These Bruises Come From?

"You can't go through treatment alone. You need your family to support you, and you also have to help yourself. You have to fight your cancer. Don't give up!"

—Justin, brain cancer survivor

When we're going through cancer treatments, we can end up looking like we've been in a bad fight. The problem? Blood platelets that just don't want to stick together. In other words, a shortage of clots.

Usually, if you're injured, platelets in your blood stick together to help form a clot and stop the bleeding. Certain chemotherapy drugs, however, can inhibit or even reduce the number of those platelets — by affecting the bone marrow, where platelets are produced—making your blood run more "freely" than usual, so to speak.

Consequently, if an injury crushes the small blood vessels under your skin, they break open and leak blood more than usual, creating a bruise. Cuts bleed longer and more profusely as well.

"If the skin is thin enough," says Dr. Dattner, holistic dermatologist, "I would use protective measures. Say the skin on your shins is very thin, and if you bang into a coffee table you take weeks or months to heal; then it would make sense to get some hockey shin protectors to protect yourself."

Aside from the unsightliness of carrying around a collection of bruises, reduced platelets increase your risk of dangerous complications from what would otherwise be considered "common" cuts or accidents, like nicking yourself shaving or banging your elbow against the wall. Talk to your doctor, as he or she may have medications to help blood clot more readily.

If you find yourself bruising easily and often while going through treatment, you may also want to avoid aspirin (and other NSAID anti-inflammatory

drugs) and certain vitamins or supplements that may increase your susceptibility to bleeding. (These may include garlic, bromelain, gingko, don quai,
and others.)

If you do get a bruise (or several), what can you do about it? Try applying ice to the area for twenty to thirty minutes, which will help shrink the
blood vessels that may be bleeding. After forty-eight hours, switch to heating compresses, which will help the body reabsorb the blood. You can also
try applying ointments containing Arnica, which may help lessen bruising.
Use acetaminophen to handle any pain. If you cut yourself and the bleeding
hasn't stopped after five minutes, go directly to the doctor.

In the meantime, take a few precautions. Avoid sharp tools and objects
until your platelet count comes back up. Use a very soft toothbrush, avoid
forcefully blowing your nose, use an electric shaver instead of a razor, avoid
tampons or suppositories, and take a break from contact sports or other
activities that may cause injury.

Above all, watch yourself. If you experience any of the following, get to
your doctor right away: a) unexplained or unexpected bruising, b) bleeding from your gums or nose, c) reddish or pinkish urine, d) unusual vaginal
bleeding, e) a warm or hot area on an arm or leg.

The Injection Site Hurts—What Can I Do?

Chemotherapy is most often administered by injection, which can result
in an irritating, sometimes serious, side effect: the injection-site reaction.

Two basic types of reactions can occur: an irritation (or local allergic
reaction called a flare reaction) and an extravasation (leakage of medication)—or in normal language, minor and major.

A minor reaction causes redness, itching, tenderness, and perhaps swelling, and is usually the result of an allergic reaction to the injection. Certain
chemo drugs cause this type of reaction. Usually it goes away fairly quickly.
In the meantime, you can apply ice or cold compresses to the area.

A major reaction starts out looking like a minor one, but then can
become blistered and painful, even potentially causing severe skin damage
in a matter of days. This is usually the result of chemotherapy medicine
leaking from the blood vessel to the area under the skin near the injection
site. You may not notice any effects for six to twelve hours after treatment,
and the severity of your reaction will depend on the type of drug used, the
dosage, and how quickly the problem is treated.

When I was getting chemo through an IV, I experienced a minor reaction to the nitrogen mustard medication. It swelled my arm intensely and irritated and burned the IV area. They took me off the IV right away, and I think they gave me an antihistamine and an antibiotic. They didn't want to take any more chances, so they booked me for surgery the week after for a port-a-cath, and I never had chemo through my arm again.

As far as preventing such a reaction, it's kind of up to your nurse! He or she needs to be well trained in injections, so you may want to strike up a conversation before treatment to try to determine his or her expertise. It can also depend on the drug and the condition of your blood vessels. Some drugs that are more likely to cause extravasation will be administered in larger blood vessels in the torso rather than the smaller ones in the arms to help prevent reactions. Whatever your case, if you do notice anything hurting or swelling, be sure to speak up and bring it to someone's attention.

Other options to reduce your risk of injection-site traumas include the following:

1. **PICC Line:** A long plastic catheter is placed into one of the larger veins of the arm and then used for multiple short infusions. It is temporary.

2. **Tunneled catheter:** These are placed through the skin in the middle of the chest, then "tunneled" through the tissue between the skin and muscle into the vessel at the entrance of the right atrium of the heart. They can be left in place for months or years to reduce incidence of infection, but they require dressing changes.

3. **Port-a-cath:** This is like the one I had. It's similar to the tunneled catheter, but is a more permanent option and involves no "tunneling." Rather, the device is positioned under the skin on the chest and the catheter inserted into the vessel at the entrance of the right atrium of the heart. It can last three to five years and requires less maintenance.

Any of these options can decrease your risk of injection-site irritation or infection. If you do experience pain or discomfort at the injection site, be sure to tell your doctor immediately. If you were the victim of extravasation, physicians will try to remove as much of the leaked medication as possible, apply ice or heat, and administer an antidote.

Some chemo drugs are more likely to cause extravasation than others, so ask your doctor about your risk before starting treatment, so you can be more aware.

This Wound Just Won't Heal!

Chemotherapy, radiation, and lack of nutrition during cancer can cause delayed wound healing, where typical cuts, scrapes, scratches, and punctures—particularly surgical incisions—take much longer than normal to repair themselves.

Radiation, because it damages healthy tissues as well as cancer cells, complicates wound healing. Chemotherapy, because it targets rapidly dividing cells, interferes with wound healing as well, since it can kill immune

Metal Taste

Taste distortion is not a side effect to take lightly, as it can lead to malnutrition. Researchers have found that for as many as 20 percent of cancer patients, the primary cause of morbidity was malnutrition, not malignancy.

During treatment, you may not be able to taste or perceive odors, or you may find that things taste and smell differently than they did before.

Tell your doctor; he may decide to employ alternative methods to be sure you're staying nourished. Then, try these tips:

- Avoid red meats and eat more chicken, dairy, and casseroles.
- Try tart foods like yogurt and lemon-based items.
- Avoid drinking juices or soft drinks from metal cans. Use glass bottles instead.
- Suck on hard candies or chew sugar-free gum between meals to take away bad tastes.
- Maintain good oral hygiene.
- Eat smaller meals in pleasant surroundings.
- If hot foods are unappealing, try cooling them to room temperature or refrigerating.
- If food smells bad, try bland items like cottage cheese, applesauce, and sandwiches.
- Eat with plastic utensils to avoid metal mouth.
- Suck on ice chips between bites to help numb taste buds.
- Don't force yourself to eat foods that are unappealing. Find things that taste good.

cells involved in tissue repair. Finally, 40 percent to 80 percent of cancer patients are clinically malnourished, which makes them increasingly susceptible to infections and delayed healing.

What can you do? Researchers recommend delaying radiation treatment for a minimum of three weeks *after* surgery to give surgical wounds time to heal, so if you're scheduled for radiation, you may want to talk to your doctor about the healing of any surgical incisions.

Since chemotherapy drugs create so many varying effects on different individuals and at different dosages, it's more difficult to give a blanket recommendation. Timing, dosage, and type of drug used can all make a difference, so it's best to monitor yourself carefully as you go and report any difficulties to your physician.

There is one area where you can take more responsibility for your own health: nutrition. Though it's best to seek the help of a naturopath or nutritionist to target your particular nutritional needs as you're going through treatment, below are a few general recommendations (always check with your doctor before using supplements during treatment):

- Make sure you're getting adequate calories and protein.
- Vitamins C and A optimize healing and recovery.
- Vitamin E supports wound healing.
- Zinc deficiency impairs protein production; restoring zinc to healthy levels returns wound healing to a healthy rate. (Take extra zinc only if you are deficient—excess zinc can be detrimental.)

Other tips for wound care include:

- Wash your hands thoroughly before and after changing dressings.
- Remove dressings carefully (to avoid reopening the wound).
- Clean wounds daily (don't rub).
- Always use new dressings and bandages.
- Don't pick at scabs.
- Eat vitamin-rich foods like citrus fruits, leafy vegetables, whole grains, lean meats, fish, and eggs.

Dry Mouth

"I had extreme dry mouth; cracks in the side of my mouth. I used tons of lip balm."
—Karen, thyroid cancer survivor

In the medical world, it's called "xerostomia" (pronounced zeer-o-STO-me-uh). In the cancer world, it's more likely referred to as, "What the devil happened to my saliva?"

A common side effect of cancer treatments, dry mouth is more than just an inconvenience. Saliva normally keeps acid levels down in the mouth, protecting teeth. Without it, teeth are more susceptible to decay and gums at a higher risk for disease.

Saliva also does other great things, like break down foods for easier digestion, assist in swallowing, help us talk clearly, protect the inside of the mouth and throat, and enhance our ability to taste.

If you've got dry mouth, you probably already know it, but here are a few signs: The mouth feels dry, like you've been in the desert for days; the saliva you do have may feel thicker than normal, or ropelike; your tongue

Could Your Toothpaste Encourage Mouth Sores?

Many toothpastes contain triclosan, an antibacterial that's been shown to be a hormone-disruptor in tests on animal and human cells. (Read labels to see if your toothpaste has it.) On top of that, sodium lauryl sulfate (SLS) is in many brands to encourage foaming, but is a particularly harsh detergent that can irritate tender gums (especially when you're going through chemotherapy).

Scientific research has suggested that SLS can increase your risk of mouth ulcers. Study participants who brushed using SLS-free toothpaste reduced their number of canker sores—by as much as 81 percent. You definitely don't need more mouth sores during treatment, so if your brand has this ingredient, throw it out!

Another harsh ingredient is hydrated silica. A "whitener" in toothpastes, it's abrasive and can wear down our naturally protective tooth enamel. If you've got sensitive teeth and gums, avoid this one.

Other toxic ingredients like parabens and propylene glycol may also be present in your formula. Colored pastes often contain dyes that have the potential to cause headaches, allergic reactions, and fatigue.

Shop for brands that stay away from SLS, silica, and triclosan.

may feel sore; you may be more sensitive to acidic and spicy foods; and you may have trouble swallowing.

There are a lot of things that will lessen discomfort and prevent damage.

- First of all, take care of your teeth. Brush at least twice a day, and use a fluoride rinse or gel to strengthen enamel. If your mouth is too sensitive for brushing, use foam pads. Ask your dentist about mouthwashes, toothpastes, and moisturizing gels that are made for dry mouth. (Avoid mouthwashes with alcohol; they can cause additional dryness.)

- Ask your doctor about artificial saliva products, or you may find some over-the-counter rinses or sprays. There are also drugs available that increase saliva.

- Carry water with you so you can sip on it almost constantly, and keep a glass or bottle by the bed. You may want to try adding vanilla extract or a few crystals of drink mix to the water.

- Suck on sugar-free candies, ice chips, and sugarless gums to stimulate saliva flow.

- Wet your foods down with gravies, sauces, light creams, and butter, and choose lukewarm and cool foods over hot.

- Avoid salty, dry foods like cookies, chips, and dried fruit, and stay away from drying alcohol and caffeine drinks.

- Use a humidifier in your bedroom. It moistens the air, reducing the dryness that occurs when you sleep.

- Consider acupuncture. A recent small pilot study showed great promise for acupuncture's ability to reduce the symptoms of dry mouth.[8]

- Other options: Echinacea dropped in juice, evening primrose in a capsule, red pepper added to foods, and multiflora rose tea.

Mouth Sores

"I had more mouth sores with my second chemo. More on my lips because of the dry skin. I have canker sores on the outside and I haven't had canker sores forever."

—Jody, breast cancer survivor

You may have had them before. They're called "mouth ulcers" or "canker sores," and some people are prone to getting them, even without

Oral Thrush

During cancer and cancer treatment your immune system takes a hit, leaving you more at risk for oral thrush. This is an infection in the lining of your mouth that creates white lesions on your tongue or inner cheeks. (It's caused by the fungus Candida albicans.) Sometimes it spreads to the roof of your mouth, your gums, or the back of your throat. In severe cases, the infection can spread down the esophagus.

These lesions are painful and can cause bleeding and loss of taste. If you develop one, see your doctor right away. He or she may recommend antifungal medications or other drugs to control the infection.

You can also try eating unsweetened yogurt or taking acidophilus supplements, as they can help restore the normal bacterial flora in your body. Keep your mouth clean. If it's too tender, use foam brushes or non-alcoholic mouthwashes and warm salt water. Finally, limit your intake of sugar, which can encourage the growth of the bacteria.

cancer treatment. A little salt-water rinse or numbing gel usually gets rid of them within ten to fourteen days. If you've had one, you know how painful it can be.

Unfortunately, some cancer treatments can damage the cells in your mouth, creating mouth ulcers, or causing the ones you used to have to appear more often. Severity can vary, from a small burning pain to a more relentless discomfort that can make it difficult to eat or drink.

Swishing ice chips in your mouth while receiving chemotherapy may protect it from the drugs. (Cold temperatures slow blood flow, making it more difficult for the blood to carry drugs to cold areas.) It may be wise to get a dental checkup before starting treatment, to make sure your mouth is as healthy as possible to start with.

Drink plenty of water, eat a balanced diet, and get into a steady, thorough mouth-care routine (if you don't have one already). Avoid alcohol-based mouth rinses. Choose those with natural ingredients, or try saltwater or baking soda and water (½ to 1 teaspoon in 8 ounces).

Rinsing *before* a meal may soothe your mouth enough to make it easier to eat. Cold popsicles before a meal can also help numb the pain. Your dentist may also have a pain-relieving rinse you can use. Cut your food into smaller pieces, and remember—the sores will go away after your treatment ends.

Healthy lips will help promote a healthy mouth, and since lips tend to get dry and chapped during treatment, be sure to keep them moist. Avoid products with chemicals and go for natural and organic brands. (Refer to Appendix VII for websites that carry these.)

If you do form mouth sores, tell your doctor. There are some treatments available, such as medications that coat the inside of the mouth or topical painkillers. Avoid acidic and spicy foods, caffeine, alcohol, and sugar. (Sugar coats the inside of the mouth and makes it easier for bacteria to grow.) Try comfort foods like yogurt, macaroni and cheese, mashed potatoes, applesauce, baby foods, and foods with bland sauces and gravies.

If a toothbrush hurts, ask your dentist for foam swabs, which are more comfortable. If your sores start to bleed, become infected, cause you difficulty swallowing, or are so painful you start losing weight, you may need to stop treatment for a while until you recover. Ask your doctor for his or her advice.

Dry, Itchy Eyes

Some cancer treatments can cause dry, gritty, sensitive eyes that water and itch, often creating blurry vision. Not a *horrible* side effect, but certainly one that can interfere with your daily activities, restrict your use of contact lenses, and screw up your makeup in a big hurry.

Unfortunately, besides using rewetting drops, there's not much you can do about contact irritation. If they're too hard to put up with, try wearing them for just a few hours at a time, or go with eyeglasses.

To relieve discomfort, as always, ask your doctor—he or she may have some lubricating ointments you can use at bedtime. Your eye doctor can also prescribe artificial tears that you can use throughout the day. (Don't confuse these with formulas that just reduce redness—they don't address the cause of dryness.) You can also try herbal eye drops.

To help rejuvenate your eyes at night—and to avoid that burning, sticky sensation in the morning—try hydrating goggles. You can find kits online that include goggles, foam pads, and a travel case. With these, you soak the foam pads in water, put them on your eyes, and wear the goggles over them, to help seal in moisture and prevent the evaporation of natural and artificial tears.

To protect your eyes during the day, sunglasses are a must. Choose those that form a seal around your eyes and really cut down on the wind and grime that can get into them. Stay away from smoke and wind whenever possible, and use a humidifier at night.

Another trick: consume more omega-3 fatty acids. (This supplement is so helpful during cancer treatments!) One study showed that women who had the highest levels of omega-3 fatty acids in their diets reduced their risk of dry-eye syndrome by 20 percent.[9] Eat more fatty fish (salmon, sardines), nuts, and flaxseed oil, or try fish-oil supplements.

Do you have to go without eye makeup? Makeup that flakes can increase irritation, so women who use it may want to avoid powder eye shadow and glitter makeup for a while. As mentioned in Chapter Six, apply mascara only to the tips of eyelashes, and refrain from using any on lower lashes.

Remove makeup as soon as you can, rather than waiting until the end of the day. Avoid waterproof formulas; the rubbing required to remove them further irritates your eyes. Use organic, toxin-free eye makeup remover for sensitive eyes. Above all, don't leave makeup on the eyes overnight, and replace makeup products frequently to avoid chance of infection.

Night Sweats

Some types of cancer and cancer treatments can cause night sweats—severe hot-flash type sweating that drenches sleepwear and sheets, may be accompanied by a flushing sensation or chills, and isn't related to an overheated environment.

I remember having these before I was diagnosed. I would have to change my nightclothes up to three times a night because they were so wet it would wake me up.

Medically termed "nocturnal hyperhydrosis," night sweats can be caused by Hodgkin's disease (like I had) or other forms of cancer. Lymphoma is one type that may cause night sweats in many people. Breast cancer drugs like tamoxifen, as well as certain types of chemotherapy (if they drain the body of estrogen), can bring on menopausal symptoms like night sweats as well.

Scientists aren't sure what causes night sweats, but speculate that cancer cells release certain hormones during sleep that trigger the reaction. Medications can also interfere with the body's natural temperature regulation.

If it's possible you're experiencing menopausal symptoms as a side effect of cancer treatment, your doctor may have medications to help. You can also do some things at home. Consider sage tea before bedtime. A 2005 study found that sage and alfalfa reduced hot flushes by 60 percent compared to a placebo.[10]

Avoid caffeine or alcohol for about three hours before bed, cut down on spicy foods, keep your bedroom cool (consider a fan near the bed), drink water if and when you do wake up, and incorporate a relaxing routine at night that includes meditation and deep breathing or yoga (*not* vigorous exercise). Research has shown that acupuncture may also help.[11]

Finally, I have two other interesting products you may want to try. One is called the Bedfan. It's a little gadget that sits at the foot of your bed and provides a breeze between your sheets and along your body. Check it out online. Another is moisture-wicking sleepwear, which helps you stay more comfortable overnight. These are made from lightweight materials that wick the moisture away from your skin so you're less likely to wake up in the middle of the night.

I'm Soooo Tired

"I had this overwhelming feeling of exhaustion. There were some days after treatment that I'd get up and feel good and take a shower and have to sit back down. I can't remember ever in my life feeling that exhausted. The only thing I could do was sleep. You feel like you lose days."

—Rayette, ovarian cancer survivor

Fatigue is one of the most common side effects experienced by cancer patients. Unlike just feeling "tired," cancer-related fatigue results in a lack of energy that can last for days, weeks, even months. It feels like a whole-body tiredness that is not relieved by sleep.

When I was going through cancer, I remember that no matter how much I slept, I still didn't feel rejuvenated. Even though I was only sixteen years old and my body had all the resilience of youth, I felt like I was always dragging. I had to miss school on some days and say "no" to participating in some activities because I just wasn't up to it. My father also went through debilitating fatigue; he made it a habit to sleep Friday, Saturday, and Sunday so he could maintain his schedule at work by going Monday through Thursday. If he didn't sleep those three days, he couldn't make it through the other four.

"When my body said, 'You've got to relax,' I would just lie down and sleep, or watch TV, or try to read something," says Chris, non-Hodgkin's lymphoma survivor. "I didn't have the energy to do anything."

Fatigue can be one of the hardest side effects to deal with, as it can make you feel worthless. When all you can do is lie around and sleep, what are you accomplishing? It is during these times that you need to be kindest to yourself.

"Fatigue is probably the most debilitating side effect of chemotherapy and radiation," says Jarrod, Hodgkin's lymphoma survivor. "You can't even get off the couch or out of bed. You don't have energy to cook or work. Forcing yourself to walk and be as active as possible does help a little."

Causes of fatigue are varied. Drugs, radiation, bone marrow transplants, decreased nutrition, reduced blood counts, nausea and vomiting, depression, anxiety, and more can all play a part.

Though much of the time you will need to be patient and kind with yourself and allow yourself to sleep—you are fighting a serious disease, after all!— there are some ways my dad and I found to help better deal with this side effect:

- Keep a journal or chart showing when you feel more energy. It will help you to see that you're not "always" tired and will help you schedule activities for those times of day when you feel more energy.

- Pace yourself. Try to rest before you become overly tired.

- Avoid extreme temperatures, as they can tire you more.

- Prioritize your activities. What can you delegate to others? Remember: Job #1 is to take care of yourself so you can get well. Ask for help.

- Try to get enough calories. Even if it's tough to eat, find things that appeal to you. (Many cancer fighters like ice cream and protein shakes.) Protein helps repair damaged tissue and is especially important.

- See a nutritionist or naturopath to help you get the nutrition you need. Some survivors have had great luck with juicing as a way to increase energy.

- Try to keep a regular exercise schedule. Exercising a little on most days of the week can help stimulate energy. Even if all you can do is a ten-minute walk, do it.

- Adjust your expectations of yourself. You're not going to be able to do as much as you did before. Pare down your "to-do" list to include only three to five things a day, rather than ten or more.

- Work on *relaxing*. Stress and anxiety further depletes your energy stores. Try meditation, deep breathing, music therapy, and time with friends—whatever helps put you at ease. Even a gentle stretching routine can help you feel more alive.

Joint Pain: I'm Aching in My Bones

Perhaps one of the most difficult side effects of cancer treatment is the pain that can settle into your muscles and joints. Caused by chemotherapy drugs, it can leave you feeling stiff, uncomfortable, and older than your years.

When looking for joint-pain remedies, you're likely to be overwhelmed with options. First of all, ask your doctor. Joint pain can come from cancer that has spread, so it's important to rule out this possibility. Before you talk to the doc, keep a diary for a few days so you can accurately describe the pain. When and where does it occur? How bad is it, and how long does it last? Is it interfering with your activities?

Next, incorporate a low-impact exercise into your day. It helps lubricate joints with synovial fluid and maintain your ability to function. Try walking, swimming, or yoga. Yoga requires deep breathing and stretching, which increases circulation, helps you relax, and loosens your muscles—all great ways to relieve joint pain.

Of course, you can try over-the-counter pain relievers like aspirin or ibuprofen, but it's not good for your liver or your stomach to take these long term, so be sure to seek out other solutions. Glucosamine, for instance, has a long and impressive record. It stimulates the production of proteins important to the makeup of cartilage, which provides joint cushioning. The latest research shows that glucosamine in liquid form is most effective, so look for a quality brand that gives you at least 500 mg per dose, and take up to three doses a day.

According to a news release from the Washington University in St. Louis School of Medicine, patients experiencing joint pain and stiffness often had suboptimal levels of vitamin D in their blood.[12] Once they started taking supplements, the pain went away. B Vitamins and omega-3 fatty acids also help reduce inflammation and pain.

Naturalists suggest rubbing the painful area with "arthcare oil," arthcare being a powerful antioxidant. Boswelia has shown promise in scientific studies and is included in many joint-care supplements. SAM-e (1,000 mg daily) and cancer-fighting turmeric (1,500 mg daily) can also help, as might massage and heat therapy.

You may also want to experiment with your diet. Try cutting back on sugar, dairy products, red meat, and vegetable oils, which have a reputation for making joint pain worse. Whatever you do, don't stop trying, and don't lose hope. This side effect, like most, will eventually subside or disappear altogether.

Other Side Effects

I'll talk about some of the other side effects that attack the hands and feet in an upcoming chapter. However, if you find yourself experiencing some discomforts or problems we haven't covered here, be sure to ask your doctor about them. Never be afraid to bring something up.

I've talked with so many survivors who realized after the fact that there was something that could have helped them feel more comfortable, but they weren't able to take advantage of it when they were going through it because they felt they were supposed to just buck up and deal with it on their own. Looking back, they all say that with hindsight, they would do all they could to alleviate their discomfort.

It's kind of like a new mother, you know? I have two friends, for example, who went into that first round of childbirth with an idealistic point of view. They insisted on going totally natural and refused any help or assistance in dealing with their pain and discomfort. Some women continue with this method for the second, third, and fourth child because of dearly held principles, but for most women, when that second child comes, they're happy to receive any help they can get! My two girlfriends realized halfway through their first births that all they were doing was draining themselves of the energy and strength they needed to get through the birth and care for their children afterward, so guess what? They asked for the epidural right then and there, before it was too late.

I hope you won't wait until you're looking back on your cancer experience to get the help you need. Remember: Cancer is *not* something you should do alone! You have many doctors and nurses on your team. Use them. You have the Internet at your disposal, and many helpful books. There are a myriad of resources out there. If you're too tired to do the research yourself, enlist the help of friends.

Suffering more than you need to may be considered by some to be brave, but it could also hinder your chances of healing as well as you might. Your body needs strength to get through this, and the more you suffer, the more you sap yourself of that strength. If you can bring yourself some comfort, some ease, some relaxation—even some *sleep*—you'll be helping yourself and your body, and increasing your odds of beating this thing. At the very least, you'll be making yourself a little easier to be around for a while!

"When you start getting that pit in your stomach, and your thoughts snowball in the wrong direction, take five minutes and you can change that. Focus on the things you're grateful for. Some days it may be that you're still alive. Or that you still have your loved ones around you. It's a process and you have to learn how to do it, but the benefits are huge."

—Donald, five-time cancer survivor

Let's Review

- When your body is feeling pain and discomfort, it's more important than ever to be kind to yourself and encourage positive emotions as often as possible.

- While going through treatment, change your bathing and hygiene habits to those that are more gentle and kind to your fragile skin. Choose products that are nontoxic, fragrance-free, and full of nourishing ingredients.

- There are natural ways to ease side effects like nausea, dry skin, radiation burns, bruises, lasting wounds, dry mouth, mouth sores, dry eyes, night sweats, fatigue, and joint pain. You don't have to simply suffer; there are many things you can try to ease your discomfort.

- Being strong is admirable, but don't be afraid to seek out solutions for your pain and discomfort. The more you can put your body at ease, the more resources it will have to heal itself. Don't try to be the strong and silent type; speaking up is much better for your prognosis.

Goals

When I feel uncomfortable side effects, I'll work toward redirecting any negative thoughts to more positive and nourishing ones.

Instead of	Try
I'm going to feel this pain forever.	This pain is temporary. It will go away.
There is no way to relieve this discomfort.	There are a lot of natural remedies I can try; if they don't work, I can check with my doctor for other options.

I feel so discouraged—I am always tired.	I may feel tired more than usual, but I will be loving toward myself and get the rest I need, and enjoy the moments when I do have more energy.
I'm so angry with my body—it's always hurting me.	My body is fighting this disease as best it can. I'm going to help it by generating loving energy for myself.
I hate how I feel. Why can't things be how they used to be?	Cancer changes things. I'm learning to accept that, celebrate the good moments I have, and keep faith that I can make it through this.

Personal Affirmations

I take excellent care of my body.

I accept where I am today.
I listen to my body and take care of my needs.

8

Complementary Therapies: Massage, Yoga, Reiki, and More

"I would say to other fighters to invest in getting massages throughout your treatment. There's something about the physical way it gets the blood flowing. A friend stood at my bed and massaged my feet one day at the hospital and it was awesome. It removes your focus from the fact that you have pain in your chest and drains coming out and changes it to 'Oh, my feet feel so much better!' Those kinds of things can make you feel better. I always come to a massage more than anything, even a head massage, neck, or hands. Schedule something like that at least once a week."

—Jody, breast cancer survivor

DO YOU FIND YOURSELF FEELING DOWN MORE THAN UP lately? Are you obsessing more and more about your treatments, and less likely to find any joy in your day? Are you consistently self-conscious about your appearance, criticizing your skin or your lack of hair? If so, you've probably been neglecting yourself. It's time to even out the scales between the challenging experiences and the restorative ones.

Hopefully some of the suggestions we've been talking about so far have helped you to regain some sense of control—if not of your cancer, at least of your daily existence. Now, however, I'd like to talk about doing something proactive. Something that, regardless of whatever side effects you may be experiencing, is an action you take for yourself, to encourage your own well-being.

Consider making an appointment strictly for *you*. An appointment that will help you relax, reconnect to your inner self, and recharge, body and spirit. I'm talking about a trip to the spa, an appointment for a massage, a yoga or tai chi class, or an acupuncture treatment.

All these things have been shown to help relieve side effects and in many cases, boost the immune system. We'll talk about that as we go over each one. But more importantly, these are all things *you* can control, that will help *you* feel better. You may even find, after going a few times, that you become almost addicted to these therapies, because of how good they make you feel, and that's great, because you need to be doing things that help you feel good!

"But I can't afford it," you might say, or "I can't do all that for just *me*." We're not talking about a selfish indulgence here. This isn't a luxury, but a part of your recovery treatment. Your body needs all the nurturing it can get. We're talking about putting back some of that energy and vitality that the cancer and the treatments are sucking out of you every day. If you don't put some good stuff back in, you're lowering your chances of getting well.

As for affording it, there are many cancer centers, spas, hospitals, and other organizations that provide free services and/or discounts for cancer patients and survivors. It just takes a little looking to find them, or you can ask your oncology nurse. Cancer center spas, alternative therapy spas attached to hospitals, and even some private spas all cater to cancer patients. Check with your local hospital, or go to my website (www.cincovidas.com) for a list of cancer center spas around the country that offer not only massage, but Reiki, reflexology, acupuncture, and more.

The more relaxed, happy, and at peace you feel, the better your body can fight this thing, and the more capable you'll be of handling each challenge as it comes along. Putting energy and love back into your body and spirit is also key to balancing your emotions, which becomes more critical the longer you're in treatment.

Let's just brainstorm about some ways you can be proactive in giving back to yourself. Here are some of my ideas, and then I hope you'll add some of your own.

- Buy yourself some flowers. I buy white roses weekly and put them in my room and in the living room. It's something I invest in because it brings me peace of mind, calmness, and a bit of nature in my New York apartment. Plus the aroma is glorious.

- Get yourself something you've wanted for a while. A book, CD, or set of sheets. A tool, techy gadget, or jacket. Buy it without guilt. Just enjoy the experience.

- Take a long walk somewhere you haven't been in a while. Stroll by an old elementary school, around the river or lake, or through the trees at the edge of the forest.

- Go on a retreat. There are many retreats made specifically for cancer patients that can be very rejuvenating.

- Go get that certain candy or dessert you've been craving for months, sit down, and thoroughly enjoy every bite.

- Make a list of every good quality about yourself, from your perfectly shaped ears to your ability to make people laugh.

- Take a short holiday. If you feel well enough, get out of town just for the weekend. Drive a short distance to a mountain cabin, or even just a hotel by a creek. A little time in a beautiful place can do wonders for your spirit.

- Go see a performance you'd really like to see—a play, a concert, or a comedy show.

Okay, your turn. Add some of your own ideas here—ways you can infuse joy and energy into your spirit.

_____

_____

_____

I hope you'll make a point to do at least one of these things every week from now on!

Now, let's look at some other things that not only boost your energy and well-being, but have been shown through scientific studies to be beneficial to your health during cancer. We'll review each one, and then you can decide which you'd like to try.

Take a Healing Trip to the Spa

The power of touch can be so healing while we're in treatment—a hug, a neck or back massage, even a facial. When we're trying to heal, these little touches provide hope, love, and strength.

Vicky Weis, founder of Faye's Light, a nonprofit organization providing free spa services for cancer fighters and caregivers, understands firsthand. "There are so many benefits of touch. It can help relieve pain, get circulation going, and relax pinched muscles. After a few spa treatments you can just see patients open up. Fear and anxiety melt away."

If you're considering touch therapy, Weis suggests looking first to the people around you. Those who feel comfortable hugging or holding hands may be more than willing to give you a neck rub or hand massage with some natural lotion. "It's a time to be together, to talk, and to bond," Weis says. "It's free, and it benefits both of you."

Professional spa services are often complementary or available at a discounted price at many spas, and some hospitals and cancer centers offer them for free. If you can't find one near you, Weis strongly suggests looking for someone certified by the American Massage Therapy Association (AMTAMassage.org) and has experience in treating cancer patients. "Make some phone calls and ask some questions. I have cancer—do you have products that are fragrance-free, made without harmful chemicals, and that are good for sensitive skin?"

Mórag Currin, LA, CMLT, and president of Touch for Cancer Online, suggests that you ask if the person is certified in oncology esthetics (have they done massage on cancer patients before?), or knows anything about cancer or cancer treatments. If not, find another therapist to work on you to ensure your safety.

Massage: The King of Relaxation Methods

"When I was getting chemo they were giving me reflexology and massage. It was just awesome! To say that while you're getting infused with chemo, that's something! I was so relaxed. It was so calming. My husband learned how to do it so he could do it at home. I would highly recommend it."

—Joanna, breast cancer survivor

"In the world we live in," says massage therapist Jean Lazar, "we're so full of stress. To feel good has become the exception rather than the norm."

If you're going through cancer treatment—or caring for someone who is—you may find "feeling good" to be a rare experience. Yet it's during challenging times that feeling good becomes even more important. If all you come in contact with day after day are doctors, hospitals, medications, treatments, traffic, news, work, and responsibility, how can you hope to sustain health and happiness in your life?

"Stress is the biggest killer," says Lazar. "The body has the ability to heal itself, but stress hinders that ability. Muscles tighten up, trap toxins, and create painful knots in your neck, back, legs, and feet. Massage loosens the muscles, releases toxins, and when you drink water, flushes those toxins out. In essence, it gives you back the strength you need to heal."

By increasing circulation, boosting the immune system, easing the breath, reducing pain, and shutting down stress and anxiety, massage strengthens your body's ability to fight disease. But it's not just about the end result.

"We've been hearing so much about living in the 'now,'" says Lazar. "To be truly happy, we're learning to savor the moment, to find joy in the present." However, when going through cancer, we often resign ourselves to feeling miserable, hoping for some day in the future when the disease will be gone, the tumor healed, and our bodies returned to "normal."

This kind of thinking steals our lives away from us. By living for some unknown time in the future, we neglect today. It's like we're not really here. On some days when your treatment is particularly difficult, you may wish you were somewhere else, and that's understandable! However, if you find yourself endlessly wishing for it all to be over, you're neglecting yourself. None of us can predict the future, but we can find happiness today. Lazar, with over ten years of experience, has seen massage create that kind of happiness time and time again.

"I worked with a man in his sixties who had been exposed to Agent Orange in the Vietnam War," she says. "It caused cancer and totally messed up the nerves in his feet. He could barely walk; he described the sensation as walking on needles and pointed rocks. I spent an hour with him, giving him a foot and leg massage. The next week when I arrived for his appointment, he was ecstatic. He told me he had gone from walking on rocks to 'walking on cotton,' and the effect had lasted for two days."

A few years ago, the Memorial Sloan-Kettering Cancer Center did a study on massage and symptom relief in cancer patients. Over a period of three years they studied nearly 1,300 patients, and found that symptoms were reduced by approximately 50 percent, even for patients with more severe symptoms, and benefits lasted for at least two days. "These data indicate that massage therapy is associated with substantive improvement in cancer patients' symptom scores," said the researchers.[1]

Some patients are concerned that massage will "spread" the cancer around

Tips for a Safe and Comfortable Massage

Studies abound on the benefits of massage for cancer patients, and many old fears about "spreading" the cancer have been put to rest by scientific studies. However, there are some precautions you'll want to take to ensure your safety.

Choose an experienced therapist. Make sure your therapist is either certified in oncology esthetics or oncology massage, or has experience working with cancer patients. "There is a strong possibility of harm," says Mórag Currin, LA, CMLT, and president of Touch for Cancer Online, "if the person is not educated. They could create pain, dislodge a port, or induce swelling in fragile lymph node areas. If they don't have experience, find someone who does."

Avoid aggressive therapies. Deep tissue massage, sports massage, hot stone massage, Shiatsu, Rolfing, trigger-point therapy, or any massage that is aggressive needs to be off your list until you're done with treatments. "Not all types of massage are good for someone going through treatment," says Mórag. "Anytime you're working with someone with a health challenge, you have to use a lighter touch."

Stay away from compromised areas. If you have wounds that haven't healed, painful surgical incisions, new scar tissue, or other areas of the body that are sensitive, ask your massage therapist to stay away from those areas until they have healed. If you've had lymph nodes removed, be sure you go to a certified oncology massage therapist who knows what he or she is doing. The incorrect method of massage may increase your risk of lymphedema—a devastating, lasting condition where lymph accumulates in tissues and causes swelling. A knowledgeable therapist administering the proper technique, on the other hand, can help drain lymph (waste fluid) away from the surgical area.

Ask for clean, simple products. Make sure your therapist knows that you want safe, gentle products used on your skin. Ask about the ingredients, and avoid parabens, fragrances, and harsh acids (like salicylic and glycolic).

Communicate! The most important thing to ensure a comfortable, enjoyable spa experience is to trust and respect your own feelings. If something hurts, speak up! Nothing should cause you pain. "Sometimes people are nervous to speak up," says Mórag, "and they really need to. Nobody else can tell how you're feeling. Tell the therapist so he or she can make adjustments."

the body and so fear making an appointment. You don't have to worry—this is an outdated fear that has been put to rest. In fact, the fear is so outdated that today's studies focus exclusively on the benefits of massage to cancer patients. Debra Curties, RMT, a massage therapist since 1984, says in her book *Massage Therapy and Cancer,* "Fears about the risks from increased circulation of blood and lymph are . . . unfounded. [T]he effects of massage therapy may well mitigate against the survival of cancer cells moving in these media."[2]

Of course, you do need to take some precautions with massages for your own safety. Deep tissue massage, for example, is not recommended for cancer patients because the body is so tender. It's also very important to be sure your therapist has experience with cancer patients, so she doesn't do anything that could hurt you. (See sidebar, "Tips for a Safe and Comfortable Massage.") However, massages are just wonderful, and I highly recommend you try one, at least once. Make the effort to make the appointment and go. You'll be amazed at how much better you feel.

Reflexology: A Foot Rub and So Much More

"When we were getting our chemo treatment, there was this group of people who did reflexology on our legs and feet. They could tell from my feet that my cancer was in the kidney area! They worked with the feet and talked and it was very soothing and very comfortable. I was there for a good six hours for my treatment—they put your feet up and do this on your legs, and you could sit back and almost fall asleep while you're having chemo."

—Chris, non Hodgkin's lymphoma survivor

Who doesn't enjoy a nice foot rub now and then? It's soothing and relaxing, and can ease aching muscles and joints and relieve stress. However, according to researchers, a certain type of foot massage—called reflexology—can do a lot more than that.

One study, for example, found that reflexology had a positive effect for cancer patients experiencing pain,[3] and another found that following foot reflexology, patients with breast and lung cancer experienced a significant decrease in anxiety and pain.[4]

A third study found that compared to regular foot massage (in which reflexology pressure points weren't stimulated), reflexology improved quality of life in 100 percent of the participants, compared to only 33 percent of the regular massage group. "Not only did the patients in this study enjoy the intervention," said the researchers, "they were also relaxed, comforted, and achieved relief from some of their symptoms."[5]

In Australia, ten minutes of reflexology treatments helped provide cancer patients with relief from pain, nausea, and anxiety. The results were so positive the researchers recommended further study with larger numbers of patients.[6]

What exactly is reflexology? The therapy operates on the theory that following illness, the body is in a state of "imbalance," with vital energy pathways blocked. Reflexology restores and maintains the body's natural equilibrium and encourages healing.

A reflexologist uses his or her hands to apply pressure to the feet, working on certain points of imbalance to release blockages and restore free flow of energy to the whole body. Pressure may also be applied to the hands and the ears, and is believed to send signals through the peripheral nervous system. Practitioners may use specific pressure points on the feet (similar to acupuncture), which are thought to correspond to certain parts of the body.

Reflexology isn't only used to relieve cancer symptoms. Back pain, sports injuries, migraines, digestive disorders, and sleep disorders can all benefit from the treatment. However, if you're going through cancer treatments and haven't tried reflexology, now might be a good time.

It's a relaxing, balancing treatment for the body," says Mórag Currin, LA, CMLT, and president of Touch for Cancer Online. "If someone is nervous about being touched for fear of pain or for other reasons, reflexology is often a great alternative. The feet are typically far away from any sensitive areas like surgery incisions or ports, but yet massaging them creates a huge benefit."

Sessions range from thirty minutes to an hour and are usually very relaxing, with the potential to relieve symptoms and side effects. Check with your cancer center for alternative therapies, or look to area spas that may offer reflexology as part of their massage services. Of course, if anything hurts or feels uncomfortable, be sure to let your reflexologist know.

Reiki: Realign Your Skewed Energy Centers

"I've done Reiki. I'm going for another one next week. They have a typical spa where you go. They have music going and [the practitioner] does it over your head, with her hands. It was relaxing."

—Dee, breast cancer survivor

During cancer treatments, you're constantly losing your energy to treatments, anxiety, stress, and fatigue. Reiki (pronounced "ray-kee") is an ancient healing practice that originated in Japan, with a foundation in Tibetan Buddhism. It's used to promote health and well-being, or to ease disease-related symptoms or side effects. The word "Reiki" is derived from two Japanese words: *rei*, or universal, and *ki*, or "life energy."

Benefits of a Hand Massage

If you're not ready to try it yet or you don't have time for a full-blown regular massage, you can get many benefits from a simple hand massage. In fact, one study found that hand massage had a positive effect on pain and depression in patients with cancer.

Most anyone can give you a hand and arm massage. You can go to a professional or ask a friend or loved one. You don't have to worry too much about technique. The power of touch along with the massaging motion can help increase circulation, relax muscles, and help return flexibility to the hands and wrists. If you use lotion, it's also a great way to rejuvenate the skin.

Reiki is based on the idea that there is a universal (or source) energy that supports the body's innate healing abilities. Practitioners access this energy, helping it to flow into the body to facilitate healing, often through twelve to fifteen basic positions or energy centers in the body (chakras). They direct Reiki energy through the palms of their hands to the patient, who normally sits or lies down fully clothed. A treatment can last anywhere from thirty to ninety minutes.

At the time of the printing of this book, the National Center for Complementary and Alternative Medicine (NCCAM) is funding research on the effectiveness of Reiki on cancer-related side effects and symptoms. As of 2001, 47 percent of U.S. state nursing boards recognized providing alternative therapies, including Reiki, as being within the scope of nursing practice.[7] A pilot study with twenty volunteers found that Reiki helped reduce pain, including pain caused by cancer.[8]

Jean Lazar, who also practices energy medicine through therapeutic touch and Reiki, says, "We have energy fields inside, around, and through our physical bodies. When we are balanced and in harmony with our energies, we will defuse illness and disease."

If you've been feeling a little "off" lately and you can't really put your finger on the cause, Reiki may be the solution for you. The American Cancer Society cites anecdotal support that some patients going through chemotherapy find that Reiki even reduces the intensity of nausea and vomiting. More research needs to be done, but Reiki is already used in many cancer centers and hospitals. Many provide sessions on site, or have recommendations for practitioners.

For practitioners near you, look for alternative healing clinics in hospitals, ask a friend for a referral, ask your nurses, or check my website (www. cincovidas.com). The International Association of Reiki Professionals (IARP) provides a locater page as well.

When you do find a practitioner you're considering, ask questions like these:

- How long have you been practicing Reiki?

- What qualifications do you have? (Look for completed classes, membership in Reiki organizations, and/or time with a master. Currently there are no certifications.)

- How long will each treatment take? How many treatments do you recommend?

In the end, go with the person who feels right. What matters is that you feel better—without more drugs.

Acupuncture: A Proven Remedy for Many Side Effects

"I would definitely put more alternative methods in my program if I were to go through it again. The one I would use right off the bat would be acupuncture for nausea and for hot flashes."

—Jody, breast cancer survivor

I know what you may be thinking—needles. Ugh! You probably don't want to even think about more needles, especially after being poked and prodded during hospital visits and chemo treatments. Yet acupuncture has been shown in many studies to be helpful at lessening the side effects of cancer treatment. If you're not a needle person, is it worth the anxiety?

First of all—I would *not* describe acupuncture as painful. According to practitioners, it's "virtually painless." I started using acupuncture for stress relief and was amazed at how balanced, calm, and restored I felt after just two treatments. In fact, most patients experience acupuncture as relaxing. The needles are extremely thin—about the width of a hair—and flexible. Nothing like those shot needles you may be thinking of.

Sensations vary from person to person, but can include an initial pinch when the needle is first inserted (like someone pulling on a hair). Depending on the location and the insertion technique, however, you may not feel anything at all.

Once the needle penetrates the skin, any such pinch should stop. (The depth the needle penetrates depends on the location and the problem being treated.) Once the needle is at its proper depth, sensations may include tingling, numbness, a slight heat or ache, a "fizzy" sense of nerve stimulation, or nothing. If the patient feels a numb sort of heaviness—called "deqi" by acupuncturists—it's a sign the treatment is working.

If a needle is uncomfortable, just say so and your acupuncturist will reinsert it in a slightly different location. According to most acupuncturists, most patients experience little to no discomfort at all.

"I found out about a local acupuncture school that had a free program for cancer patients," says Alli, ovarian cancer survivor. "For a year and a half now I've been going once a week. I can really tell a difference. I can be tired or have trouble breathing and the headaches are pretty intense, and when I leave there it's alleviated. Treatment is anywhere from thirty minutes to an hour. Sometimes I'll fall asleep; sometimes I can just meditate. It's a safe place for me."

Acupuncture has been proven in studies to be an effective way to deal with cancer side effects. The National Institutes of Health says that, based on a review of thirty-three controlled trials, there is clear evidence that acupuncture helps with chemo-related nausea and vomiting.[9]

The Memorial Sloan-Kettering Cancer Center found that acupuncture improved post-chemotherapy fatigue by over 30 percent.[10] Researchers in France found that acupuncture decreased pain intensity in cancer patients.[11] And for those of you going through early menopause because of treatment, acupuncture has been found to help reduce the frequency of hot flashes.[12]

In fact, Eleanor M. Walker, M.D., of the Henry Ford Health System in Detroit, reported that acupuncture was as effective for reducing breast-cancer-treatment-related hot flashes as the medication Effexor.[13]

How does acupuncture work? Chinese doctors believe the body has many energy-carrying channels and that the needles help lift disruptions in these channels, rebalancing the body's "qi" (pronounced "chee"). Western doctors are more likely to talk about how needles stimulate muscle and sensory neurons, sending messages to the central nervous system and releasing endorphins (natural painkillers) and other chemicals that modify nerve impulses.

If you have pain or discomfort that's not responding to other treatments, I highly recommend you try acupunture. Ask your doctor for

Might Ayurvedic Medicine Help?

An ancient system of medicine that originated in India over 5,000 years ago, ayurveda (meaning science or knowledge of life) is a holistic way of diagnosing illness and bringing the body and mind back into balance to help restore health.

Treatments and techniques can include special diets, medications, detoxification, herbal medicines, massage, meditation, yoga, and breathing and relaxation techniques.

I spent some time learning about ayurvedic medicine and have incorporated certain practices and diet changes as a result. I learned that my body tends to get overheated (Pita constitution) and that eating cooling foods makes me feel more comfortable. I also do self-massage before I shower, which helps me relax and contributes to ridding my body of waste. Learning more about yourself in this way helps you feel more empowered about your health.

Some studies on particular aspects of ayurveda—such as extracts like curcumin and boswellia, and therapies like massage and yoga—have shown some promise in protecting cells and DNA and alleviating treatment side effects. Other common ayurvedic remedies, however, such as some herbal and cleansing treatments, have had harmful effects. Check with your doctor first; then, for a list of qualified practitioners in your area, go to the National Institute of Ayurvedic Medicine (NIAM) and ask them for a list.

There are no licenses offered in the U.S. to practice ayurveda, but several institutions have educational programs that issue certificates. Many practitioners educated and licensed in India come to practice in the U.S. as well.

recommendations, look to see if your hospital has an alternative healing clinic, or look up the American Academy of Medical Acupuncturists (AAMA) or acufinder.com for a practitioner in your area.

Choose one who's been certified by the National Commission for the Certification of Acupuncturists (they usually have the title Dipl. Ac. after their name), and one who is a member of AAMA. Don't be afraid to ask questions, like how long the doctor has been practicing, where she received her training, and the length and type of treatment she recommends. Most importantly, let her know that you have cancer and ask if she's worked with cancer patients in the past.

Before your first treatment get a good night's sleep, and go in with a positive attitude—it can make a difference. Eat something light two to four hours beforehand (don't go on an empty stomach), and dress comfortably; needles may remain inserted for thirty minutes or more, so you want to be able to relax. Finally—very important while your defenses are down—make sure your acupuncturist opens a new pack of needles before treating you (they are sterile and disposable) and disinfects your skin with alcohol before insertion.

Yoga: Relieve Muscle Tension and Return to the "Now"

"A friend took me to a class in Los Angeles. I went and felt amazing afterwards. I felt super vibrant and healthy and alive. I thought, 'Wow, I want to keep doing this!'"

—Laura, breast cancer survivor

Want a new treatment for side effects like insomnia, mood swings, constipation, "chemo fog," and other aches and pains? Never mind the drugs. Your body has had enough. Instead, try taking yourself to a yoga class.

"Something magical happens when you do a total and complete class," says certified yoga teacher, therapist, and cancer survivor Laura Kupperman.

Particularly if you go to a class for cancer survivors (recommended), you'll enjoy a unique camaraderie you'll be unlikely to find anywhere else. If you've just been diagnosed, you may meet up with someone who's already been through the treatment, or someone who's survived for years.

"There's a great sense of acceptance," Laura says. "Everyone's been through something. But it's not a support group. There's no complaining about what's going wrong. People rally around doing something healthy and positive for their bodies." In other words, attending a yoga class is a proactive move on your part that will help you reconnect to that powerful person inside. Plus, learning a new skill and increasing your physical activity is always good for your brain and overall energy level.

I regularly go to yoga classes, and I walk out feeling better every time. There are many kinds to choose from. If I really need to nurture myself, I'll go to a restorative class, whereas if I need to connect and ground myself, I go to a kundalini class. If I need to stretch, I'll go to a vinyasa class. Not only do they all help me better manage everything else I do in my life, they encourage me to breathe deeply and to quiet my mind. Truly, yoga is a form of meditation. When I start getting into obsessive thinking, I know I need to go to a yoga class.

Yoga also addresses specific physical problems. Laura explains: "If you've had a bilateral mastectomy, for instance, you're going to have scar tissue. It's your body's way of guarding the injured area, but it causes the chest to get tight. Pretty soon the whole front of the body is rounded forward, weakening the upper back and shoulder muscles, compressing the breath, and often causing back pain. Certain yoga poses gently open up the front of the body and strengthen the back, making it easier to breathe full, deep breaths, increasing energy, and reducing aches and pains."

Studies support Laura's findings. An early study found that cancer patients participating in two ninety-minute yoga sessions a week reported improved appetite, sleep, bowel habits, and feelings of peace and tranquility.[14] A more recent study found that yoga helped cancer patients walk longer with a lower resting heart rate.[15] Another showed that yoga helped patients feel less stress,[16] and a fourth found that restorative yoga helped breast cancer patients feel less fatigue.[17]

"They had a yoga program for cancer patients," says Alli, ovarian cancer survivor. "All of it was done sitting on a floor or on a chair, and it was gentle stretching. I felt relaxed. My muscles weren't as tight, and that helped me physically be more relaxed."

Besides the physical benefits, yoga can provide many emotional benefits, too. "When you have any illness or huge stress in your life," Laura says, "it's so easy to think about all those scary 'what-ifs.' Like, what if the test results come back positive, or what if this cancer is going to spread all over my body. All these things that aren't actually happening, but you have these fearful thoughts that snowball into each other.

"Yoga opens you to the peace of mind that's available if you can be in and accept the present moment. Through focusing your breath or focusing on your body being in a particular posture—really paying attention to how you feel and what is in the moment right now—you give yourself a break from worrying about what could be and open up to what is. And you realize that where you are might be a pretty okay place."

Since yoga requires a steady focus on the breath, it tends to quiet the mind. "My students tell me, 'I come to yoga, and it's so nice, as I have to stay focused on what's going on, so I can't think about all the other stuff,'" Laura says. "Through yoga practice, we learn to be more present in the moment, which is so helpful in all areas of our lives."

Many yoga poses can help minimize the side effects of cancer and ease the symptoms of chemotherapy. In addition, various postures rebuild muscle strength, create energy, and bring back range of motion. Best of all, yoga is something you can do for yourself. On those days when you may not

Have You Tried the B.E.S.T.?

The Bio Energetic Synchronization Technique (or B.E.S.T.) is a hands-on procedure that works with the energy centers in your body to encourage healing potential. Developed during the mid-1970s by chiropractor Milton Ted Morter, Jr., B.E.S.T. uses a nonforceful chiropractic technique to help remove "interference" from the nervous system, correcting physical, nutritional, and emotional stresses.

In essence, B.E.S.T. seeks to balance the body's physical, mental, emotional, and spiritual energy fields, to help promote optimal health. I regularly go to my B.E.S.T. practitioner to "realign" my energy, and I always walk away feeling more centered and vital. If you'd like to try a treatment, look for a qualified practitioner in your area, or go to www.morter.com to locate a practitioner near you.

be able to get an appointment for a massage or acupuncture treatment, you can go home and practice the poses that feel good to you.

"You learn lifelong tools that will help you when you need them," says Laura, "even beyond treatment."

Laura recommends looking for a good class to get the full benefits. (Be sure to check with your doctor before starting.) Classes specific to cancer fighters and survivors are best. Yoga classes for cancer fighters are much more mainstream today than they were a few years ago, and many yoga centers around the country offer them. (Search the Internet for "yoga and cancer centers" or "yoga for survivors" and you'll find dozens of listings.) If you don't find one offered in your area, try to find an instructor schooled in working with cancer patients. (Check out the International Association of Yoga Therapists, or YogaClassSearch.com.)

"Yoga gives you this great toolbox of things you can use to feel better," Laura says. "It teaches you to say, 'Here's how I feel right now, in this moment, and here's what I need to do to take care of it.'"

If you're worried you won't be able to do it, put it out of your mind. Yoga practice is about no one but you, and classes are not competitive.

"After being poked and prodded through treatment," Laura says, "yoga is a yummy way to celebrate, and to say, 'I'm still alive and I'm still breathing and I can still do things that feel good.'"

Tai Chi: Controlled Movement that Improves Health

Historically, tai chi chuan (translated as "supreme ultimate fist") was a form of self-defense in which the practitioner neutralized his opponent's use of force before applying a countering force of his own. Students learned how to efficiently transmit energy, relax the mind, and control the breath. Such skills translated into other areas of their lives, promoting health and well-being.

Today, many people find health benefits from daily practice of the graceful exercise of tai chi, and many of those are cancer survivors. Tai chi can ease pain and stiffness, build muscle strength, improve coordination, balance, and flexibility, and improve sleep. Studies suggest that it may enhance the immune system and reduce blood pressure.[18]

A small study of breast cancer survivors showed that the women in the tai chi group had improved flexibility, strength, and aerobic capacity.[19] The slow, graceful movements accompanied by deep, mindful breathing help increase circulation and promote relaxation. Practitioners claim that it balances the flow of vital energy (called qi or chi), which helps improve health and extend life.

The nice thing about tai chi is that the movements are gentle, so if you're going through cancer treatment and/or recovering from it, this exercise can be the perfect way to help maintain or regain your flexibility and strength with a low risk of injury. Slow, precise movements are good for muscle control, while deep breathing creates a meditative serenity that can help ease stress. Of course, talk to your doctor first to discuss any limitations you may have before starting.

To find a class in your area, check your local health clubs, schools, YMCAs, and recreational facilities. You'll find a lot of books and DVDs out there for self-teaching, but as a cancer fighter or survivor, you're safer with an instructor. He or she can show you how to practice safely to help avoid injury and derive maximum benefit. You'll want to learn the fundamentals well, so choose someone who has received good instruction. The *T'ai Chi Magazine* is also a good source for instruction.

Once you get started, you may become addicted, as this exercise is not like your usual aerobic pounding. Instead, your feet are always firmly on the ground, and the movements have symbolic meaning, with names like "Wave Hands Like Clouds" and "Grasping the Bird's Tail." Like yoga, your focus is on the breath, and as you move gently and slowly, you may find cancer is the last thing on your mind.

Walking: The Simplest Form of Restorative Movement

"My main source of exercise is walking. It gives me time with God."

—Joanna, breast cancer survivor

We've been talking about forms of exercise that may help you feel better during cancer treatment, but there's one very simple one you may not have thought about—just going out to take a walk!

Some days all you may feel you can do is get up and walk around the block. But hey, even that can have great benefits. One study found that a twelve-week home-based walking intervention was safe and effective at helping breast cancer survivors to regain physical activity.[20] Another found that exercise improved breast cancer patients' well-being,[21] and yet another found that walking helped improve cardiorespiratory fitness and physical function in prostate cancer patients, and also reduced the sensation of pain.[22]

Walking is so effective that researchers outline how patients can—and should—start their own program. "Unnecessary bedrest and prolonged sedentarism can contribute significantly to the development of fatigue and may result in rapid and potentially irreversible losses in energy and functioning," say researchers.[23] They suggest starting at a low intensity, keeping a walking diary, and monitoring pulse to regulate pace.

When my father was the weakest in his cancer journey, walking helped him get out of his head and into his body. The fact that we lived near the ocean helped as well. The sound and smell of the water was very healing, so we walked along the seawall whenever he could. Sometimes it was too much for him, but when he felt up to it, he often felt better afterwards and slept very well.

Harvard researchers found that breast cancer survivors who engaged in regular physical activity—including walking at an average pace for one hour—were 50 percent less likely to have a recurrence of their cancer than women who exercised less than an hour per week.[24]

"I would at least do a walk, do something," says Jody, when speaking about her own battle with fatigue.

"Every day I try to exercise," says Justin, brain cancer survivor, "like treadmill walking, very slowly, or a brisk walk. It helps a lot."

Walking is something you can always do. You don't need a class, an appointment, or money, unless you want to buy a pedometer, which can be a good motivator. Ask your doctor about your limits, and then put on a good pair of supportive shoes and head out. Ten minutes is better than nothing. Try it and see!

Let's Review

- It's very important to do something for yourself during cancer treatment—something that will give you back some of the relaxation, energy, and vitality that cancer and cancer treatments take away.

- An appointment for a massage, a spa treatment, or acupuncture can help you relax, reconnect to your inner self, and recharge, body and spirit.

- Massage can help reduce the pain of cancer treatments. Choose a therapist experienced with cancer patients, preferably someone with an oncology certification, and avoid any aggressive massages. Ask for a light touch.

- Reflexology can help relieve pain, nausea, and anxiety.

- Reiki may help relieve pain and realign your energy centers so you feel more alive.

- Science has found clear evidence that acupuncture helps reduce nausea and vomiting from chemotherapy. It may also help relieve pain, fatigue, and hot flashes.

- Yoga classes for cancer patients provide camaraderie and a positive place to interact with other fighters and survivors. Yoga may also help restore flexibility and strength and help you sleep better.

- Tai chi is a gentle form of exercise that may improve flexibility, strength, and aerobic capacity. The slow, graceful movements accompanied by deep, mindful breathing can help increase circulation and promote relaxation.

- Walking is an easy form of exercise that you can do any time, anywhere, and that may improve well-being, fitness, and physical function. It may even help reduce your risk of recurrence.

- Other forms of alternative medicine like B.E.S.T. and ayurvedic medicine, may help you heal and reduce the severity of side effects—without more drugs.

Goals: Alternative Medicines for Me

To take proactive steps toward your own healing and well-being, circle the alternative medicine types that you are willing to try within the next month.

Massage   Spa Facial   Acupuncture   Yoga

Tai Chi   B.E.S.T.   Ayurvedic Medicine   Walking

Reiki   Other: _____

Personal Affirmations

*I deserve to feel good, and I enjoy taking time for myself
in ways that restore my spirit and help me to feel more
comfort and solace in my own body.*

I am worthy and deserving of every healing process available to me.

9

Hair, Wigs, and Scarves

"After my second chemo my head got really tender to the touch. I could feel every hair follicle on my head. I asked my sister to shave it for me. I had a really hard time with that. I felt like I lost myself. I had had long hair since I was sixteen years old. I was like, 'I don't even know who this is. Who are you?'"

—Karen, two-time thyroid cancer survivor

WHEN I WENT THROUGH CHEMOTHERAPY, MY DOCTOR assured me my hair was going to fall out.

I was devastated.

Hair loss typically starts two to three weeks after chemotherapy starts. For many patients, it's not until after the second treatment that they really start to see the effects. My long, brown hair—which I loved and took for granted—started to rapidly thin after my first treatment. I got it cut short, because the doctor told me it would be easier for the hair to come out in short strands than longer locks. I still remember feeling like I was losing a part of myself.

In fact, losing my hair at that time seemed worse to me than getting the disease itself. Granted, I was naïve about cancer at age sixteen, but the impact of losing my hair was very clear to me. When it actually happened, my first priority became to make sure that I looked normal. Without my hair, I looked sick, and looking sick made me feel "different."

"My hair fell out, which was the most traumatic thing for me," says Laurie, breast cancer survivor. "Your hair is part of your identity. It's what people see first—it's how you are out in the world. I'm out in the public every day. It's bad enough to have a bad hair day, but I lost sleep over this. It was more traumatic than having cancer. Cancer we can take care of, but I remember thinking, 'What am I going to wear on my head?'"

For some of us (usually more men than women), hair is just hair, and when it's gone, it's no big deal. "I lost my hair during treatment," says Justin, brain cancer survivor, "so I shaved it off. It was fine, actually." My father, who lost his hair three times during his eight-year cancer battle, also liked his bald head—he thought he looked pretty good.

But for many others—especially women—hair loss is a very difficult side effect. We have fewer bald role models to look up to, and an expectation in society that our hair will crown our look. According to Susan Beausang, president of 4women.com and author of *Loving Our Bald Selves* ("Coping," January/February 2010), hair loss can affect women down to their very core.

"At no time is love of self more important than when fighting cancer," she says. "Yet many women find their love of self becomes compromised by the emotions stirred when they find a bald, 'sick-looking' person staring back at them in the mirror."

In fact, in Susan's research, based on a sample of nearly 500 female cancer survivor survey respondents, over half said that the hardest part of hair loss was the feeling that it advertised their cancer to the public.

"When I look back on it," says Rayette, ovarian cancer survivor, "the worst thing about losing my hair was that once it happened, I knew I looked sick. Up until then I could hide it. It was like my secret. That was my big fear when I was diagnosed—I didn't want people to treat me differently. People tend to be afraid of people who have cancer; they don't know what to say. They assume that you're dying. So that was the big disappointment when I lost my hair, as then I knew that I looked like something was wrong with me."

So many things come into play when we're talking about hair loss. It goes much deeper than vanity. As it is for me and for so many other women, hair is part of our identities, our personalities—who we are to the people in our lives. "Without hair," says Susan, who went through a prophylatic double mastectomy after discovering she and her family had the breast cancer gene, and is a victim of alopecia herself, "many women feel stripped of their identity and femininity, making it even more difficult to maintain the sense of positive optimism that is so important for healing."

Meghan, three-time cancer survivor, felt awful when people would confuse her gender because of her bald head. "People mistaking me for a boy—that felt really shitty," she says. "I was like, 'Do you not see that I'm wearing hoop earrings and makeup?'"

On top of that, many women are caretakers. We have a strong instinct to care for our children, husbands, and even our parents. We want to protect them from this illness. Many women worry more about what their families will think of their hair loss than anything else.

"I didn't want my kids to be afraid of me, or not to know how to treat me," says Joanna, breast cancer survivor.

"Before a women loses her hair to chemotherapy," says Susan, "she will often put much of her energy into maintaining a sense of normalcy for the benefit of loved ones, especially children. Many women find it is their hair loss that pushes their parents, partners, and children over the edge with fear."

"It didn't really bother me," says Deb, breast cancer survivor, "but it bothered my daughter. It was a signal to her that I was sick. I have thick, dark hair. It was always long and curly. And I think for women, it's unusual to see bald women. It's one thing to see a bald man. But for women, it's such an outward symbol of being sick."

Job number one is to focus on healing. Any worries and anxieties surrounding hair loss can make it much more difficult for you to encourage the positive emotions you need during treatment. Still, you can't ignore the emotional upheaval that may accompany hair loss. You certainly must not feel ashamed or guilty about these emotions. Well-meaning friends and relatives may try to trivialize your feelings, saying that hair loss is nothing compared to a life-threatening disease, but you must always honor your own experience.

"Many women are emotionally devastated when their hair begins falling out and find that no one quite understands why they care about their hair when facing something as significant as cancer," Susan says. "If you feel devastated by your hair loss, you should know that most women do and that it is entirely normal. We live in such an appearance-driven society, where hair very much defines female beauty. Many women enjoy public attention for their style of dress, hairstyle, or smile, and no one enjoys the attention that can come with what feels like a 'cancer image.'"

You're Losing Your Hair: 5 Things to Do

1. Decide if you want to buy a wig, if you'll get by with hats and scarves, or if you'll just go all natural.

2. Shop for a wig before you start losing your hair. (Take a friend with you.) It will be easier to match your regular color and style.

3. Take your time and investigate all your resources. There may be several wig shops in your area. Find the one that will give you the best selection and price.

4. If you choose to wear scarves, check with your hospital, cancer center, and online shops for those made specifically for cancer patients. They are usually more comfortable and easier to wrap.

5. Take a deep breath and remember—your hair will grow back after treatment is over!

Processing emotions, as we talked about in Chapter 4, can help, as can finding alternative headwear options you feel good about. If you can look in the mirror while wearing a wig or a hat or a scarf and say, "Hey, that looks okay," you'll be much better able to cope with the side effect.

"Many women find that taking actions that give them a greater sense of control over their changing appearance helps to reduce their anxiety and lift their spirits," Susan says. "Having many headwear options on hand *before* hair loss begins helps women to feel prepared rather than helpless when their hair begins to fall out."

I know that once I found some wigs I liked and started playing around with them, I felt a lot better. I was still in high school, after all, and the other kids definitely noticed when my hair was gone. Putting on my wig and hats made me feel normal, complete, and very trendy. I actually had fun with them, which made such a difference in my outlook and my ability to go to school on a daily basis without feeling overly self-conscious or "different."

"Around my birthday," says Laurie, "a friend of mine gave me a shawl that was a bright orange color like my hair. I thought, 'Hey, I could wear this on my head.' I have a ton of scarves and sarongs, so I pulled out every one I owned and started wrapping them on my head, and I thought, *This is a great look. This is what I'm going to do.*"

You, too, can find ways to reinvent your look and help yourself to feel confident again.

My Hair Loss Plan

Take a moment to think about—really think about—the experience of losing your hair. It may have already happened, or it may be something you'll soon have to face. Then answer the following questions. These will help you develop your own plan for dealing with this side effect. Even if you find more than one answer that fits, circle the answer that *most* describes how you feel, most of the time.

1. When I think about losing my hair, I feel
   a. Devastated
   b. Sad
   c. Worried
   d. Scared
   e. I'm not really worried about it

2. I realize I need to process any negative feelings I have about this side effect. To get used to the idea, I'm going to:
   a. Journal about it
   b. Make a list of all my other good qualities, knowing I'm much more than my hair or my appearance
   c. Talk to a close friend
   d. Review stories of other survivors who have gone through it
   e. Other _____

3. So far in my life, my hair has been _____ to my sense of identity and style.
   a. Extremely important
   b. Very important
   c. Important
   d. Not really important
   e. I don't really think about my hair

4. My lifestyle, job, or social calendar requires me to:
   a. Look a certain way because I'm dealing with the public
   b. Look a certain way to fit into my peer group
   c. Look nice, but there are no specific standards
   d. Look casual, as everyone around me is very laid back about appearance
   e. My daily life doesn't require me to look any particular way

5. When considering my appearance, I like to:
   a. Look as stylish as I can; I hate it when my flaws show up
   b. Feel like I belong in my peer group; I don't like to stand out
   c. Look nice and presentable, but I don't have to follow the latest trends or look like I just stepped out of a salon
   d. As long as I look clean and put together I'm not too concerned
   e. I don't really think much about my appearance and I don't care what other people think of how I look

6. When I think about the options, _____ appeals to me the most.
   a. A wig
   b. Scarves
   c. Hats
   d. Going bald

Now count up your number of A, B, C, D, and E answers *only* for questions 1, 3, 4, and 5. (Use the other answers for your own information.) If you have more A and B answers, your hair is extremely important to you and you need to make it a priority to find a top-quality wig that most closely matches your real hair. If you have more C and D answers, your hair is important, but you may be able to get by with a less expensive wig, or just scarves and hats. If you have mostly E answers, you may feel fine going bald.

Whatever your answers, explore your feelings completely, honor them—whatever they are—and promise to take care of yourself by finding the option that feels best to you.

Do I Cut It or Shave It?

"When my hair started to come out in chunks, my son shaved my head for me. It wasn't so traumatic because I had a nice-shaped head and I didn't mind shaving it. My son had a bald head too, so we looked like matching pinballs, like two bowling balls only white!"

—Chris, non-Hodgkin's lymphoma survivor

Whether you cut or shave your hair probably depends on the type of treatment you're getting. Some more mild forms of chemo may only cause your hair to thin (like mine did), and you may be able to get by with a new style and some hair accessories to cover up the thin spots.

Other chemotherapy drugs will have a more dramatic effect, causing you to lose all your hair. Since it will most likely come out in unpleasant chunks, in these cases you will probably feel best if you get it shaved.

Talk to your doctor. He or she can tell you how much hair loss to expect. Expect it to thin quite a bit, however, if you go through chemotherapy. If you're a woman, I strongly suggest you get a short hairdo to avoid messy hair clumps. I remember hair showing up on my pillows, furniture, clothing, carpets, shower drain, and more. My mom remembers cleaning it up, too. She could not believe how much hair there was all over the house.

Cutting your hair short helps reduce the shedding. Then, if you need to take the next step later and get it shaved, you can. In fact, it's better to wait and shave your head after your hair has started to fall out, as then it's less irritating to your scalp. My dad let his hair thin to the point where he shaved it off. We liked his sleek look!

In the meantime, be gentle with your hair. If it's long, don't use elastics or barrettes, and wear a braid at night to limit breakage. Avoid bleaching, coloring, and perming, as all these processes involve toxic chemicals and will only weaken it further. Air dry when you can, and put away your curling irons and hot rollers.

To strengthen your hair, purchase a great deep-conditioning hair treatment with protein and commit to using it on a weekly basis. Also, your hair is most vulnerable when it's wet, so be more careful during treatment. I always use a wide-tooth comb and comb from the bottom up. In other words, get the knots out on the ends and work your way up. You can then use a paddle brush to brush the hair, but be gentle, and avoid pulling and tugging.

Invest in a satin pillowcase, which creates less friction and pull while you sleep. My mom bought me one when I was going through cancer and it really helped minimize the pulling and tugging on my hair. Use gentle, natural shampoos that don't contain irritating sulfates, fragrances, and alcohol, and use a soft, gentle brush. For dehydrated scalp and hair, try working in natural oils like jojoba and black cumin, which are nourishing and restorative.

Even if you retain some of your hair, chemo treatments may eventually cause it to become brittle, frizzy, and dry, so you can't really style it the way you're used to. Your scalp may also feel irritated and itchy, or even tender, to the point where you *want* the hair gone. Finally, shaving your head can make it easier to wear a wig.

Shaving your head can also help you feel more in control of your situation. After all, it's more empowering to shave your own head than to look in the mirror each morning and take stock of how much hair has fallen out. If you decide to do it, make sure it's cut short first. It's more uncomfortable to shave longer hair. If you're doing it yourself (or a loved one is doing it for you), use a well-maintained set of professional clippers that won't pull. Electric shavers that aren't meant for head hair may irritate tender skin on the scalp. (Definitely don't use a razor.)

Start at the back of the neck and run the clippers in rows up over your scalp to the front. Move slowly and carefully to avoid nicking the skin. When you're done, run your hands over your head to be sure you haven't missed any spots.

You can also make an appointment with your stylist and have him or her do the shaving for you. Donating your hair to an organization like Locks of Love (which makes wigs for children) or Wigs for Kids can help you to feel better about the whole experience. Then, get ready for your new look. For me, my wigs made me feel much more confident. I wouldn't have chosen to lose my hair, but after a few months I got used to what it was like to be bald, and I actually really liked experimenting with my look. Who says you have to feel ashamed about having no hair? Why not enjoy the opportunity to try something new?

Finding a Wig

"I took the route where we splurged on my wig. I think it was the best thing for me because I'm young and I'm pretty social. I was a bridesmaid three different times during chemotherapy. I wanted to feel like myself, so we went to a place before I cut my hair, took a picture, and made a wig to look exactly like my hair. People don't even know I have a wig. I would recommend that to everyone. It made me feel better."

—Jamie, non-Hodgkin's lymphoma survivor

You have several choices about how to create your new style during cancer. You can go all natural, or choose to wear hats, scarves, or wigs. Wigs are, by far, the most popular choice, probably because they're the best at camouflaging your hair loss. Wigs can also be a lot of fun!

The most important thing if you're going to wear a wig is to shop for it *before* you lose your hair. That way, the wig store can most closely match your regular color and style. I scheduled a time before my treatments started to go shopping. I took my mom and a friend and did my best to have fun with it. I remember experimenting with all the crazy colors and styles, which made my friend and me laugh. It also made my mom feel more at ease to see that the whole thing wasn't so daunting for me.

Once you've decided on a wig and scheduled a day to go shopping, you'll want to think about the types of wigs you have to choose from. Basically, they come in two kinds: synthetic and natural human hair. Synthetic is generally easier to wash and maintain, and is typically the more economical choice. Human hair is more expensive, but does give you that familiar feel, texture, and styling options. I had both kinds when I was going through treatment, and I personally preferred the human hair.

You can go for a wig they already have in the shop, or you can have one custom made for you. Ready-made wigs can be purchased immediately and shaped by your stylist later. Custom-made options are more expensive, but they can be great choices for those who feel very particular about their hairstyles. Be prepared: If you're going for this option, you'll need to shop several weeks ahead of time, as you will have to wait for the custom wig to be made.

It's not only the hair that's different between wigs. Some have the hair attached to cloth, while others ("monofilament wigs") have the hair woven individually into a gauzelike fabric. These provide good ventilation and may be more comfortable for you.

When you actually do go shopping for a wig, don't let a salesperson or wig specialist pressure you. Ask a friend or family member to speak for you if a salesperson becomes too aggressive. The trip may be emotional for you, and you don't want someone making it worse.

Go shopping on a day when you're feeling good. If you've planned it but you wake up feeling particularly anxious, postpone until another day. Set aside a good amount of time for the venture, and make sure you get something to eat before you go, as it will take a while to find a wig you feel comfortable with. You may have to visit a few different places, or if you live in a remote area, you may have to travel to find a good wig shop.

If you're feeling confused at any point during the shopping excursion, stop, step back, and walk around the block or go to lunch to give yourself time to think. Most wig salons have a "no return" policy, so it's crucial to make a decision you feel good about. Ask your friend or loved one how you look before you make the purchase, and consider viewing a photograph of yourself in the wig.

Think about your personality and lifestyle when choosing. Do you like to get ready quickly? Find a wig that will be fast and easy to style, and that

Will My Insurance Cover It?

Insurance companies are beginning to realize the necessity for a wig in cases of chemotherapy or alopecia, and many will now cover most or all of the cost.

First, get your doctor to write a letter or a prescription that includes information as to why you need it and that it's for emotional well being, not for cosmetic reasons. Insurance companies love to turn down cosmetic claims.

Specifically, ask him to prescribe a "hair prosthesis" or "full cranial hair prosthesis" instead of just a wig. It's the same thing, but to the insurance carrier, the word "prosthesis" takes your request out of the "cosmetic" realm. In that case, they'll usually cover most of the cost.

Next, fill out your insurance claim paper and get your doctor to sign it; then send it in together with your doctor's letter and/or prescription. You may also want to include a picture of yourself with your hair gone, and potentially, a letter from your employer if he or she can further support your need for a wig, as it relates to your ability to do your work.

If all else fails and your insurance won't cover your wig, you can appeal the decision and ask for a review by the medical board. In addition, many organizations offer free or reduced-cost wigs, like Locks of Love and Cancer*Care*.

Another option: Use your wig as a medical deduction on your next year's taxes. Even if you do get some coverage from your insurance company, keep your receipts, as the portion that is not covered can be deducted.

will take little upkeep. If you enjoy hair that you can play with, get a wig that has options, perhaps with more hair.

As for where to find your wig, you have many choices. You can try checking for available wigs at your hospital's cancer center, a local beauty salon, or even online. I also have a wig directory on my website (www.cincovidas.com). If you just can't afford a wig (see sidebar, "Will My Insurance Cover It?"), ask your doctor for a prescription for an "extra-cranial prosthesis"—the medical term for a wig—and submit that to your insurance company. There's no guarantee they will reimburse you, but it's worth a try.

There are also organizations that provide free wigs for cancer patients, including the American Cancer Society, which provides free wigs through their wig banks. (Visit their website for a location near you.) Cancer*Care*, Y-ME National Breast Cancer Organization, local chapters of the Susan G. Komen for the Cure, the Duke Comprehensive Cancer Center, and Wigs for Kids all also provide free wigs. Several wig shops are also willing to give cancer patients significant discounts.

You can find wig shops online, but be sure you'll have the option to try the wig before buying. You need to see how the wig looks on you. Find a place that will work with you to ensure you find the right color, length, and cut for your face. What you think will work and what actually ends up looking good could be two different things.

Caring for and Styling Your Wig

So you get your wig home, try it on, look in the mirror, and hey, it looks pretty good! You turn your head back and forth, maybe make up your face a little, and breathe a sigh of relief. Yes, you can go out with this wig and feel good about yourself. You can go back to work, out with your friends, whatever you feel like doing, and not feel self-conscious about your hair loss.

I remember feeling really good about my wigs during treatment, because they were so convenient. I could just slip the wig on in the morning and go. I saved so much time, and the style always worked. No more bad hair days! That was a definite plus. When I wore my human hair wig, I could still use styling tools to play with my hair. I took pride in making myself look good, and it felt great to be able to do so, especially when I wasn't particularly confident about other areas of my appearance.

You may find that your wig gives you a similar boost in confidence, which is certainly welcome during treatment. However, once you take it off, what do you do with it? It's your hair, but it's not *your* hair, so do you use shampoo on it, or what?

When Caring For Your Wig, *Do Not:*

1. Expose your wig to high temperatures. Hot oven doors, barbecue grills, intense sun, and hot lamps can cause wig fibers to frizz.

2. Brush the wig when wet. Always use a wide-toothed comb or brush made specifically for wigs.

3. Use curling irons, hot rollers, or blow dryers on synthetic wigs.

4. Use products on the wig made for regular human hair. Use products made specifically for wigs.

5. Use dyes or bleaches on synthetic wigs.

6. Wear your wig in the swimming pool.

Fortunately, wigs are pretty easy to maintain. Your first question is probably, "Do I wash my wig?" In general, wash both synthetic and human-hair wigs every ten to fifteen uses (more often in hot, humid climates), but be careful to use the appropriate products and techniques. Your regular hair shampoo is *not* going to work well on your wig. Wigs require specialty shampoos, combs, and conditioning sprays to stay looking good. You can usually purchase these products at the wig salon.

When you're ready to wash your wig, gently brush it first with a brush or comb designed for wigs. Your regular brush may overstretch the hair. Then immerse it for about one minute in the sink in cold water and about a tablespoon of wig shampoo. Swirl throughout the mixture. Avoid rubbing, teasing, or scrubbing your wig, as this will damage the hair. Think about when you wash your fragile clothing items by hand—it's the same idea.

Rinse thoroughly afterward with cold water, and then—if you want to—apply wig conditioner and leave for three to five minutes, then rinse again. Blot carefully with a clean drying cloth. If you have a leave-in conditioner, spray it on carefully after blotting—not too much! Wait to brush your wig until it's dry; you can damage it if you pull on the hair when it's wet. Allow the wig to air dry on something like a can of hairspray or a towel-covered shampoo bottle. If you put it on a Styrofoam head, it may stretch out the cap. You can shake the wig out periodically to speed drying.

For daily care, remove tangles with a specialty spray conditioner designed for wigs, and comb through with a wire brush starting at the ends (instead of the roots). Never use heat-generated styling tools like curling irons or dryers on synthetic wigs, and if you use them on your human-hair wig, be careful and tread lightly. Remember, your wig doesn't grow new hair like you do, so if you damage the hair, it's damaged for good.

For simple wearing, you can just shake out the wig and use your fingertips to direct the hair where you want it. Use a spray bottle with cold water to lightly spritz the hair and remove any static electricity. Resist the urge to get every hair perfectly in place—that can make the wig look less natural.

There may be times when you want to restyle your wig. Most likely your stylist (or the wig stylist) already created one style for you that you liked when you bought the wig, but what if you want to change it a little?

One option, of course, is to take the wig back to the stylist who did the original style, and let him or her adjust it for you. He or she can also show you some great styling techniques that you may not have thought about for future reference.

If you want to create a different style at home, the techniques you can apply will depend on the type of wig. Human-hair wigs can be styled much like your own hair. You can probably blow dry them, straighten, or curl them; but be sure to check with the manufacturer first, so you don't create any damage. Most recommend using a lower heat level than you may be used to (medium setting as opposed to high).

Synthetic wigs dry faster after washing, but they don't handle heated styling tools—the hair may melt! You can use liquid wig mousse to create wavy or curly styles or to lift the volume a bit. You can also use hair accessories like clips and combs to pull the hair into an up-do.

What if you want to cut the wig? Be careful. Once you cut it, most wig shops will not accept the wig back for a return or exchange. If you want to get a great style, it's best to consult with a professional stylist before you start wearing your wig. Many salons and stylists around the country cut wigs for cancer patients, and you may even have access to one in the wig shop where you bought your wig.

Finally, how do you store your wig when you're not using it? Make sure you leave it in a place that's clean and away from sources of high heat, dust, and excessive humidity. Leave the wig on a Styrofoam head (as long as it's dry) or a wire rack to help it keep its shape and to allow air to circulate around it. This helps keep the wig fresh. Finally, make sure it's out of reach of small children and pets.

If you're going to travel somewhere, place the wig in a portable travel storage container (if you're not going to wear it). It will support and protect the wig so it doesn't lose its shape or otherwise become damaged during your trip.

Can Guys Wear Wigs, Too?

Men have more bald role models than women do, so they are often more comfortable with no hair. After all, if you can emulate one of the many movie stars, rock stars, or sports stars who have gone for the slick-head look, why not, right? My dad, for example, was often told that he looked like Howie Mandel!

However, role models or not, many men don't feel comfortable going bald. It may not be part of your style, or maybe you don't like the way your head looks, for whatever reason. It doesn't matter. What matters is that you feel comfortable!

Men's wigs are also called toupees or hairpieces. They can be custom made or mass-produced, just like women's wigs. Beware of cheap men's wigs, however; they can look unnatural on you. You may also be more concerned about the wig coming lose somewhere in public. That's why it's important to take some time and find a good, quality wig that you will feel confident in.

The best advice—go to a professional wig salon, and look for one that has experience with men's wigs. They can do all the styling you need, plus make sure it's fitted right. Today's wigs are very sophisticated—they can appear like the hair is growing right out of your scalp. (These are usually called "monofilament" wigs.)

Bottom line: Don't feel that just because you're a man you can't enjoy the benefits of a wig. A well-fitting wig styled the way you want can go a long way toward helping you feel more confident during treatment.

What if the Wig Gets Hot and Itchy?

"I prefer not wearing my wig. Where it sits I get a pimple at the top, where the band is, and it's so hot. I'd rather go with nothing."

—Dee, breast cancer survivor

When I first started wearing a wig, it wasn't the most comfortable. Sometimes it felt hot and itchy. It was hard to get used to it, but within a few weeks it didn't bother me anymore.

It can take a while to get used to wearing a wig, so if it doesn't go perfectly the first day, don't worry. It will get easier with time. If you do experience some discomfort, I recommend you try the following:

- **Choose a quality wig.** If you're going to wear your wig on most days, find the highest quality one you can afford. Low-quality wigs are more likely to itch and feel uncomfortable. (Remember, your insurance may cover it.) Some survivors recommend synthetic hair over real human hair, saying they wash more easily and stay comfortable longer.

- **Rinse thoroughly.** Remember those days when your real hair went limp because either a) you didn't rinse it well enough, or b) it had too much product buildup? The same thing can happen to your wig, so after washing, be sure to rinse thoroughly. Any leftover shampoo or conditioner residue can cause scalp irritation.

Phthalates In Your Hairspray?

Phthalates are a family of chemicals that alter the characteristics of certain products. Some make hard plastic flexible, for products like shower curtains, vinyl tile, children's toys, and artificial leather. Others are used in personal care products—like nail polish, for instance, to help resist chipping; or in fragrances, to make the scent last longer; or in hairsprays, to help the product cling to hair.

Unfortunately, phthalates have been found to damage the liver, kidneys, lungs, and the reproductive system. One of these chemicals has been labeled a "probable human carcinogen" by the Environmental Protection Agency, and some are suspected of damaging sexual development in babies, especially developing testes.

Though phthalates are feared to cause the most harm in developing fetuses and very young children, women, too, are exposed to the chemical at higher levels than deemed safe. One study found that 5 percent of women between age twenty and forty had up to forty-five times more phthalates in their bodies than researchers initially hypothesized. The scientists speculated that personal care products could be one of the reasons why the women were more susceptible.

To help reduce your exposure, buy organic products, use cloth or hemp organic shower curtains, and read labels. Look for chemical names like DBP (di-n-butyl phthalate) and DEP (diethyl phthalate), often used in personal care products; DEHP (di-2-ethylhexyl or Bis 2-ethylhexyl phthalate), used in PVC plastics; BzBP (benzylbutyl phthalate) used in some flooring, car products and personal care products; and DMP (dimethyl phthalate), used in insect repellent and some plastics. Also, stay away from synthetic fragrances.

- **Plan a refresher.** If you're going to wear the wig all day, or at least for a few hours, plan to refresh your scalp several times during the wearing. Take along some organic witch-hazel and every so often, steal into a private place, remove the wig, wet a towel, cloth, or cotton pad with the witch hazel, and pass it over your scalp. It will help remove oil buildup and make you more comfortable. You can also use a natural, after-sun cooling aloe-vera spray to bring some relief and reduce the itch. You may want to take along a small bottle of your gentle, nontoxic face moisturizer or your cooling, spray toner to apply to your scalp afterward.

- **Consider a cotton liner.** A 100% cotton liner can be worn under your wig, which will help absorb moisture and heat, making your head feel more comfortable. You can get them at almost any wig shop, or go online. You can also send the wig back to the manufacturer and ask for a silk lining, which has a reputation for being the most comfortable.

- **Carefully care for your wig.** As your wig suffers some wear and tear, strands of hair can come back through the base, which can also cause itching. You can help reduce this tendency by always caring for your wig according to the manufacturer's instructions and by brushing and combing carefully.

- **Use zinc lotion for skin irritations.** If you notice bumps, redness, or irritation on your scalp after wearing your wig, you may want to try an organic zinc lotion. Zinc is a natural antibacterial and can help prevent infections and irritations. Try a natural or organic baby diaper-rash ointment—they really work!

Be Careful with Your Tender Scalp

Most of us aren't used to having bare skin on the top of our heads that we have to take care of. If you've never before taken care of the skin on your scalp, how do you go about it now?

All skin is fragile during chemotherapy and radiation treatments, and the scalp even more so, as it's probably never been so "naked" before and may be a little tender and sensitive. Forget regular harsh shampoos and opt for a more caring approach—one you would take toward baby skin.

- **Shampoos are out.** Would you wash your face and hands with shampoo? Not usually, so either skip the shampoo on your scalp as well, or find an extremely gentle formula. Some doctors suggest baby shampoo for cancer patients, which is probably okay, particularly if you have some hair left. (Make sure it's natural and free of harsh chemicals.) Another good option is the gentle cleanser you're using on your face.

- **Cover up.** You're probably already applying sunscreen to your face. If you're going out bareheaded, put some on your scalp as well. Have you ever seen a scalp-burn? (Ouch!) Even if the sun is hiding, dangerous UV rays can still penetrate skin that's not used to sun exposure, raising your risk of painful burns, skin damage, and skin cancer. You can also cover up with a hat, scarf, or wig.

- **Moisturize.** Hair conditioner helped moisturize your scalp before. Now, without the protection of hair, your scalp will need moisture more than ever. You can use the same moisturizer you use on your face on your scalp. (Make sure it's a gentle formula and free of harsh ingredients.) Apply at least two times a day, preferably more while you're going through treatment, since chemotherapy and radiation are drying to the skin.

- **Treat.** You know all those things that happen to your face that you don't like—breakouts, dry skin, oily patches? The same thing can happen to your scalp. If your scalp is having a hard time adjusting to being hairless and is challenging you with skin problems, consider a scalp treatment at your local spa. Tell them you have cancer and ask for chemical-free products, and then enjoy a nice scalp massage and possibly a light exfoliation to get rid of dead skin cells. You'll come away feeling refreshed, and the skin on your head will look healthier and smoother. If you want to do it yourself at home instead, try a gentle scrub and finish with a rich moisturizer.

- **Keep it warm.** You may have never thought about it, but without your hair, your scalp will probably feel cold on occasion. Invest in some comfortable hats—fleece material feels nice on your head overnight—and some warm pillowcases made of natural cotton or flannel. Many wig shops and hat stores also carry sleep caps.

When You're Done with Your Wig, Donate It

When you've finished with cancer treatments, your hair will most likely grow back and you'll find yourself with a wig just sitting around. What to do with it?

First, if you know someone who may need it, you can send it directly to him or her. Some of the message boards on cancer communication sites like Cancer Compass have places where you can advertise your old wig for cancer fighters who would like a wig, but can't afford a new one.

If you don't make a direct connection with someone, there are several other options. Here are just a few. Whatever you do, don't just let that head of hair sit and gather dust!

- **Local cancer centers** often donate wigs to cancer patients. Call any in your area and ask them where you can donate.

- **Oncology offices,** like cancer centers, will often take used wigs. Call your local oncology centers.

- **Cancer support groups** often know where you can take used wigs. If you took part in a support group during your treatment, contact them for information on where you may donate your wig.

- **Wig shops** often make a habit of donating wigs to cancer patients. Yours could become one of those passed on to someone who needs one.

- **The American Cancer Society (ACS)** has many local chapters that provide free wigs to cancer patients and take wig donations.

- **Cancer***Care* has offices throughout the nation and would be happy to take your wig donation.

- **University of Michigan Health Center** maintains a large collection of donated wigs. Check other health centers in your area as well.

- **City wig drives** may be occurring in your area. Watch the news and take your wig to the drop-off sites.

Donating a wig can make a big difference to someone you may not even know. It's very rewarding and will make you feel like you're helping someone—always a great feeling! It can also help you celebrate the fact that you made it through your cancer treatments and your hair is growing back! If you itemize your charitable deductions, don't forget to list the value of the donated wig on your tax return.

Scarves and Hats—They May Be the Choice for You

"I just wore scarves. I live in a very small town two hours away from Austin. I think the idea of having to drive to town and shop for a wig was something I just didn't want to deal with. I had several people stop and ask me, 'Do you have cancer?' or 'How did you tie that scarf?' I was never offended. It didn't bother me. I found most of them extremely kind. "

—Rayette, ovarian cancer survivor

Some people don't feel comfortable in wigs. For whatever reason, wigs just don't work for them. If this is how you feel, you may want to consider hats and scarves.

Scarves are generally ideal for patients who are uncomfortable in wigs, who can't afford expensive head covers, or who want their scalp to remain cool and free from irritation. They can also be incredibly chic!

You may want to try scarves even if you are wearing wigs. I would always go for my wig first, but I would sometimes use a hat or a scarf on top of it. People always complimented me on the look. You may be amazed as you get creative what kind of response you'll get!

You can wrap and wear scarves in numerous different ways and can choose different colors and prints to match your outfits. Most cancer survivors prefer the cancer-created brands of scarves because they have features like padding (to mimic the fullness hair creates) and are made with more material, so it's easier to use them to cover the entire scalp. A wide variety of companies create fashionable scarves for patients; some even sell matching earrings!

When it comes to wearing a scarf, fold it in a triangle shape, place at the top of your head, and tie at the nape of your neck to sufficiently cover your head. This is a very basic style, but you can get more creative with different wrapping techniques. Try on a variety of scarf shapes and styles before deciding what works best for you. Among the many choices are hoodlike square wraps, rosette turban scarves, and the list goes on. Many are pre-tied, which can be great if you want a quick solution. In other words, you can find ways to wear a scarf that matches your personality.

When you're shopping, look for options that are made with fabrics that won't irritate your sensitive skin. Cotton scarves are usually best; they won't build up heat or slip on your head. Wash them frequently using toxin-free detergents.

I wore regular hats that you can buy anywhere, but just like tailormade scarves, hats made by companies catering to cancer patients are often more comfortable for long-term wear. They usually come with a fleece lining that's comfortable against your scalp and are made with super-soft materials like angora, delicate silk, or workout fabrics. Other companies offer sun hats that actually have an SPF factor!

Whatever type of scarf, turban, hat, or other head covering you choose, you can experience a fun and fashionable alternative that helps you maintain your sense of style and confidence.

Going All Natural

This whole chapter has been about ways you can cope with hair loss. However, don't feel you have to choose some way to cover up your bald head. I spoke to many fighters who felt perfectly comfortable going without a wig or scarf or hat. They found the "badge" of a bald head empowering—it helped spur them on to fight the disease and win. Others simply felt most comfortable with a naked head, as coverings irritated the tender skin on their scalp.

You may find that you'd like to go without a head covering, but you're worried about getting stares and comments from other people. All of the survivors I've spoken to who chose to go bald were pleasantly surprised at the kindness expressed by strangers. Yes, people may look and they may realize you have cancer, but most are nice enough to offer encouragement or share their own cancer stories.

If you run up against some people who stare, realize that it may have nothing to do with you—they may just not know how to react. They may have an experience in their past related to cancer that saddens them. Just smile and move on.

Living as you choose to live without letting others dictate your actions can be very freeing. If "going natural" is your choice, go after it with gusto!

Let's Review

- Hair loss can be a devastating side effect. Take some time to process your feelings; then explore your personal lifestyle to determine the best way for you to cope. Realize that many people have difficulty with hair loss, and that your feelings are perfectly normal.

- If your doctor tells you you're going to lose your hair, get it cut short to help you make the transition. When your hair actually starts falling out, go to a stylist or ask a friend or loved one to shave your head.

- If you choose to wear a wig, be sure to shop for it *before* your hair falls out so you can most closely match your natural color and style. Ask someone to go with you when you shop for your wig, and take your time in finding just the right one. Check with your insurance company to see if it will cover it, and ask area cancer centers and wig shops about discounts.

- Be cautious in caring for your wig. Use products made specifically for wigs, and avoid using heated styling tools on a synthetic wig. If you want to change the style of your wig, go to your stylist, or use wig-styling products to do it yourself.

- Guys can wear wigs too, so if you want hair, don't hesitate to look for the perfect hairpiece.

- If your wig gets hot and itchy, there are several things you can do to make it more comfortable.

- As you may have never had a bare scalp before, you'll need to take some extra steps to care for the tender skin.

- When you're done with your wig, consider donating it to another cancer fighter or to an organization that takes used wigs.

- If you don't want to wear a wig, explore the many options in hats and scarves to find something that fits your style.

- Don't feel you *have* to find a head covering. Many cancer patients feel empowered going out with no hair.

Personal Affirmations

I release the need to judge myself.
I look beautiful/handsome just as I am.

I accept my present situation and find joy in this new process.

10

Hands & Feet: Care for Swelling, Fragile Nails, Numbness, and Pain

"I had neuropathy in my feet really badly. I couldn't even walk straight, and couldn't drive without coming to tears. Fortunately, that did go away about 98%."

— Jarrod, Hodgkin's lymphoma survivor

CERTAIN CHEMOTHERAPY AND RADIATION SIDE EFFECTS target the hands and feet. Since you use them so much—probably even more than you realize—having them hurt or feel uncomfortable while you're trying to go about your day can be especially frustrating.

My dad had an extreme case of hand and foot syndrome. Once, when I came home from New York to see him, I found him lying in bed, watching television, with his hands to the side and up, as though he had gotten some type of goo on them and couldn't touch anything. As I walked closer I realized they were red and inflamed.

He told me it was from the chemo and that his hands really hurt. I later realized he had hand and foot syndrome, a typical side effect from certain chemo drugs. He didn't know how to handle this side effect because neither the nurses nor the doctors had told him what to do, except to apply a generic moisturizer, which wasn't helping.

What struck me most in that moment was that my father, this man I loved, was just lying there, suffering. It made me feel sad and angry at the same time. Sad for the pain he was feeling, and angry that nothing was being done about it.

I hope that as you read through this book, you start to realize that there are *always* things you can do. I think sometimes when we get a cancer diagnosis, we think that we are doomed to suffer inordinate amounts of pain and discomfort, and we just resign ourselves to that because we think it's a "fact" and there's nothing we can do about it.

"I see people who are seriously under-medicated and do have pain," says Colleen O'Neil, RN, breast cancer survivor and peer counselor for cancer patients. "There are better ways to control pain. A good pain specialist can control it. You don't have to suffer."

I've heard survivors tell me horror stories of lying in bed for days, suffering some type of difficult pain, and then finding out later, when they told their doctor about it, that oh, by the way, there's a medication for that. Nice to know after the fact, huh?

Don't let this happen to you. There is almost always a medication, a soothing technique, a natural remedy—something.

I've had other survivors tell me that they didn't want to take the medications that could have helped them. "I was getting shots of Neulasta that would make my entire body ache really really badly," says Deb, breast cancer survivor. "So much so that if someone laid a hand on me it would hurt. Even just lying in bed hurt. The doctor did tell me they could give me something, but I was just stubborn. I don't know. In hindsight, maybe it was counterproductive?"

Deciding what medications to take or not to take is always a personal choice, and I can understand people feeling they don't want to swallow more drugs, particularly when their bodies are already full of them. But even if you don't want to take more drugs, there are often natural remedies that may help—at least to ease the situation—and in the end, is it worth it to go through the additional suffering?

When you think about it, you're in the fight of your life when you're going through cancer. Why wouldn't you take advantage of every tool at your disposal? Why would you willingly let something like pain sap you of your strength, when you need that strength to heal? Why would you allow yourself to waste away in bed when something might help you to get up and enjoy at least part of the day?

There are so many things in cancer that can wear us down: the treatments themselves, the side effects, the anxiety and worry surrounding the disease, the financial concerns, self-esteem issues, health insurance complications, and more. You need every ounce of strength you can get. Why would you allow something to get you down if you don't have to?

Suffering has a nasty way of creating a downward spiral. If you lie in bed for days in pain, what's going to happen? You're going to gradually feel worse, and you may become depressed. Your depressed emotions will further depress your immune system. You'll start to feel worse, which will further depress your emotions, and further depress your immune system…you get the idea. In the end, you're sabotaging your own efforts to beat the disease.

"The upside of getting rid of pain," Colleen says, "is that your mobility is improved, so you're going to move better, which is going to reduce your chances of getting pneumonia or circulation problems. You're going to sleep better, eat better, and take in more fluids. This is all going to help you heal faster. You also do better because you're not so fearful. Pain makes you feel vulnerable; you're afraid it's going to get worse and you're going to die. If you don't have pain, you're more optimistic."

The point I've been trying to make throughout this book is that you need to feel *good* as often as you possibly can. Those good feelings are key to getting through this. Yes, there may be some side effects that don't respond well to medications or even to natural remedies, but I hope on the whole, you'll realize that there's always *something* you can do to lessen the severity, or even just get your mind off it.

Don't fool yourself into thinking that if you can't completely erase the pain, it's not worth the effort to lessen it. You need to take pain seriously, because it erodes your efforts to heal. One study found that cancer patients with pain had lower levels of emotional functioning and higher levels of depression than those without pain.[1] Furthermore, those patients who had continuous pain had higher levels of depression.

Researchers wrote, "Cancer pain has a significant impact on the overall quality of a cancer patient's life by influencing physical, psychological, and spiritual aspects."

Another study found that depressive symptoms are more frequent in patients with pain than those without pain.[2] And get this. A study in the Netherlands found that the more patients catastrophized about their pain—in other words, the more they let themselves get down about it and allowed negative thinking to rule the day—the more that pain affected their quality of life.[3]

That's why I'm telling you that doing something—even if it's just to get your mind off the pain—is worth the effort, as it will help you better cope with the situation. It will help you get some of your control back. You don't have to sit and suffer. You can *do* something. You can ease the pain, relieve the tension, cool the burn, relax the muscle, tame the nausea, or even get a foot massage to get your mind off your upset stomach. Whatever it may be, you can help yourself feel better. So please, don't ever just sit and assume you have to suffer!

Researchers from the first study wrote, "It is important for clinicians to make every effort to prevent cancer pain and to relieve pain effectively and promptly. Pain therapy that addresses the multidimensional aspect of pain by relieving the patient's physical burden, psychological disturbance, and emotional distress are more likely to lead to long-term benefits."

Check with your doctor. Get your loved ones to help. Try alternative medicine. Watch a funny movie. Put on some soothing music. Use every tool at your disposal. You're not being a baby, here. You're taking care of yourself at a critical time when you absolutely need to be doing so!

That day at home with my father, I flew into action. Luckily for us, my neighbor had an aloe plant. I got a cool washcloth—I mean, cool, cool, cool—put some aloe on it, and wrapped it around his hands. He relaxed and said, "Oh, that feels so much better!"

I realized then how severe these side effects can really be. Sometimes because it's a side effect, you think you have to endure it to survive. You don't think there are options. But there *are* options, and you are promoting your survival by trying them.

Hand and Foot Syndrome

Much of the time, sore hands and feet are the result of a side effect called "hand-foot syndrome," or palmar-plantar erythrodysesthesia (PPE). Certain types of chemotherapy drugs cause the condition by leaking out of small blood vessels (capillaries) in the palms of the hands and the soles of the feet. The leakage results in redness (like a sunburn), tenderness, numbness and tingling, and sometimes peeling.

If your hands and feet are exposed to heat or friction (like the soles of your feet rubbing against flooring or the bottom of shoes), even more of the drug can leak into them.

This is what my father had when I put the aloe on his hands. He also had it in his feet, so he took to wearing comfortable shoes whenever he could. It was particularly hard for him to walk at times.

You can take steps to try to reduce your chances of ending up with PPE. These mostly involve avoiding heat and friction, particularly for about a week or so after getting a chemotherapy treatment. If you're taking oral medication, it pays to be cautious on a day-to-day basis.

- Avoid warm or hot water as much as possible. Wash your hands in lukewarm water, and stay away from long, hot baths. Take short showers in tepid water instead.

- Avoid activities like washing dishes, housecleaning, or gardening for a week after treatment. You might think rubber gloves would help, but they actually hold heat against your palms and fingers, so don't use them.

- Avoid vigorous exercise like jogging, aerobics, and long walks until the week is over. After that, make sure you have comfortable shoes and absorbent socks.

- Avoid squeezing your hand on things like screwdrivers, garden tools, pliers, jars, and knives.

- Moisturize hands and feet regularly with a nourishing formula.

Another tip: Ask for help. My father would regularly ask us to open jars for him. It's a small thing, and people are happy to help—why not let them and lower your risk of a difficult side effect?

If you do develop PPE, try these natural remedies to ease your symptoms:

- Cool the area with a cold compress, cool washcloths, or frozen veggies wrapped in a soft cloth. Avoid extreme cold, however. Alternate on and off for fifteen to twenty minutes at a time.

- Try applying after-sun spray to the hands and feet, then pat in some lotion and put on gloves and socks.

- Soak hands and feet in lukewarm water and Epsom salts to help alleviate pain.

- Dry hands and feet by patting with a towel. Don't rub!

- Slip gel insoles from the freezer into your shoes.

- For cracking and peeling, apply a thick, toxin-free gel that's been cooled in the refrigerator. Aloe creams are great options here, as are those that contain calendula. However, don't rub the product in—pat gently.

- Swab hands and feet with heavy cream, then slip on soft gloves and socks (preferably cotton) for thirty minutes to an hour, or overnight. (Make sure you wash the socks and gloves after every use to avoid infection.)

- Wear shoes that fit well. Women, especially, need to be more cautious than usual when choosing footwear. There are many styles and fashions that look great, but aren't great for your feet. See a podiatrist if you need to, get some cooling insoles, and choose brands that are well-made and well-ventilated.

- Take additional vitamin B6 (100 mg/day). Studies have shown it helps reduce the intensity of hand-foot syndrome.[4-5]

- Try over-the-counter pain relievers like acetaminophen and ibuprofen.

- Some reports have mentioned that COX-2 inhibitors (pain relievers) are promising in treating PPE. Ask your doctor.

If none of these suggestions brings relief, be sure to check with your doctor. Watch out, too, for any peeling or open wounds, as these can be entry places for germs and bacteria. If your symptoms continue to get worse, your doctor may elect to hold off on treatments until they improve. Just don't neglect to let him or her in on what's happening!

Edema and Swelling: My Shoes Don't Fit

PPE isn't the only cause of cancer-related sore feet. Edema, or swelling, is another, caused by fluid buildup in the body. It usually occurs in the feet and lower legs, but can also show up in the hands or even in the abdomen.

Edema usually occurs as a result of the medications used in cancer treatments. Steroids are known for causing "puffiness" in the face and body and contributing to weight gain. Swelling can also come about as a result of an allergic reaction, where fluid in the cells leaks into the layers of the skin. In these cases, swelling may show up in the eyelids, lips, and tongue, even the airway.

You probably already know if you are suffering from edema, but sometimes you may not have realized that this is what you have. Some telling signs include: your hands feel tight when you make a fist; your rings feel too tight; your feet and lower legs seem larger when you sit or walk; your abdomen feels distended.

If you experience swelling in the lips, eyes, tongue, or airway, take an antihistamine right away and check with your doctor immediately, as an allergic reaction can be dangerous. However, if you have swelling in your hands and feet, here are some things you can do:

- Elevate your feet as often as possible. Put your feet up in a recliner, or on a stool with a pillow.

- Avoid standing for long periods of time.

- Again, be sure you have comfortable shoes. Some cancer patients have to go up a shoe size after treatment.

- Use compression socks for more severe swelling in the legs.

- Avoid tight clothing and don't cross your legs.

- Reduce your intake of salt—it can contribute to fluid retention.

- Check with your doctor. In more serious cases of swelling he or she may prescribe a diuretic to help your body get rid of the extra fluid.

- Consider talking to a nutritionist. Making modifications in your diet can help control edema.

- Try a massage. Slow, light-touch, rhythmic massage can help the body process the extra fluid. Reflexology, in particular, has shown in studies to help reduce edema around the feet and ankles.[6]

Finally, if you gain five pounds or more in a week, the swelling moves up your arms or legs, or if your hands or feet feel cold to the touch, get to your doctor right away.

Neuropathy: I Can't Feel My Fingertips

Another side effect that can hit the hands and feet is called neuropathy, or nerve damage. Certain chemotherapy medications damage the nerves that take signals from the brain and spinal cord to other peripheral parts of the body, such as the hands and feet. The breakdown occurs on the nerve endings (axons) that send sensations to the brain and sometimes to the coating of the nerve fibers (called myelin).

This all affects the transmission of pain signals—as if the wires were down, so to speak—creating pain signals for no reason, burning pain (especially at night), numbness, tingling (feeling of pins and needles), extreme sensitivity to touch, even loss of sensation to touch or of positional sense (getting off balance).

Some patients have difficulty picking things up, buttoning clothes, or performing other everyday tasks like opening doors or carrying bags. Usually neuropathy afflicts the hands and feet—fingers and toes—though the bowel, face, back, and chest can also be involved.

My dad had this sort of nerve damage in his hands and feet. He would ask my mom and I to help him button his shirts before he went to work or to assist him in opening cans and jars. He even had trouble dialing the phone sometimes.

We don't realize how much our nerves are involved in these tasks until something happens to them. Remember that feeling you have after you've gone to the dentist and gotten a novacaine shot? You know how you can't even drink a glass of water without spilling it all over yourself? It's similar with neuropathy—numb fingers and toes become clumsy.

Several chemo drugs can cause neuropathy, as can drugs used to treat cancer, hormonal therapies, certain types of radiation therapy, and surgery. You may be more at risk if you're having more than one type of drug or treatment that can cause nerve damage, if you've had previous anti-cancer drugs that cause it, if you have low levels of nutrients like vitamin E and B, or if you drink too much alcohol.

So far, there aren't many options for preventing neuropathy before it occurs, but things are constantly changing and improving. Ask your doctor about the chemo meds he's going to use, and if the drugs are known to cause neuropathy, ask him if there are any preventative options. The minerals calcium and magnesium, given as part of hydration during chemo treatments, can help, as can vitamin B1 tablets, which naturally support nerve function.

If you're noticing signs of neuropathy, tell your doctor right away, as he or she may be able to adjust your medications to help. Symptoms usually go from mild to more severe, advancing with each treatment, so it's best to mention it as soon as possible. Pain may be treated with certain types of drugs, by injecting anaesthetic around the damaged nerve, or through electrical nerve stimulation (TENS). Acupuncture has also shown in studies to help reduce symptoms.[7-8] If you're having trouble with coordination, muscle weakness, or balance, your doctor may refer you to a physical therapist.

Making Movement Easier

Neuropathy can make many everyday tasks more difficult. Here are some tips to help:

- Purchase easy-open bottles and containers.
- Wear zip-up or Velcro rather than button-up shirts and jackets.
- Take your time when performing difficult tasks; be patient with yourself.
- Consider getting custom-made orthotics for your shoes to help increase comfort and balance.
- If tying shoes is difficult, purchase shoes with Velcro fasteners or elastic stretching laces.
- Supportive sandals (*not* high heels!) may be more comfortable than regular shoes.
- Wear thick, fluffy socks to provide more cushioning.
- If sheets and blankets are irritating, use a footboard or hoop (in medical supply stores) to raise the covers.
- Really *look* to make sure you have a good grip on things.
- Use a cane to assist in balance.
- Install a grab bar in the shower.
- Try a massage.

As for self-care, here are a few things you can do:

- Keep your hands and feet warm. Wear gloves and warm socks.
- Avoid sharp objects and use working gloves when needed.
- Use potholders to avoid burns, since you may not accurately feel the heat.
- Wear well-fitting shoes or boots.
- Avoid walking around barefoot.
- Test bath and shower temperatures with your elbow or knee before entering.
- If you're having trouble with balance, make sure rooms are well lit, keep walking areas clear of clutter, keep electrical wires hidden or

taped down, and install non-skid matting in your bathtub and shower. Wear shoes with rubber soles to help you avoid falling.

- Consider massage to relieve pain and provide comfort. Be sure your therapist is experienced with cancer patients, and speak up if anything hurts.

- Try deep breathing, meditation, and guided imagery to help with emotional stress.

- If you're experiencing neuropathy-induced constipation, exercise at least thirty minutes a day, eat foods high in fiber, and drink at least eight glasses of water or juice a day.

- Talk to your doctor about taking higher doses of B vitamins.

- Consider nerve-support formula supplements made for diabetic neuropathy.

- Your doctor may have medications you can try.

- The coolness of the "Chillow Pillow" may help you sleep, particularly if you have restless legs and feet. (You can find it online.)

- If you can, turn to swimming for exercise so you can get the pressure off your feet.

Brittle, Cracked Nails—Have You Bought Cotton Gloves?

"My nails split and cracked and broke. I used tea tree oil on my nails to deal with the fungus. I used olive oil and a salve I had made out of beeswax and olive oil around my nails and cuticles to keep them from cracking. I think shea butter would be good for that as well."

—Karen, two-time thyroid cancer survivor

We talked in an earlier chapter about how chemotherapy attacks the fast-growing cells in the body. The skin contains these types of cells, as does the hair and the inside of the mouth, which is why we have dry skin, hair loss, and mouth sores.

Chemotherapy also attacks the fast-growing cells in our nails. Have you ever kept track of how often you have to trim your nails? These cells are always rapidly reproducing and replenishing themselves to continue growing your nails, so naturally they are affected by chemotherapy.

Cancer treatments left my father's nails discolored, grooved, and brittle. He had extremely dry cuticles that caused hangnails, and if he hadn't been careful, they could have led to infection. Sometimes his nails separated from the nail bed, turned black, and fell off. It took a while; the nail would gradually weaken and started to loosen up from the nail bed as the drugs took their effect. If this is happening to you, you can tell by the way the nail looks. That's why it's very important during this time to be extremely careful with your feet and hands. You don't want to rip off a nail that is weakened and loose.

If you're a woman, your first instinct may be to get your nails fixed. A wrap. Acrylic nails. Anything to make them look better. However, I would strongly recommend you stay away from acrylics until you're finished with treatment. The space created behind acrylic nails and wraps often harbors and traps bacteria, which can lead to an infection—the last thing your body needs.

Fortunately, there are many things you can do. First, keep your nails short and filed smooth. Next, wear gloves, wear gloves, wear gloves! If you're concerned about PPE, use soft, breathable cotton ones. Around the house, they'll protect against accidentally hitting something and ripping a nail, and will help protect your hands from germs. Household gloves also protect from excess water, which can be drying. Nails actually absorb water even more quickly than your skin does, so constantly wetting and drying them out over and over again can contribute to dryness, cracking, and tearing.

Avoid chemical cleaning products. If you simply *must* clean the house yourself, use natural cleaners to lessen your contact with toxins that can cause skin reactions. If you don't have PPE, feel free to wear rubber gloves. Otherwise, stick with soft, cotton materials.

Buy another pair of gloves to wear outside. They'll help shield against the elements, particularly from wear and tear when you're gardening or doing yard work. They'll also help protect you from germs, as you're more susceptible when your cuticles are weakened.

Next, switch from regular soap to a sulfate-free moisturizing hand wash and avoid soap bars, as they are very drying. Look for "made for dry skin" on the label of your hand soap and avoid any possible chemicals, including triclosan, which is usually found in antibacterial soaps. (See sidebar, "Avoid Germs, but Ditch the Triclosan.")

Dry by patting with a towel. Don't rub, tug, or pull, to help protect your nails. Even if they are starting to fall off, you can avoid bleeding and pain by protecting them as long as possible.

Avoid Germs, but Ditch the Triclosan

Most soaps that boast germ-killing powers contain "triclosan," an ingredient that kills bacteria, but has no effect on viruses. Since most common illnesses, like colds and flus, are caused by viruses, antibacterial ingredients don't prevent them, so we're not really protected as much as we may think. Even the FDA reports that there is no evidence that antibacterial products protect people any better than regular soap. The fact that we're using them so much could also lead to new superbugs—germs resistant to current treatments.

Triclosan's chemical structure is remarkably similar to dioxin, a class of super-toxic carcinogenic chemicals formed as byproducts of the manufacture of chlorine-containing products. A recent study already found that when triclosan was exposed to ultraviolet light, a type of dioxin formed. Besides the dioxin fear, triclosan has already found its way into human breast milk and urine, and has been shown to be an endocrine disruptor in tests on animal and human cells.

It's important to avoid infection during cancer treatments. Antibacterial wipes can really help if you're traveling or going shopping or cleaning off utensils in a restaurant. However, when washing your hands, there are lots of triclosan-free options. Look for "organic" and "natural" on labels. (Always read the ingredient list!)

After every wash, my father applied lotion and vitamin E cuticle oil, then reapplied as often as needed. At night he slathered his hands and feet with a rich aloe vera cream, applied his cuticle oil, and then slipped on cotton gloves or socks. Cotton gloves can be purchased from your drugstore for a few dollars, or go to Amazon.com to see a full selection.

You can also try getting more calcium, protein, and iron in your diet—all nutrients that nourish nails. Consider taking a multivitamin, and eat calcium-rich foods like spinach and yogurt; protein-rich foods like lean meats, beans, eggs, and fish; and iron-rich foods like beef liver, sardines, shrimp, turkey, and clams.

Here's something else you may want to try: Keep your fingers in ice water or immersed in a frozen bag of vegetables during your treatment. Some studies have shown that keeping nails cool during sessions can help reduce damage, as it makes it harder for the drugs to reach them.

Remember: taking extra care of your nails is helpful not just for vanity, but most importantly, to avoid infection and keep your fingers and toes protected and healthy. You want to avoid as much pain and discomfort as possible.

What About How My Nails Look?

"My nails got pretty flimsy. They were pretty short. They let me get a manicure, but I couldn't allow them to cut the cuticles. I could get them filed and polished, though."

—Jamie, non-Hodgkin's lymphoma survivor

Our hands are nearly always exposed. We use them to greet one another, through handshakes and waves. We use them when we're talking, to help support our expression. And we use them to express love and tenderness when we touch another person.

Is it any wonder, then, that the appearance of our hands becomes so important to us? I even use anti-aging products on my hands to reduce the appearance of wrinkles. I also put sunscreen on them, and I'm constantly lathering up with lotion to keep the skin moist and supple. To top it off, I like to have manicured nails. Manicures help me feel pretty and feminine, and the process of getting one is often very relaxing and rejuvenating. Pedicures, as well, give me that feeling of being put together and well-groomed.

It's not only women who benefit from nail care. Men, too, often take advantage of manicures and pedicures these days, especially if their profession requires them to meet a certain standard of appearance. Sometimes just the experience of getting a spa treatment is beneficial to men, just as it is to women—a chance to sit back, relax, and let your concerns drift away.

As you're going through chemotherapy and side effects start showing up on your nails, you may be tempted to turn to chemical treatments to hide them. Unfortunately, many nail products and processes can do you more harm then good. That doesn't mean you can't take advantage of the restoring experience of having your nails specially cared for. As long as you take a few precautions, you can reap the benefits without the dangers. Let's look at each of these processes.

Care for Your Nails but Avoid Infection

As I mentioned earlier, chemotherapy raises the odds of infection. It taxes the immune system and makes patients more susceptible to bugs and germs everywhere.

If you're going through treatment, be hypervigilant about cleanliness, and avoid crowded and busy areas that may harbor extra bacteria. Did you know one of those places is the nail spa? It's true: Spas can be teeming with germs. Many people have suffered infections as a result of going to a spa that didn't follow the proper disinfecting procedures, and they didn't have immune systems compromised by cancer!

The bugs that can live in footbaths are commonly found in dirt, dust, and water supplies—but they're nasty little critters. California has had several outbreaks in which people suffered pus-filled sores all over their lower legs. (The infection had to be treated with strong antibiotics.) The breakout looked something like insect bites, or pimples, that gradually grew in size and severity. The cause was traced back to bacteria from pedicures performed weeks or even months before the sores showed up. Nearly 200 people were affected, and similar problems have now shown up in other states, including Georgia, Illinois, Oregon, Texas, and Arizona.

It's not just that technicians aren't cleaning the spas. Sometimes they may not, but most of the times, they're not cleaning then *correctly*. Proper cleaning involves several steps that include draining the tub, rinsing thoroughly, cleaning with the right surfactant, and disinfecting with a hospital-grade disinfectant. A more complete cleaning should be done every night (to clean filters), and thorough disinfecting every couple of weeks. Companies should keep logs to be sure the cleaning is completed as intended and should be sure they're using the right cleaners for the types of foot spas used. Unfortunately, this isn't always happening.

If you're going through cancer treatments, to safeguard your health, I'd suggest avoiding pedicure salons altogether for now. If you get a pedicure from a loved one, be sure that your spa is very clean, and don't shave beforehand. Tiny nicks and cuts are perfect entryways for bugs. Even if you have insect bites, wait until they've healed.

As for manicures, at-home is best, but if you're really craving a salon treatment and feel your white-blood cell count is strong enough, you may still enjoy one without increasing infection risk. First of all, don't allow the technician to cut off your cuticles. They protect the nail bed from germs. Cutting them away leaves you open to infection and puts you at risk from sharp cutting tools. So allow pushbacks only, with a soft instrument.

Second, steer clear of artificial nails for now. They carry more germs than natural nails (which have enough by themselves), because the space behind the acrylic nails and wraps harbors and traps bacteria. These bacteria are known to stick around even after careful hand-washing, so spice up your own nails and leave the fake ones alone.

Next, invest in your own tools and nontoxic polishes, and always take

Safer Manicures & Pedicures

Here are some quick tips to help you avoid infection and toxic chemicals and still enjoy having your nails look good.

- Avoid spa pedicures during treatment. Footbaths may contain harmful germs.

- Avoid clippers; use a file.

- Don't cut cuticles; just push them back.

- Choose nail polishes that are free of harsh chemicals like formaldehyde, toluene, and DBP. There are many brands available now that pride themselves on making safer polishes.

- Be wary of alcohol-based nail polish removers. Alcohol is drying and could make your nail condition worse. Choose a gentle, nourishing remover.

- When going to a spa, check the bathrooms and the stations for cleanliness. Watch how the technicians clean up after a customer. Take your own tools to help avoid infection.

- Tell the spa technician that you have cancer and need very sensitive treatment. If anything hurts, speak up.

them along! Avoid nail clippers completely, as they harbor a lot of germs and may cut open the skin. Stick to a file. Pack your own cuticle pusher and buffer as well, to protect yourself from community germs.

Don't forget the polish. Most nail spas pay little attention to the toxic chemicals present in polishes and polish removers—plus the bottles themselves can harbor germs—so purchase safer brands.

What about the spa? Most of us go to the one most conveniently located, but it's wiser to do a little research to make sure you're going to a quality place. If it looks dirty (check the restrooms and workstations), go somewhere else. Make sure state licenses are in plain view, and watch to see how frequently and thoroughly technicians sanitize their tools—and their own hands.

Baths and sinks should be thoroughly cleaned with antibacterial products and plenty of water after every customer, or they can harbor germs, pieces of skin, and hair. Typically, those salons that are professional looking with licensed cosmetologists are safer than drop-in corner shops, but use your own judgment.

Finally, respect how you feel during the manicure or pedicure. If anything hurts or stings, speak up. Don't allow the technician to use *anything* sharp on you, including razors, blades, or callus files. Ask for those specialists who are particularly gentle, and mention your need for sensitive care. If you don't feel comfortable at any time, ask for another technician, or find another salon.

Of course, you can always set up your own manicure at home with a friend or loved one and enjoy the same benefits!

Nail Polish May Expose You to Harsh Chemicals

Having manicured nails is a great way to look put together, but how many of us like the smelly fumes and toxic chemicals in the polish?

That sharp odor comes from a mix of alcohol, solvents, and resins that gives polish its ability to adhere to the nail, deliver the pigment, and resist chipping and peeling. Unfortunately, with repeated exposure, several of these ingredients are toxic as well as pungent, especially to sensitive and compromised nails. But since treatment may be leaving your nails brittle and discolored, you'll probably want to cover up with nail polish. Is there an alternative?

Browse the nail polish aisle and you'll find a lot of pretty names, like Siberian Nights and Shanghai Shimmer, but the words in the ingredient lists are significantly less flattering. Many brands contain chemicals like toluene and formaldehyde, and some still contain dibutyl phthalate (DBP)—though the European Union has banned it from their cosmetics. Fortunately, many major manufacturers are beginning to create formulas without this toxic ingredient.

Toluene, when inhaled in large doses, has been reported to cause extreme fatigue, mental confusion, nausea, headache, and dizziness. As for formaldehyde, the National Institute for Occupational Safety and Health (NIOSH) recommends it be handled as a potential occupational carcinogen.

And then we have the polish removers. Full of things like acetone (known to irritate the eyes and lungs) and ethyl acetate (highly flammable, can lead to neurological damage), they tend to dry skin and nails, making your hands look worse.

Thankfully, we can avoid these chemicals and still have pretty nails. As long as your nails aren't broken or exposing wounded skin, I encourage you to use nail polish, but opt for safer formulas. Gentler products do exist, and they're usually labeled "water-based" and/or claim to be free of these dangerous chemicals.

To determine the toxic rating on your favorite polish, check out the Safe Cosmetics listing of many popular brands (www.cosmeticsdatabase.com). If you're getting your nails manicured, make sure to take your gentler polish and remover with you—you're more likely to avoid infection and stay safe. (See Appendix VII for websites where you can purchase toxin-free, safe nail polishes.)

If One Doesn't Work, Keep Trying

While my father was going through cancer treatments, I was always on the lookout for things that would help him. We are all different, both in how we respond to treatment and how we respond to solutions. Aloe may help the burning in your hands, but it may not work at all for someone else.

If something doesn't work for you, please don't get discouraged. There are always options. This is why I don't recommend specific brands, but instead give you places to look for solutions. Not every product will work for every person. Finding the best thing for your particular symptom may require some trial and error. That doesn't mean that you have to suffer without help—it just means you have to look a little more.

Don't give up! Some of the creams the nurses suggested for my father, for example, didn't work at all for him, but then I would find something that would. Enlist your friends and loved ones in your search if you need to. I'm hoping this book will give you several options you can try, but you can also do more research on your own for remedies.

Above all, listen to your body and keep your doctor informed of what's going on. Cancer is not about suffering in silence. It's a disease, and that's all. Use everything you can against it. That includes every pain-relieving solution possible.

Remember—your job is to take care of yourself and get well!

Let's Review

- Cancer treatments can result in side effects that specifically target the hands and feet.

- Pain is destructive to your body and spirit. Finding solutions that either relieve or lessen pain and discomfort help you stay positive and support your body's own efforts to heal.

- Hand and foot syndrome creates symptoms like burning, tenderness, and peeling on the palms and soles of the feet. There are several remedies you can try at home. You should also tell your doctor so he or she can monitor the severity of the problem.

- Edema and swelling can be relieved by putting your feet up, avoiding salty foods, and getting light massages. Your doctor may also have medications to help control it.

- Neuropathy is the nerve damage that can occur in hands and feet. Symptoms include numbness, tingling, pain, and even loss of balance. There are many things you can try to cope with the effect. If the pain gets worse, check with your doctor, as he or she may choose to delay further treatments.

- Brittle, cracked, and broken nails may result from the use of some chemotherapy drugs. Use lots of cuticle oil and constantly protect hands with gloves and feet with socks.

- Feel free to use some nontoxic polish on your nails, but be cautious about infection. Avoid clippers and other sharp tools, and thoroughly inspect any spas you go to for cleanliness and adherence to disinfecting standards.

Personal Affirmations

Every day I feel better and better.

My body heals rapidly.

11

Treatments Are Over,
but Things Aren't Normal

"My husband and I went on a holiday. I said, 'Okay, I'm discharged. Great. We're going on a holiday.' I was able to lay out in some warm weather and get back to feeling really good about myself, knowing the cancer was gone. I went swimming and walked around on the beach. It was wonderful."

—Chris, non-Hodgkin's lymphoma survivor

NOTHING MATCHES THE FEELING OF THAT *LAST* TREATMENT. Whoo-hoo, it's all over! No more drugs, no more radiation, no more needles, no more nasty side effects, right?

"The last day I had twelve of my closest girlfriends in my chemo room," says Jamie, non-Hodgkin's lymphoma survivor. "We annoyed everyone because we were so loud. They had this bell you rang at the end of your treatment, and when I rang it we got it on video. Everyone brought cookies and cakes and cupcakes, and we had a little mini-party. The next day we all went and got our nails done."

On your last treatment day, I hope you celebrate. When I had my last chemo, I felt so relieved, as if the hospitals trips, the side effects, and the stress my parents had endured—it was all over. The fight had finally ended. I could move on to being a normal teenager again in my new life as a "survivor." Talk about a load off my shoulders!

You, too, have made it through a big chunk of your journey, and you're still here! You're probably much stronger now than when you started out—spiritually, if not physically. You're wiser about a lot of things, and you've gathered a lot of experience that one day down the road may help someone else. You're holding in your hands right now the culmination of my father's and my experiences—who knows what you may do with yours?

So celebrate. Go do something fun. Pamper yourself. Mark this important occasion of your life. Too often we let big events like this slide by without much attention. Take this opportunity to pat yourself on the back for what you've survived. Take time to enjoy those people who have been on the journey with you, supporting, loving, and helping you along the way. Most of all, take a moment to thank God or whatever spiritual power you believe in that you're still here!

When the excitement dies down, however, get ready to be patient.

"Prepare for a different phase of life," says Jody, breast cancer survivor. "The adjustment period is similar to the one women go through who have had children. Their doctor says to them, 'It took you nine months for your body to do this thing. You're not going to be your pre-baby self tomorrow.' It's the same for us. You're not going to be your pre-cancer self immediately. It's a time of adjustment. Prepare for that."

Yes, treatments are over. But that doesn't mean that everything will return instantly to the way it was before. Yes, the side effects are going to fade away. You *are* going to feel better. Your body is going to recover. But all this is going to take time.

"When you're through the crisis," Jody says, "there's this expectation that you're going to go back to normal, but you don't feel that way. It's a time that needs a lot of TLC. You need to be very, very patient with yourself. If you have a grandmother, find her. You need someone strong and loving to nurture you through this."

Does it surprise you to read this? Maybe you thought that once you got through that last treatment, your job was over. Back to life as usual, right?

Well, not if life as usual means ignoring the care you need. Yes, treatments are over, but your job of extreme self-care is not.

Let's take a moment to do a reality check. I bet you haven't really taken stock of what you've gone through. We often tend to downplay our own accomplishments and experiences. So for a moment, imagine everything has happened to someone else besides you. A really good friend, perhaps. This will help you to gain a realistic perspective on your experience.

Okay. Imagine everything that's happened to you has happened to someone else whom you know very well. Then answer the following questions. Use an extra sheet of paper if you need to.

1. What is the name of your good friend? (Choose any name you like.)

_____

2. For how many months and weeks has he or she gone through serious treatment, whether chemotherapy, radiation, or other?

_____

_____

3. What side effects did he or she go through? (Including nausea, PPE, neuropathy, constipation, mouth sores, etc. Please list them all.)

_____

_____

4. How many medications did he or she have to take? (Try to count them all, including pain relievers.)

_____

_____

5. What emotions has he or she gone through during the course of treatment? (Anger, frustration, depression, despair, etc.)

_____

_____

6. What other crises have occurred during this treatment time? (Loss of a relationship, loss of a job, cutback in hours, loss of material possessions, missed opportunities, financial troubles, family issues, etc.)

_____

_____

7. What changes has he or she experienced in the body? (Changes in appetite, weight, hair, skin, energy level, and overall appearance.)

_____

_____

8. What other physical challenges has he or she faced? (Extra time in the hospital, severe side effects, delay of treatment, dental problems, nutrition issues, post-op infections, the flu, or other.)

_____

_____

9. What other treatments did he or she have to go through, if any? (Stem cell transplant, reconstructive surgery, other surgeries.)

_____

_____

10. What health issues is he or she still dealing with? (Surgical wounds, mastectomy drains, limited movement from surgery, loss of function somewhere in the body, etc.)

_____

_____

Now, take a moment to review your answers. Still expect you can bounce back in a matter of weeks? You have been through a lot, don't you think? Can you be compassionate with yourself? How about your body, which has worked so hard to get you to this point?

It's going to take some time, but that's okay. You've shifted from the period of poisoning the cancer to the period of rebuilding the body. In the meantime, most likely you're going to have a few lingering effects from all you've been through.

The important thing during this time is to _be patient_. You may find it frustrating if you're body isn't exactly as it was before cancer. If these feelings come up, return to Chapter 4 and use some of the tools there to process and release those feelings. It was important to keep your spirits up during cancer treatment, but it's also important to keep them up during your recovery time.

Each time my father completed treatment, he had a side effect that stayed with him. Sometimes it was nerve damage, other times it was chemo brain. Sometimes it was thin, baby hair, and other times it was scars from surgeries. He was frustrated at times, but he also had the most wonderful attitude about it. For him, these things were *reminders that he had made it through!* They were souvenirs from the battle he had fought, and reminders that he had won, and was still alive and enjoying his family and his work!

Can you view your lingering side effects this way? Can you use them to remind yourself of just how strong you've become?

"Keep up with your positive self-reminders," Jody says. "It's better to be here and be adjusting and becoming yourself again, because that's what it is. It's a function of returning."

Roadblocks on the path to returning include several of the following potentially longterm effects. I'll walk you through each one and discuss how you can deal with it. In the meantime, keep encouraging positive thoughts. It may not all happen immediately, but you're on the road back to health!

Surgery Scars: Keep Moisturizing!

"To this day my doctor recommends that I continue moisturizing the radiation site because it can get tight. I still do it every day, and it will be three years this summer."

—Deb, breast cancer survivor

Young boys love to brag about their scars. "Here's where I got hit by a baseball," they'll say, showing you a dark line about the eyebrow. "I got this in my bike wreck," referring to the long scar down the shin. Scars can be badges of honor, evidence of battles fought and won, of adventures taken and conquered.

Cancer scars can have a similar "I've-been-there-and-survived" quality, but they can also be tight, painful, and embarrassing. I still have my scar, for example, where my port was put in and taken out on my left collar area. To this day there's scar tissue left that can be painful when I'm getting a massage. I always have to let the therapist know ahead of time—even now, eighteen years later! I also have to make sure to cover it up with sunblock or clothes when I'm out in the sun, because it's still very tender and can get burned really easily.

Scar tissue is the body's natural reaction to healing damaged areas. It's like a latticework laid down over the injured area—which can be anywhere on or in the body—through which new connective tissues are woven. (Think of a scab over a wound on your arm.) These tissues are usually denser and thicker than surrounding tissues, however, so they are more limited in movement, circulation, and sensation.

Though scars on the skin usually pale and fade without further irritation, larger scars from surgery—particularly from mastectomy or other significant surgeries—can create limitations in movement and may become so stiff that they cause pressure or pain.

If you have stiff movement because of a scar, you can try physical therapy or gentle stretching exercises like those in yoga. "Certain yoga poses gently open up the front of the body and strengthen the back," says Laura Kupperman, yoga instructor, "making it easier to breathe full, deep breaths, increasing energy, and reducing aches and pains."

What else can you do about thick, uncomfortable scar tissue? I used vitamin E and cocoa butter on the area every day, which helped soften the tissue. Massage can also help. Mórag Currin, LA, CMLT, and president of Touch for Cancer Online, says that massage can loosen up scar tissue, but to always listen to your body, and if anything hurts, tell your massage therapist right away: "If scars are not painful, you can massage and soften them. There are estheticians and massage therapists who are trained to help stretch them out, which can help you regain movement and flexibility. However, if the skin is still compromised or the wound hasn't healed, it could be extremely uncomfortable."

Other options for treating scar tissue include:

- **Surgical treatments** – For serious, stubborn scars, surgical options are available that can reduce (but not completely remove) the scar.

- **Microdermabrasion and chemical peels** – These procedures remove the top layer of skin, allowing new skin to grow and reducing scar tissue.

- **Needling** – In this process, the affected area is "needled" to allow formation of collagen, which helps remove scar tissue.

Though all these may be effective, you may want to try natural remedies first, to see if you can reduce scar tissue without the side effects of other treatments. Some home remedies from other cancer fighters include lemon juice (applied to the scar), sandalwood paste (applied on the scar and left overnight), fenugreek seeds (washed on the scar once a week), and oil massage (with lavender, olive, cod-liver, coconut, and vitamin E oils).

Finally, if you feel a "lumplike" scar in an area where you had surgery, you may want to insist on thorough investigation to make sure it isn't another tumor, an abscess, or something similar that requires attention. You know your body best, so listen to your own intuition; if something doesn't feel right, be sure to have it thoroughly checked.

What are These Dark Spots on My Face?

Sometimes, as a result of acne, dry skin, or radiation treatments, you may be left with dark areas on your face or on other parts of the body. It's called hyperpigmentation, and basically it means the skin gets darker in places. This darkness can remain after treatments are over—not a serious lasting side effect, except when you look in the mirror. Usually the darker skin doesn't occur all over, like a nice tan, but in unattractive blotches and spots.

Scientists aren't sure why chemotherapy causes hyperpigmentation. It may have something to do with inflammation, stimulation of skin-color cells, or toxicity. (If you had acne rashes, that could also cause it.) Radiation, of course, can cause it at the treatment site.

Like most side effects, hyperpigmentation typically fades within ten to twelve weeks of the last treatment, but sometimes it becomes a long-term, unwelcome guest. This is no fun after treatments, when your hair is growing back and you're trying to regain your former appearance.

First of all, now that you are no longer undergoing treatments, gradually add exfoliation back into your daily routine. You need to loosen up the dead cells on the top layer of skin so that new, younger cells can come forward. Try natural facial scrubs from reputable manufacturers, products that have ingredients like pumpkin and enzymes and other exfoliants from nature.

Once your skin has recovered from treatment, you can also try microdermabrasion. In this process, you or a technician will mechanically remove the uppermost layer of dead skin cells from the face, neck, and/or hands. You can enjoy the treatment at your local spa or try an organic home version. A spa technician will use a power device to spray microcrystals of aluminum dioxide across the skin's surface, blasting away the dead cells. If you use the at-home version, you may use a power device that stimulates a sandy cream on your skin, accomplishing the same outcome.

Microdermabrasion leaves skin with a more glowing look and can also help your skin care products penetrate into the deeper layers of skin to help build collagen and elasticity. As always, be careful. If it feels too aggressive and your skin is still too sensitive, speak up so the technician can proceed at a more gentle speed.

Next, become obsessed with protecting yourself from the sun. UV rays trigger the production of melanin, the pigment that produces skin color—and darkened areas are particularly susceptible—so cover up with clothing and physical sunblock, like zinc and titanium oxide. Apply sunscreen every day, rain or shine, as UV rays still penetrate through clouds, and one day of exposure can ruin all the lightening effects you've been working so hard to accomplish.

All these efforts will help renew, refresh, and protect your skin, but to get rid of those dark areas, you'll need a little more help. Unfortunately, many "lightening" creams include the bleaching agent "hydroquinone," basically because it does work. However, the Environmental Working Group has assigned a "hazardous" warning to this ingredient. It has shown mutagenic (potentially cancer-causing) activity in lab studies[1] and has been banned in the European Union and in Japan. It increases sensitivity to UV rays and may cause the degeneration of collagen and elastin fibers, which would only hasten the aging process. In rare cases it can lead to a skin disease called ochronosis, and prolonged use can thicken collagen fibers and damage connecting tissues, making your situation worse.

Instead, try one of the many hydroquinone-free products out there, most of which use kojic acid, alpha-hydroxy acids, vitamin C, arbutin, and niacinimide (a form of vitamin B) to lighten. Make sure to choose toxin-free versions.

As I said earlier, be patient! Give any product two to three months to work. In the meantime, use the makeup tips we spoke about in Chapter 6 to cover up the dark spots. If, after that time, you're still not satisfied, you may want to consider more aggressive facial peels or laser therapy, but be sure to wait until your skin has fully recovered from treatment, which is at least six months.

Facial peels that help with hyperpigmentation often include alpha-hydroxy acids or heavy exfoliating ingredients like glycolic acid. Check with your dermatologist. Laser treatments like FotoFacials and others (administered by a doctor or nurse technician) have also been shown to significantly reduce hyperpigmentation. I've undergone a series of five for sun damage and I was amazed with the results! However, there is some risk of scarring with these treatments, so be sure to gather all the information you can before proceeding and select your medical spa or doctor very carefully. Most likely, some good creams and concealers might just do the trick and will give you the smooth look you're going for.

I Keep Forgetting Things—Is That Normal?

"With chemo brain, you forget stuff. We still joke about it. It's a different state of mind. You're kind of in a daze, but not. You go through every day, but you're treating this cancer and the treatment itself has an impact on your thought processes."

—Laurie, breast cancer survivor

It's not all in your head. If you find it hard to focus, remember things, retrieve words, analyze difficult data, or multitask like you used to before cancer treatment, you may have chemo brain.

Doctors used to shrug off patient complaints about foggy thinking and forgetfulness, but finally science is catching up with what patients have long known. Just like chemotherapy can cause problems in the rest of the body, it can do so in the brain as well, and these problems can last well beyond treatment conclusion.

"I still forget things," says Justin, brain cancer survivor. "It's hard to focus, get my mind back on track. Not frequently, but sometimes I have memory loss. Sometimes it happens."

"I think I have chemo brain all the time!" says Rayette, ovarian cancer survivor. "I didn't know if it was just an old wive's tale, but I forget things, things I can't recall."

Chemo brain definitely affected my father. Sometimes he would speak about two different things in one conversation. He would talk about one subject, and then in the middle of it, he'd switch to something else. We'd interrupt him with a puzzled, "What?" Seeing our confusion, he would stop and ask, "What's wrong?" We'd tell him that he'd just switched conversations! He'd say, "Oh, okay," and go back to his original train of thought.

My dad was also forgetful. He would forget if he'd paid a bill, or where his keys were. These things were no big deal, but it became more serious when he forgot whether or not he'd taken his medications. Overdosing on drugs is a very real possibility in this situation, so if you're encountering this type of memory loss, get one of those little pill containers that's labeled with the days of the week, so you'll be sure not to take more or less than you need. You may also ask a loved one to give you the pills daily so you're not worrying about whether or not you took them.

Chemo brain is real, so if you're experiencing it, relax. It's normal. After all, the chemo drugs affected the rest of your body; why wouldn't they affect your brain? Symptoms can include memory lapses, trouble concentrating, taking longer to finish things, trouble remembering common words, and inability to multitask. Sometimes the fuzziness goes away after chemotherapy ends, but for an estimated 15 percent of patients, the problems stick around.

In fact, pictures of the brain have shown changes in brain activity of breast cancer survivors treated with chemo when compared to those not treated with chemo, and the changes were still seen on scans five to ten years after treatment stopped.[2] They also estimate that up to 70 percent of people who undergo chemotherapy will experience chemo brain.

Just what causes chemo brain? Scientists still don't know. Most believe that the chemo drugs in combination with the cancer itself and other factors like patient age, stress, low-blood counts, other drugs used in treatment, infection, and anxiety have a lot to do with it. Hormonal changes as a result of therapy are also highly suspect.

If you're suffering from chemo brain, either during or after treatment, talk to your doctor. He or she may have medications that may help. Meanwhile, making some lifestyle adjustments can help you cope.

Try the following tips, and consider getting a copy of Dr. Daniel Silverman's book, *Your Brain After Chemo: A Practical Guide to Lifting the Fog and Getting Back Your Focus.*

- Write everything down—appointments, things you need to do, phone numbers, addresses, meeting notes, even movies you'd like to see or books you'd like to read. Become an obsessed list maker.

- Exercise your mind. Do puzzles, learn something new like how to play an instrument or a sport, practice sudoku or crosswords in your spare time.

- Get enough sleep.

- Get into a workout program. Regular exercise increases alertness.

- Set up routines. Pick a time to do important things each day, like feed the dog, exercise, take out the trash, mow the lawn, take medications, or brush your teeth. Designate locations for important things like keys, wallets, purses, and papers, and make a point to deposit those things in the same place at the end of each day.

- Keep a diary of any memory or mental problems you have. If they become serious, you'll have a record that may help you in treating the issue or figuring out what's triggering it.

- Prioritize. If multitasking is proving difficult, pick what's most important and do that first.

- Carry notebooks and/or sticky notes with you and use them.

- Leave messages for yourself on your own voicemail.

Yay, Here Comes My Hair! Why is it Curly?

"Things are different—my hair isn't the same. My facial hair has fallen out and come back three-four times since treatment. Not all the way, but in patches. When it first comes back, it comes back really dark and thick—and I'm Swedish blond! Then it falls out and thins out. I've just kept it shaved!"

—Jarrod, Hodgkin's lymphoma survivor

After months of treatment and wigs and hats and, of course, the endless waiting, I remember the day my hair started to grow back. *Thank God*! I thought. It was a time to celebrate!

Unfortunately, hair growth after cancer treatment hardly ever goes like you'd expect. Your locks could be thicker, straighter, curlier, even a different color than they were before.

"When my hair grew back, my stylist told me I had 'beaded' hair," says Teresa, colon cancer survivor. "When cancer patients grow hair back we get these little beads on the end of the hair. It's like your new hair is coming back, and it beads up. It's a good sign. Your new hair is starting to grow through."

As your hair struggles to set up house again on your head, keep in mind that it's still in a state of transition. The chemo (or radiation) affected the hair follicle, and it will take time before it regains its health and strength. Be ready for a change, and perhaps even more than one shift in texture or color.

Because weaker hair follicles are often killed off completely while stronger ones recover, you may have hair growing out strong on the top of your head, but thin on the sides. Your hair may be a different color or tone as strands die out. It may be kinky after radiation treatment because of uneven damage to the follicle, which causes the hair grow at an angle, making it curl.

This happened to me when my hair started growing back. Here I was, waiting for it to be thick and full and shiny like it was before, and instead it came in curly. I mean, my hair was so straight before, perms wouldn't hold for more than a couple of weeks. The texture changed too, to something quite fine and fragile. As the years have gone by, I've learned to manage hair that once used to be as strong as a rope. I've learned to accept my fine hair and take care of it and nurture it.

The important thing to remember is this: Be gentle. New hair is fragile—like baby hair, starting all over again. Think of the strands like baby sprouts on your spring plants, and you'll get the idea of the tender care they need! It's best to use a gentle shampoo and conditioner and avoid any processes like perms or colorings for at least six months.

However your hair reacts after treatment, you can count on one thing—it needs moisture and nourishment to make it stronger. For moisture, you can find a lot of solutions right in your own kitchen. See sidebar, "Homemade Moisturizers for Hair," or try some nontoxic deep-moisturizing conditioners or hair oils. Use these treatments once or twice a week. Once your hair has gained some strength and shine, you can back off to once weekly.

Make sure you're getting a good supply of B vitamins and omega-3s, either through your diet or in supplements, and drink plenty of water. Consider a multivitamin and perhaps an extra supplement of B vitamins, which are known to be good for hair. Other good nutrients include zinc, magnesium, and beta-carotene. Since hair is made of keratin and protein, a diet rich in protein will promote healthy growth. For more nourishing tips, see sidebar, "Natural Nourishment for Hair."

Homemade Moisturizes for Hair

- Mix honey with warm water and apply it after shampooing to create more shine. Leave on 5-10 minutes and rinse.

- Mix egg yolks in warm water and apply after shampooing. Leave on for 3-5 minutes and rinse.

- Mix a mashed avocado with coconut oil and leaving on the hair for 10-15 minutes.

- Create your own conditioner by mixing olive oil, sandalwood, rosemary, and aloe vera gel. Leave on the hair for up to an hour, then wash off.

- Apply jojoba oil to the hair and let sit before shampooing, or sleep overnight in it. Adding lavender or tea tree oil to the mix helps stimulate the scalp.

Foods for Healthy Hair

If you want to eat your hair healthy, what foods should you choose?

- As with skin, omega-3 fatty acids moisturize and nourish from the inside out. Eat more salmon, sardines, almonds, flaxseed, beans, and walnuts.

- Be sure you're getting enough protein, in the form of beans, white meats, and vegetables. The hair is made of protein, so these foods give it fuel to grow.

- Calcium is also an important mineral for hair growth, so get some low-fat milk, yogurt, and/or cottage cheese daily.

- Low iron levels can lead to hair loss. Women are usually more likely than men to be iron deficient, so ladies, beef up on foods like egg yolks, dried fruit, whole grains, spinach, broccoli, and turkey.

- Zinc is also important in retaining strong hair strands for both sexes. Sources include oysters, nuts, beef, and lamb.

- Surprisingly, coconut is considered an excellent "hair food." Add it to desserts, salads, fruits, and rice.

- Spices like cumin, tumeric, and black pepper are also hair friendly.

- Drink plenty of water.

The skin of your scalp remains sensitive as well, and is best not exposed to strong chemicals. Stay away from potentially harmful and drying ingredients like mineral oil; DEA, MEA, and TEA (hormone-disruptors); fragrance; phthalates; sodium lauryl sulfate; parabens; and betaine. Try not to wash it every day if possible (so your own natural oils can moisturize the strands), wear a cap when swimming, and use only a wide-toothed comb when combing wet hair (as this is when hair breaks most). Never tease or rat tender strands; it causes breakage. You may even want to use heated styling tools like curling and straightening irons and hair dryers more sparingly, as they can easily damage new hair.

Don't forget to protect new hair from the sun (resurrect your favorite hats and scarves!), and go for natural styles that won't require a lot of manipulation. You may also want to try scalp massage. It feels great, and it improves circulation, supporting hair growth.

What if your hair isn't growing back? Talk to your doctor. He or she can rule out causes like treatment-induced low levels of zinc or iron, thyroid problems, or stress.

Natural Nourishment for Hair

- Mash up an avocado and mix it with 3 tablespoons jojoba oil to help strengthen hair and moisturize.

- Massage can help encourage better circulation and hair growth, so try a scalp massage with a soothing essential oil like Brahma.

- To fortify weak, fragile hair, try simmering geranium leaves in water for fifteen to thirty minutes, then rinse with the water twice a week.

- Drink a glass of alfalfa juice (combined with carrot if you like) to help nourish hair roots and prevent hair thinning.

In the end, use the patience you've learned through the whole cancer process, and remember that the whole experience has given you something not a lot of people have: an appreciation for your own hair!

Where Did All Those Drugs Go?

After cancer treatments you may feel a little "muddy" inside. Your body has been hit with so many drugs and perhaps radiation—is it possible some residual waste may still be hanging around inside you?

If you're having digestive problems, fatigue, stomach bloat, headaches, muscle aches, poor memory, a suppressed immune system, even bad breath, then yes, these could be the result of excess toxins in your blood and tissues.

There's a cleansing process that goes on in your body every day. The intestines, liver, and kidneys are all involved, whisking away toxins from the environment, stress, drugs, and the food you eat, and flushing them out where they can no longer pose a threat.

If you've been going through chemotherapy or radiation treatments, however, most likely your system is overloaded with waste products. There were so many, your body may not have been able to handle them all. Chemotherapy drugs fill the body with toxins, radiation can damage healthy cells and create toxic buildup, and even cancer cells themselves become toxins as they wither up and die.

If you'd like to help your body clean house, try these suggestions.

Detox Baths: An Epsom salts bath is one of my favorite ways to detox. Hot water opens the pores, allowing perspiration to take toxins away, as well as increasing absorption of nutrients such as magnesium and sulfate (in the salts), which help generate enzymes that clean up the body. Adding ginger to your Epsom salt bath will open pores of the skin and further aid in eliminating pain. Baking soda helps neutralize the effects of radiation, sesame is great for de-stressing, and vinegar helps sooth joints and tendonitis.

Water: It's the most natural way to flush toxins out of your body. Drink at least seven to eight glasses a day, preferably purified.

Live Juices: I've made it a daily habit to have fresh-squeezed green juice every morning. Live juices can rejuvenate, heal, and help flush away toxins. Fruits and vegetables help energize and regenerate your body. My favorite combination is kale, celery, romaine, spinach, cucumber, and a bit of ginger, parsley, and lemon.

Exercise: It gets the heart pumping, which circulates blood, moving toxins out of the body. It also encourages perspiration, which decreases toxins, and makes you thirsty, so you'll drink more water. Be gentle with yourself at first, then gradually increase time and intensity; but no matter what, try to get your body moving daily.

Fiber: It "sweeps" the digestive tract clean and speeds up elimination, which means waste products are in your body for a shorter amount of time. Eat more fruits, vegetables, and whole grains.

Dandelion: Many herbs are known to stimulate detoxification in the body. Dandelion is one, used in traditional Chinese medicine as a powerful liver tonic. Try a daily cup of dandelion tea, some dandelion greens (full of nutrients), or mix some dandelion in a smoothie or in your fresh-squeezed juice. Other foods that support healthy liver function include lemons, apples, beets, and carrots. (Note: Don't use dandelions you've picked from a chemically treated lawn!)

Contrast Therapy Shower: Take a hot shower for one to two minutes, then turn the hot water down (or off) and stand under the cold water for ten to twenty seconds. Follow this with one to two minutes of hot water, then another ten to twenty seconds of cold water. Repeat once more, ending with cold water, step out, and dry vigorously.

Saunas and Steam Baths: Increasing our body temperature leads to increased sweating, which helps clean out the dirt and impurities from the skin, opening the pores to eliminate other toxins. The warmth also increases our blood circulation, enhancing the flow of toxins for elimination. A nice side benefit—it relaxes your tired, strained muscles!

I Still Feel Tired and Sore

"I'm definitely weaker. I was pretty athletic, but I don't have the muscles I used to. My energy was really down through chemo, too, and it took a while, but I got it back."

—Jamie, non-Hodgkin's lymphoma survivor

The previous sections have covered the main side effects that may stick around for a while after you've finished treatment. However, you may also have some others. PPE and neuropathy, for instance, can sometimes take months to gradually subside, so you may need to continue with the coping techniques we discussed while you're recovering.

Fatigue is another side effect that seems to hang around after treatment is over. Check back to Chapter 7 to review some coping techniques, and consider talking to a naturopath about dietary measures that may help you. Dr. Donielle Wilson, ND, for example, says that balancing blood-sugar levels is key following cancer treatments.

"When we're under elevated stress from cancer," she says, "we're constantly stimulating the adrenal glands. They produce cortisol and adrenaline in response to stress, and they also have to moderate blood-sugar levels. So when we eat foods high in carbohydrates and sugars, we're requiring them to do more—namely, to release insulin to process the sugar and bring blood-sugar levels back to normal." Results are often reduced energy, a depleted immune system, mood swings, fatigue, sleep disturbances, weight gain, and slow release of toxins.

Dr. Doni says you can start feeling better by making some simple dietary changes: "Eat every three to four hours, and every time you eat, have a protein." Proteins naturally slow the body's breakdown of sugars, which eases the load on the adrenal glands and helps naturally balance blood-sugar levels. Try a few nuts with lunch, a boiled egg, some lean meats like chicken and turkey, or vegetarian proteins. Decrease your consumption of carbohydrates, and add in some healthy fats like olive oil, flaxseed oil, and omega 3s from fish and nuts.

Exercise can also help you rebuild your body and ease away the side effects of treatment. You may not feel like it, but start small. A daily walk for fifteen minutes, for example, can turn into thirty minutes a day of brisk walking, which fits the recommendations for regaining health and vitality.

You may also want to try some of the other exercises mentioned in Chapter 8. Yoga and tai chi can be very gentle on a recovering body and can also become more challenging as you get stronger. Look for classes in your area tailored to cancer patients and survivors.

Some chemotherapy drugs have been known to raise your risk of carpal tunnel syndrome. If you suspect you may have it (symptoms include burning, tingling, or itching numbness in the palm and the fingers, especially the thumb and the index and middle fingers), check with your doctor. Several nonsurgical treatments are available, like anti-inflammatory drugs, corticosteroids, or natural solutions like stretching and strengthening exercises, acupuncture, and chiropractic care. Surgical options may also be considered for more severe cases.

Your skin may also remain dry. My father continued to have rough, cracked hands and feet well after treatment was over. This can lead to itching, irritation, flakiness, and possible open wounds. Keep using the coping techniques we talked about earlier—lots of moisturizer, and wear gloves and socks to protect yourself. If your nails still haven't grown back to their former strength, keep using the cuticle cream, and file them regularly.

Whatever side effects may still be hanging around for you, keep your doctor in the loop, and don't give up on seeking out ways to deal with them. Remember: Your body has been through a lot. Be patient, and most importantly, be gentle with yourself.

Get Back into Life—On Your Terms

"I had a boyfriend who for three years was with me through cancer. He wasn't bad, by any means, but while I was sick I saw how he reacted; how he went through the motions and wasn't really there. It made me realize that our relationship wasn't what I wanted—that I wanted someone who could handle things like this, who could let me cry when I needed to."

—Jamie, non-Hodgkin's lymphoma survivor

My cancer experience definitely changed me in a lot of ways, but when I was first done with treatment, I didn't really realize it. I was desperate to get back to how I was before the diagnosis. I think most of us feel this way. We all think, *Let's get the cancer out of the way so I can get back to being 'me.'* What we may not realize at first is that our old selves probably had some unhealthy habits—working long hours, making poor dietary choices, failing to exercise, and taking on too much stress.

"I think of myself as the rat on the wheel," says Karen, two-time thyroid cancer survivor. "I'm working, I'm going, I'm moving. But cancer knocked me off. After treatment I wanted to get myself back together and get back to work really quickly. But the second time I got cancer, I took a leave of absence from work. I went through a lot of struggles about, 'If I'm not a dental hygienist all the time, who am I?' I had been doing that for twenty years. But it was a blessing in disguise. The sun still comes up every day when I'm not doing that job. All the people I thought I had to take care of are still my friends. I had this strange work ethic and an unrealistic view of what made me 'me,' and I was sacrificing my health and my family to do that instead of taking care of what I should have been taking care of."

Instead of leaping full-force back into everything you were before cancer, why not take some time to digest the experience and reflect on who you are *now*? Your body needs time to recover, and you need time to reflect on everything you've gone through. You need to see what it all means for the person you are today, and who you will become tomorrow.

"Cancer is almost like a high in a way because there's so much attention on you," says Dee, breast cancer survivor. "What do you do when it's all gone? I've always felt in the last few years like I wasn't in the right spot, like I should be doing something different. I hope something comes along and shows me my new direction in life."

After my father's third diagnosis, he went through some real changes. He started to slow down, work less, and instead of always saying "yes" to everything, he would turn down certain commitments. He would say, "I can't run myself into the ground anymore."

I'll talk more about coping with the aftermath of cancer in the next chapter. For now, I'm just hoping you'll take a deep breath, step back, and look around. While you're deep moisturizing your hands and feet, taking a detox bath, getting a soothing massage, or trying a new yoga class, feel how it feels to be who you are, now, in this moment. This person may not want to rush around ninety miles an hour anymore. He may need time to process everything at a much slower pace. Maybe she wants to write about her experiences. Maybe he would like to change jobs.

Don't make any rash decisions, but allow yourself the time to reflect. This isn't the time to jump backwards. Treatments are over. You're moving forward. And it's going to be a time of discovery to figure out just where your next destination may lie.

Let's Review

- It's important to celebrate when your treatments are over, but realize that it will take time for your body to recover after everything you've been through.

- Surgery scars can cause tightness, limited motion, and pain. Try rich moisturizers and gentle stretching through physical therapy and yoga. Go to a masseuse familiar with surgery scars or oncology massage, and consider other options if your scar doesn't loosen up.

- Cancer treatments and side effects can result in hyperpigmentation, or dark spots on your face, hands, and other parts of the body. Step up your exfoliation, and consider non-hydroquinone lightening creams.

- If you're forgetting things more often than usual or having trouble multitasking, you could be experiencing chemo brain. Check with your doctor, and adopt some coping techniques like making lists, leaving yourself messages, and setting up regular routines.

- When your hair starts growing back, it may be a different color and texture than it was before. Apply more moisture and nutrients, limit the use of heated styling tools, and treat new hair growth gently, as if it were baby hair.

- If you're still experiencing things like fatigue, headaches, and digestive problems after treatments are over, your body may still be fighting with all the toxins of treatment. Try some at-home detox methods to help flush out the waste.

- For other lasting side effects, check with your doctor, and continue to experiment with things like exercise, diet, moisturizers, and other options.

- Take your time with your recovery. As your body gradually gains strength, allow your mind and emotions to reflect on your experience. Process emotions as you need to, and resist the temptation to try to be who you were before. You're different now. You've gone through an experience that has forever changed your life.

Personal Affirmations

I continue to be gentle with myself every day.

I am willing and committed to taking good care of myself.
I am my number-one priority.

12

Your Prevention Plan:
Tips to Lower Risk of Recurrence

"Before cancer, I barely went along. Now I try to find something good about the day. I'm always grateful for what God has given me. He's given me a second chance in life to go and see and do things I haven't done before. I find the little things in life I didn't notice before are now so much sharper and clearer."

—Chris, non-Hodgkin's lymphoma survivor

THERE ISN'T A CANCER SURVIVOR ALIVE WHO HASN'T thought about it.

What if it comes back?

"It's always in the back of my mind," says Chris, non-Hodgkin's lymphoma survivor. "Like I have this cold now and my glands are swollen, and I think, 'Uh-oh. Is it back?'"

It's natural to worry about it. After you've been through so much, the last thing you want to do is go through it again. You try to tell yourself everything is fine, but there's that nagging thought in the back of your mind, scratching away like a sliver under your skin.

What if it's not all gone? What if they didn't get it all?

"When my body was trying to recover from the marathon," says Deb, breast cancer survivor, "it reminded me of when I was recovering from chemo. It makes you anxious and stressed. I think it's a part of cancer treatment and recovery. You come down with a cold and you get anxious. You have a few nights you don't sleep well. It all comes back to you and you have to put the brakes on and say, 'This is not cancer. This is not cancer treatment. It's just a cold.'"

The bottom line is, you can't control the future. Sometimes the cancer does come back, and there's nothing you can do about it. As you know, this happened to my father. He was *so* disappointed when he found out. But he picked himself back up and went on as best he could. In the end, that's all we can do—the best we can.

"The first year of treatment was okay," says Justin, brain cancer survivor, "and then it recurred. It was a surprise. I was shocked." Justin had to go through treatment again, but he made it, and he's a survivor today, reaching out and helping others going through similar experiences.

Many survivors I spoke to experienced worry and anxiety over recurrence. There's a greater sense of uncertainty and a feeling of vulnerability. Cancer robs you of that sense of control over your life. You realize that sometimes, things happen that are completely out of your control. And it can leave you feeling powerless.

"Part of the healing process is you have to learn to trust life again," says Jody, breast cancer survivor. "All of a sudden, this news came out, and you can be anxious and skeptical and expect the other shoe to drop. The deal is, if it drops, it drops. But right now, it hasn't. I don't want to live as though it's going to come down again."

If you're worried about recurrence—and if you're a human being and you've gone through cancer, you probably are—you have a choice to make. Are you going to live in fear, or are you going to do what you can do to raise your odds of staying well, and let God (or whatever power you believe in) handle the rest?

It really all comes down to one thing: fear, and how you're going to handle it. You can't stop the thoughts from coming up, and you probably can't stop yourself from worrying now and then. However, you can do things to quiet that worry when it happens, and you can definitely do a lot of things to help you regain a sense of control over your life.

It's your choice. Will you allow your life to be ruled by worry, anxiety, and fear, or will you take steps to regain your confidence and control? Will you allow depression and stress to wreak havoc on your body and mind, or will you make changes in your life to promote health and well-being?

Eight Tips to Help You Stay Well

You don't have to run a marathon or become a vegetarian to significantly lower your risk of recurrence. Little things you do every day can significantly boost your immune system and help you stay healthy.

1. **Walk.** Exercise—even without weight loss—has shown in studies to help reduce risk of cancer. The American Cancer Society recommends 30 minutes a day of aerobic activity. You can accomplish this with a 30-minute walk, or try swimming, jogging, playing tennis or raquetball, or anything that gets your heart pumping. NOTE: If you're over 45 years old, try adding 45 minutes twice weekly of strength training to fend off muscle loss.

2. **Take it off the grill.** If you blacken your beef, chicken, or fish, you're increasing the amount of heterocyclic amines (HCAs) in the meat—compounds that have been linked to cancer. Keep the heat low, use aluminum foil on the grill to protect the goods, flip burgers often, and choose medium over well-done.

3. **Relax.** We all know that too much stress can weaken our immune systems. If you feel yourself getting riled up, take deep belly breaths, think about your favorite place, and write down the things you're grateful for. If you have a little more time, try some meditation, read a joke book, or strike a few yoga poses.

4. **Eat some dark chocolate.** Yes! It's full of powerful antioxidants that maintain normal functioning in your body's cells. Watch the calories, but don't be afraid to indulge in a bit now and then.

5. **Spice things up.** An Indian spice called turmeric has shown in studies to kill cancer cells and prevent more from growing. Add it to your relishes and soups or sprinkle it over pasta.

6. **Choose a safe sunscreen.** Avoid chemical-based options and choose those made with zinc oxide.

7. **Take a multivitamin and mineral.** Supplements are no substitute for healthy foods, but as we all miss our five servings of fruits and vegetables on some days, a multivitamin and mineral can help fill in the gaps and give us a good dose of cancer-fighting antioxidants.

8. **Buy organic.** Pesticides have been linked with cancer in several instances. Organic produce has consistently tested lower in pesticide content than regular produce.

Take a deep breath. Treatments are over. You're now a survivor. Congratulations! You've shifted from one place in your life to another, and now you have a new set of challenges to face. I have confidence you can face them, and in five years you'll look back on where you stand today and feel a great sense of pride and satisfaction in how far you've come.

Conquer Your Fears about Recurrence

"I finished treatment in 2002. Certainly the fear is there that it will come back. It's always hanging around in the background. But I think, I want to be around to see my daughter's children grow up. What am I going to do to get there? When you look at the things you need to change, it's not really that hard."

—Chris, non-Hodgkin's lymphoma survivor

Worrying about recurrence is all about fear. Mastering your anxiety around recurrence means you must learn to live with fear, and to overcome it. My father always told me that fear is an illusion—only in our heads—but that it can become a real obstacle if we buy into that illusion. His way of facing it was to feel it, but to go forward with his life anyway, doing what he wanted to do and refusing to let fear hold him back. You may recall I mentioned in the introduction that his favorite book was *Feel the Fear and Do it Anyway*. It's a must read!

"Fear is imagination-based for the most part," says Jacqueline Wales, author of *The Fearless Factor* and life coach. "It leads you to imagine the worst. You're going, 'Oh no, I'm going to lose my looks and feel all this pain and what about my family and I could die and...' On and on with the worst-case scenario."

The problem here comes back to what we talked about in Chapter 4: What are you thinking about? Thoughts create fear. Most of the time we don't feel fear until our conscious mind thinks a thought that creates the fear response. There may be nothing going on at the moment that's threatening us, but one thought can take on a life of its own in our heads, until we feel like there really is something to be afraid of.

If you're walking in a dark alley in a not-so-nice neighborhood and the hair stands up on the back of your neck, you're probably sensing the presence of some questionable character you can't see—a true reason to be afraid! The instinctual part of the brain reacts first, telling you you're in danger. The body picks up the message and pumps adrenaline through your limbs to prepare you for flight.

Most of the time, however, we don't have such immediate physical dangers we have to worry about. It's our minds creating the havoc for us. I notice myself blowing things out of proportion now and then, reacting like everything is an emergency, even feeling like I have to respond right away to an email! Of course, I know I can take my time and write back when I get a moment, but instead I get all worked up about it. My body then believes it's an emergency too, and starts spewing stress hormones all over. The good news is, we can manage these thoughts when they arise and thereby reduce our own suffering.

"Don't listen to the gremlins in the mind," Jacqueline says. "Reverse it. Say, 'I can see a picture of me healthy, cancer-free, and I'm thriving.'"

As I mentioned in Chapter 4, my father told me to talk back to my "fear/ negative chatter box" by saying "Stop." *What if the cancer comes back?* Stop! *What if I went through all these treatments for nothing?* Stop! He reminded me constantly that I am the only thinker in my mind. No one can tell me what to think. I have control over my thoughts, and I can change them.

If you trace the feeling of fear back to its origin, most likely you'll find the thought that caused it. Let's imagine a person who, like Deb, finished running a marathon. We'll call her Peggy, and imagine she's sitting down somewhere after the race, out of breath, head over her knees, muscles trembling.

Peggy is exhausted, totally spent, and her stomach is upset. At first, she's just recovering from the run, letting her body come back from the exertion. But then, somewhere in her mind, the thought occurs: *Hey, this feels like the third day after chemo.*

Suddenly everything changes. Peggy is no longer just recovering from her run. Now she is in potential danger. Sparks dart down her arms and legs, and her heartbeat increases. Her mind continues with the thought train: What if the cancer has come back? What if this is more than just exhaustion from the marathon? Are other people reacting like this? Am I the only one? If so, what does that mean?

As the thoughts continue, Peggy feels worse. Oh, there's a pain in her knee. Is that from the run, or something else? And by the way, she's incredibly thirsty even though she just drank a bottle of water. In fact, her throat is extremely dry. Surely that can't be normal. And she feels like she wants to throw up. She's been training for months, so why would that happen now?

As one thought grows into another, the whole negative scenario gains power, like a growing storm. Peggy has the ability, however, to stop this particular thought train and get off.

"Always question yourself," says Jacqueline. "If you slip into negative thinking, ask, 'Is that really the truth?' The mind is always chattering, but most of it is gibberish. I call it the 'yada-yada radio.' It's on 24/7, and it brings you down with every negative thought possible. Quieting that chatter is paramount to strength and healing."

Let's say Peggy does just that. She's named her negative doomsayer "Nelly," so she says, "Nelly, I hear you, and I appreciate you trying to protect me, but I'm okay. Now go away. I'm choosing to think positive and nourishing thoughts. "

Then replace your negative thoughts with something like: *I'm doing my best. Life is taking care of me.* Next, bring yourself back into the moment—into the *right now*—where nothing is wrong. If you're feeling fear, chances are you're somewhere in the future or the past. Remember that fear-based and negative thoughts are just thoughts, most likely from old conditioning. They are not real. Replace them, and come back to the moment.

"A lot of what fear is about," says Jacqueline, "is we don't trust we're going to get the right kind of outcome. Try not to get ahead of yourself. Trust in whatever power you believe in, and live in the present. You'll get to the future in plenty of time, and by then, the answers and solutions will have all become clear."

Of course, if you really feel something is wrong, you must trust yourself and your body and check with your doctor. I have spoken with many survivors who knew something wasn't right, and it was their diligence and trust in themselves that got them the care they needed and saved their lives. Yes, sometimes it was recurrence, but their persistence in getting it treated as soon as possible often made the difference in their survival.

You can discover what your fear is really about if you take a moment to question yourself. Is your fear well-founded, because something is really wrong? Or is this just fear talking?

Stop the Fear in its Tracks

Next time your worries about recurrence come up, take the following steps:

- Stop—and notice the fear. Sometimes we fail to recognize what we're actually thinking in the moment, which allows the mind to continue on until we're feeling physically unsettled. At the first sign of worry, anxiety, or fear, stop where you are and realize what's going on.

- Take a deep breath and exhale through your mouth, blowing all the air out of your lungs.

- Check your body. Where do you feel tense or tight? What feels off?

- Check your mind. What were you just thinking about?

- Continue back in time. Retrace your steps. What was the original thought that started the ball rolling?

- Once you find that thought, ask yourself: Is this really true? Do I have solid proof of this?

- Next, ask yourself where your thoughts are at the moment. Are you trying to live in the future, or the past?

- Bring yourself back to the present. Where are you right now? What do you need to do in the next hour?

- Realize that right now, everything is fine. Return to what you had originally planned to do. Bring yourself back into the present by rubbing your neck, getting something to eat or drink, or realizing what you're holding in your hand at the moment.

- Once you've brought yourself back into real time, make an appointment with yourself to process your feelings of fear, using whatever method is best for you. (Review Chapter 4.) Some options to try: Write about it or call a friend to share about it.

- Take another deep breath, know that everything is okay, and go on with your life!

Going through a process like this helps banish negative thoughts, bring you back into the moment, and restore your sense of control. Fear is about lack of control. When you feel in control again, fear disappears.

"Know that you have choices," Jacqueline says. "You didn't choose cancer, but you can choose how to deal with it every day. When you're feeling really anxious, sit down and take a few deep breaths. Concentrate on the breath, not the muddled thinking in your head, and choose to see an image of yourself as a healthy, whole human being."

Whatever your fear is about, you can always deal with it much more effectively when you're feeling calm and in control. Take steps to get yourself into that place of relaxed well-being, and then you can make any decisions you need to make with confidence.

Five Ways to Reduce Your Risk

"I never did watch what I ate. I just ate whatever I wanted to and nothing bothered me. I didn't really think about the food part of it—since I was exercising and losing the calories, I could eat whatever calories I wanted. I did eat out a lot and did the fast-food crap and all that stuff. Now I know."

—Teresa, colon cancer survivor

Once you've learned to conquer your fear about recurrence, you can take steps to reduce your risk. You'll be amazed at how much better you'll feel when you're actually doing something to help yourself stay healthy. Taking action makes you feel empowered!

I'm not talking here about things that *might* help, but things that have been shown in scientific studies to reduce your risk of recurrence. Yes, there are such things, and they're not all that complicated. You can work them into your daily routine as you gradually rebuild your life.

The top five methods for encouraging a strong immune system and reducing your risk of disease are:

1. Eat a Healthy Diet
2. Exercise
3. Practice Regular Stress Management Techniques
4. Reduce Your Toxic Exposure
5. Feed Your Soul

That's it. It's not complicated, and it's not too hard to do. It does take effort, and it does take time, but I'll bet, like most cancer survivors, you're now more than willing to put your health first.

I know after I survived cancer, I became really interested in nutrition, vitamins, and exercise. I didn't really care about any of this before. I was into competitive sports at school, but for the game, not for the health benefits. My experience with cancer changed that. I became more interested in my health and in doing everything I could to preserve it. So I went on to study nutrition and became a certified aerobics instructor. I worked with supplement companies as a wellness consultant and taught aerobics in my early twenties.

I still live this way today. I know how much of prevention has to do with what I eat, how I digest my food, how much I exercise, and what I think about all day long. I now see my cancer diagnosis as a wakeup

Six Immune-Power Foods

Though there is no one magical food to help keep cancer at bay, many have proven strong against cancer cells in the lab and in human studies. Here are some with encouraging studies behind them. Of course, all fruits and vegetables contain powerful antioxidants and phytonutrients known to boost the immune system.

- **Bitter Melon:** A tropical fruit, this cucumberlike treat is great in stir-fries, soups, and tea, and has been shown in studies to stop cancer cells from multiplying.

- **Broccoli:** Along with similar vegetables like kale and cabbage, broccoli contains a compound called "indole-3-carbinol (I3C)" valued for its anti-cancer properties. A 2004 study found that women who consumed broccoli were less likely to get breast cancer.

- **Green Tea:** Sip from 3-5 cups a day and you could be inhibiting the growth of cancer cells. Green tea has even been shown to help cancer patients reduce their risk of recurrence.

- **Mushrooms:** Excellent sources of nutrients like potassium, riboflavin, niacin, and selenium, mushrooms are showing powerful cancer-fighting properties. The fresh button mushrooms we use in our salads have been shown to reduce the risk of breast cancer and prostate cancer, and to decrease tumor size.

- **Pomegranate:** Several studies have shown the cancer-fighting properties of this tasty fruit. The best way to add this to your diet is through quality juice with low levels of added sugar.

- **Walnuts:** Full of omega-3 fatty acids and antioxidants, walnuts have shown the potential for reducing breast cancer.

call—an alert to the importance of taking care of my health. So far so good, as I have been cancer free for twenty years.

You may be thinking, "But those five things can't be that big a deal." If you mean we've heard a lot about them, you're right. If you mean we've been told for years we need these things to be healthy, you're right. So how come this is the same message when it comes to increasing the risk of keeping cancer at bay?

Reason one: These things reduce your risk of disease in the first place.

Reason two: These things have actually shown in some studies to reduce recurrence, specifically, from certain types of cancers.

Right there, you have two very strong reasons to make some changes in your life (if you haven't already) and start regularly doing the things that are likely to keep you healthy. It's the best way to take your power back—not to mention make you feel great. Let's go over them, one by one.

1: Nutrition and Power Foods

"I drink more green tea and only a few cups of coffee a day. I don't drink beer. I drink wine instead. I eat more fruits and vegetables, and I don't overdo on junk food."
—Vel, thyroid and ovarian cancer survivor

The link between diet and cancer is a strong one. According to researchers in a 2002 review, "Dietary factors are thought to account for about 30% of cancers in western countries, and thus, diet is second only to tobacco as a potentially preventable cause of cancer."[1]

Again and again, things like obesity and high intake of red meat and alcohol are associated with a higher risk of cancer, whereas a high intake of fruits, vegetables, and fiber is associated with a lower risk.[2] Dietary changes have resulted in a widespread decline in stomach cancer.[3] A meta-analysis showed that high intake of red meat contributed to a higher risk of colorectal cancer.[4] (It was more about eating red meat and processed meats than it was about overall meat intake.)

Obesity increases risk of breast cancer in postmenopausal women by 50 percent.[5] Risk of endometrial cancer is three times higher in women who are obese than those who are not.[6] Diets high in saturated fat have been linked to an increased risk of various cancers, including breast, colon, prostate, and possibly pancreas, ovary, and endometrium.[7] And diets high in sodas have recently been linked to pancreatic cancer: researchers found that two or more soft drinks per week were related to an 87 percent increased risk.[8]

Meanwhile, diets high in fiber are associated with a reduced risk for cancers of the breast, rectum, oral cavity, pharynx, and stomach.[9] Higher fruit and vegetable intakes were associated with lower risks of lung cancer in women.[10] A high-fruit, low-meat diet appears to be protective against colorectal cancer,[11] as does a high-fiber diet.[12] One study even found that

Herbs to Reduce Your Risk of Recurrence

Early scientific studies in vitro and/or in animals have found that several herbs have anti-cancer properties. Seek the advice of a naturopath, find quality products, and check with your doctor before trying the following herbs for their health benefits.

- **Essiac:** An herbal combination developed by a Canadian nurse, Essiac is a combination of four herbs (burdock, Indian rhubarb, sorrel, and slippery elm) that have shown anti-cancer activity in independent tests.

- **Sweet wormwood:** Terpenoids and flavonoids from this herb have been shown to have toxic effects on human tumor cells. Two of the plant's components have been studied as anti-cancer treatments.

- **Mistletoe:** Mistletoe has been shown to kill cancer cells in the laboratory and to boost the immune system. Animal studies have shown that it may be useful in decreasing side effects of chemotherapy.

- **Barbat skullcap** (Scutellaria barbata): This herb has shown anticancer activity and the ability to inhibit tumor growth—both in vitro.

- **Oldenlandia:** Famous for treating snakebites, this herb is most commonly used in traditional Chinese medicine for treating cancer. It has been studied with cancer in animals and on human cells in vitro.

women who had, during adolescence, a higher consumption of eggs, vegetable fat, and fiber had a lower risk of breast cancer, whereas risk of breast cancer was increased among women who consumed more butter.[13]

I could go on and on, but you get the picture. Diet definitely has an effect on the body's ability to resist disease. What about recurrence? Science supports a healthy diet there, too. One study found that higher levels of fat intake appeared to increase risk of recurrence and/or shortened survival following the diagnosis of breast cancer.[14] Another found that women diagnosed with early-stage breast cancer might improve overall survival by adopting more healthy dietary patterns.[15] A third found that a low-fat diet reduced breast cancer recurrence,[16] and a fourth found that patients with a higher body mass index (BMI) have a higher risk of recurrence.[17]

Of course it's not just breast cancer that's affected. Increased calorie and fat intake and low fiber intake were related to recurrent colon cancer,[18] and high saturated fat intake is associated with a lower survival rate in prostate cancer.[19] Whatever type of cancer you had, researchers stress the importance of nutrition and weight control.

"Cancer survivors represent a growing population at high risk for recurrence and other co-morbidities. [Basically, this means that cancer survivors are at a higher risk for other diseases, like heart disease and diabetes.] Evidence continues to accumulate regarding the importance of weight management, and a healthful diet (plant-based, low saturated fat) in improving the overall health and promoting disease-free and overall survival in this population."[20]

The bottom line: What you eat on a day-to-day basis can significantly improve your chances of keeping your body healthy and strong. Fortunately, all these studies show that you don't have to do anything overly complicated. You don't need fad diets, you don't need strict food plans, and you don't need to break the budget buying exotic items. All you have to do is incorporate some basic, healthy habits into your everyday meals.

What are those habits? Below is an itemized list. If you can reach these goals on a regular basis, your body will respond by becoming stronger and more resistant to disease.

Basic Dietary Recommendations for Survivors

"I quit using as much sugar and I replaced it with agave. I'm not really good about eating fruit, so I bought a juicer and I make sure I juice. I try to eat more broccoli. I've started taking turmeric because that's something we don't get a lot of in our diet. I drink three cups of green tea a day. The simple stuff like that anyone can do."
—Rayette, ovarian cancer survivor

To help reduce your risk of recurrence and increase your chances of feeling energetic and healthy, follow these tips. Like many things in our lives, eating a healthy diet can lead to other healthy habits as well. Start eating healthy, and who knows what other benefits you may experience!

EAT MORE
Fruits and Vegetables. Try for five or more servings a day.

- Throw in some fresh berries or banana slices in your cereal.
- Think of meat as a side dish, and fill at least half to three quarters of your plate with vegetables. Opt for brightly colored veggies or dark green leafy ones.

- Order a side salad instead of fries when dining out.

- Use fresh fruits in your desserts.

- Snack on fruits or veggies with yogurt-based dip or hummus instead of cookies or chips.

- Keep fruits like apples, pears, and oranges out on the counter to make it easier to grab one when you're hungry.

- Stack your freezer with frozen vegetables. They're quick and easy.

- Eat a dark-chocolate-covered strawberry instead of a candy bar.

- Have fun making salads. Start with romaine lettuce; then get creative. Try cucumbers, sprouts, beans, broccoli, spinach, asparagus, beets, fruit, and more.

- Add extra vegetables to your soups and stews. Pile the tomatoes and lettuce onto your sandwiches.

- The possibilities are endless. Once you start, you may find yourself craving more fruits and vegetables after a few weeks, as well as losing your taste for processed foods and artificial flavors.

Fiber. The Mayo Clinic recommends men under fifty years old get 38 grams a day, and women under fifty years old get 25 grams. Men over fifty-one should get 30 grams and women 21.

- For breakfast, choose a high-fiber cereal with 5 or more grams of fiber per serving. Look for brands that have "bran" or "fiber" in the name, or use whole-grain oats or wheat. (Make sure the sugar content is below 5 grams.) You can also add a few tablespoons of unprocessed wheat bran to your bowl.

- Switch to whole grains. Read the ingredient list. The first or second ingredient should be "whole-grain" or "whole-wheat." Try brown rice and whole-wheat pastas and breads. One of my favorites is sprouted whole grain bread—no flour, 3 grams of fiber per slice, and it tastes delicious. Find it in the frozen section in your grocery store.

- Substitute whole-grain flour for white flour (or even half the white flour) when baking.

- Fruits and vegetables are high in fiber, so the more you eat of those, the more fiber you'll get.

- Eat more beans, peas, and lentils. Add beans to your soups and salads.

- Snack on low-fat popcorn, whole-grain crackers, or a handful of nuts.

Water. It flushes toxins out your system, carries nutrients to your cells, and keeps your energy levels high. Try for eight to nine cups a day; more if you exercise.

- Drink water instead of soda or other sweetened drinks.

- Take a BPA-free water bottle with you and sip regularly all day.

- Don't wait until you're thirsty; drink on a regular schedule.

- When you exercise, drink more. If it's hot or humid outside, drink more.

- Drink a glass of water thirty minutes before each meal and between each meal. This will also help keep you from feeling hungry.

- Substitute sparkling water with lemon for alcoholic drinks at social gatherings.

Spices. Many spices have proven to have anti-cancer and immune-boosting properties. Choose garlic, ginger, turmeric, basil, rosemary, and coriander, and use them more in your soups, salads, casseroles, stews, and other meals.

EAT LESS
Processed Food. Limit these to less than two per week. We're talking white bread and pasta, non-whole-grain cereals, packaged meals, canned foods, and boxed dinners.

- These foods are typically high in salt, chemical preservatives, and additives.

- They're also typically high in fat.

Salt. Limit your intake to 2,300 mg/day; 1,500 mg if you have high blood pressure, kidney disease or diabetes, or if you're middle-aged or older.

- Eating fewer processed foods is the best way to cut back on your sodium intake.

- Look for low-sodium soups and condiments like salad dressings, dips, ketchup, mustard, and soy sauce.

- Substitute a spice mix for your tabletop instead of salt.

- Limit salt in your recipes. Use other spices and herbs instead.

- Switch to sea salt as opposed to table salt. Sea salt is created through natural evaporation of seawater and retains trace minerals, which add flavor and nutrients. Table salt is heat-blasted and chemically treated, so is stripped of all minerals except sodium and chloride.

Sugar. Studies are finding some evidence that certain types of sugars are good for cancer cells. For example, recent research found that cancer cells can readily metabolize fructose to increase proliferation and suggested that reducing the intake of refined fructose (e.g., high fructose corn syrup) could disrupt cancer growth.[21]

Sugar is everywhere, and we're all eating far too much of it. It requires the body to produce more insulin to regulate blood sugar levels, contributes to obesity, takes up calories that could be spent on nutritious foods, and saps energy. Women should limit intake to 100 calories a day (about 6 teaspoons) and men to 150 (about 9 teaspoons).

- Cut out sugary sodas. Drink tea and water instead, and invest in a juicer to make fresh-squeezed veggie and fruit juices.

- Read labels. Added sugar can appear in cereals, condiments, soups, juices, canned goods, yogurts, and more. Always look for the lower-sugar option.

- Cut back on cookies, pies, cakes, candies, and other high-sugar items. Enjoy them once in awhile, but fill most of your diet with healthier items.

- Try honey, stevia, or agave as a sugar substitute.

Alcohol. Limit your intake to one glass a day, or avoid it entirely. Choose red wine over mixed drinks, for its health benefits.

Red Meat. It's been linked with cancer, so cut back and have red meat only occasionally.

- Choose leaner meats such as fish, chicken, and turkey. Buy organic when possible.

- Avoid processed meats like hotdogs, sausage, deli meats, and salami.

- Reduce the portion of meat in each meal (enough to fit in your hand), and fill your plate with fruits and vegetables.

- Add beans and other plant-based proteins (like tofu) to your meals.

- Free-range eggs are another great source of protein.

"Bad" Fats. Saturated fats and trans fats are the unhealthy ones. Unsaturated fats (like omega-3s) are the healthy ones.

- Cook with olive oil or coconut oil instead of vegetable oil.

- Avoid everything with hydrogenated or partially hydrogenated oils.

- Trim the fat off meat, and choose non-fat dairy products.

- Eat fish once or twice a week (more if you can).

- Limit fast food, fried foods, and packaged foods.

2: Get Moving—Exercise is a Magic Bullet!

"I do have stress in my life, but the walking and exercising releases my stress. When I have those endorphins flowing through my body, I can solve the whole world's problems!"

—Chris, non-Hodgkin's lymphoma survivor

If you've had a hard time getting motivated to exercise in the past, here's a real inspiration for you: Exercise can help lower your risk of recurrence. Studies have found that survivors who engage in routine physical activity have significantly lower risk of developing disease or dying, compared with those who were physically inactive. "Overall," say researchers, "these results significantly strengthen the evidence for the role of exercise for cancer survivors after the completion of primary treatment."[22]

Another study found that physical activity seemed to reduce the risk of recurrence and mortality in patients with colon cancer.[23] Higher physical activity was also associated with lower risk of death from breast cancer.[24] (Walking three to five hours a week resulted in the greatest benefit.)

And it's not just about reducing your risk of recurrence. Exercise improves your quality of life. You just feel better when you're physically active. A study of women with breast cancer found that those who exercised had improved quality of life, improved physical functioning, and reduced symptoms of fatigue.[25]

After my cancer experience, I became obsessed with exercise. I went on to do triathlons and marathons in college. Today I exercise three to four times per week and incorporate yoga to help me deal with stress. I can't imagine handling all of life without exercise! Those endorphins and all that great oxygen coming into my body always helps me feel so much better about my day. As a cancer survivor, it's become a regular part of my life, like brushing my teeth. I'm committed to it because I know it's a primary component in reducing my risk of disease, but also just because it makes me feel so much better.

"It's important for cancer survivors to get strong," says Starr Cleary, cancer exercise specialist and Pilates instructor. "The average person loses between 6–12 percent of lean muscle mass every decade as they get older. If you've been through cancer treatment or surgery, within six weeks your muscles begin to weaken and atrophy (lose muscle tone). The longer you go without working them, the mushier they get."

What kind of exercise are we talking about? The majority of the studies were done on aerobic exercise—things like walking, biking, running, and swimming. (In other words, taking the occasional flight of stairs or a short walk to the office isn't good enough.) If you can fit in at least thirty minutes of real, dedicated exercise five days a week, The American Cancer Society estimates you could be reducing your risk of disease. But just how do you do that?

Starr recommends calling it something besides exercise, like power movement, socializing, getting out, playing a game, antistress time, self-care to keep yourself healthy, or what we like to call it—your daily dose of preventive medicine. Call it anything that brings up positive, good feelings. "I'm rollerblading with June today" sounds a lot more fun than, "I have to exercise at one-thirty."

Join a class and you'll be more likely to stick to your commitments. "Sorry, I have to get to my salsa class" is the perfect excuse for getting out of other tasks. You can do the same with sports, if you're on a softball, volleyball, bowling, tennis, racquetball, or soccer team.

The number one recommendation? Brisk walking. It has many benefits, is easy to do anywhere (especially if you've just finished cancer treatments and don't have a lot of energy), and you can do it alone or with friends. Take your headphones and listen to your favorite music or an audio book. Get outdoors and enjoy the fresh air; you'll find yourself feeling more energized. Try it on your lunch hour (grab a few colleagues and call it a business meeting) or first thing in the morning.

Starr recommends you try Pilates, as it involves slow, powerful movements that are less likely to lead to injury, especially when you're starting

Do You Need Supplements?

The American Cancer Society says that cancer survivors may be at increased risk for second cancers and so recommends they eat a variety of antioxidant-rich foods every day. Antioxidants include vitamins C and E, carotenoids, and phytochemicals.

Though it's best to get the nutrients we need from healthy foods, it can be difficult on some days to eat right. This is where supplements can help. Always check with your doctor, but then consider taking a multivitamin and perhaps some extra key nutrients to help your body stay healthy.

Certain nutrients, for example, have been shown in studies to help prevent cancer. Researchers believe that if we had the right amounts of vitamin D in our blood, for instance, we could prevent 75 percent of colon-cancer deaths. (Shoot for 2,000 IU a day and/or fifteen minutes of sunscreen-free exposure to the sun on your arms and legs.)

Calcium supplements have been shown in some studies to reduce the risk of breast cancer. Researchers think it has something to do with enhancing DNA repair activity. Having too little folate in your diet may increase your risk for colon and breast cancers, and having too little B vitamins in general may increase the risk of cervical cancer. However, taking large amounts of these vitamins in supplement form can also be dangerous to your health, so it's best to stick with a quality multivitamin, healthy foods, and perhaps an extra vitamin D and calcium supplement.

out in a weakened condition. "A lot of patients are apprehensive coming into my class because they're afraid they're not going to be able to do what we do," she says, "but Pilates allows you to start at any fitness level. We can adapt the movements as we need to for anyone's level of fitness. Some patients start by doing movements in a seated position."

Yoga is another gentle exercise you can try to start rebuilding muscle strength. Laura Kupperman, certified yoga teacher and therapist, says yoga is also a great way to start recovering after treatment: "If you're through with cancer treatment, you're often in this place of 'Now what?' You're used to getting your treatments and going to see your doctor regularly, and all of a sudden you're thrown out of the plane without a parachute. Yoga gives you a feeling of power and control. You realize there are some healthier decisions you can start making in different areas of your life. It feels good to take back control, which most cancer survivors feel they have lost."

For me, it's more about my commitment to being healthy than it is about my free time. I find a way to make exercise a priority. Get clear on what's stopping you; examine the evidence. When you think about it, a half hour is really not that much. What kind of exercise appeals to you?

Try scheduling it for next week and get started. Even if you only do fifteen minutes a day, that's better than nothing, and will likely grow into thirty as your body starts to crave it. Better yet, get an exercise buddy or join a walking group, that will help hold you accountable when you're just starting out. Once you get in the habit, you'll find you miss it when you don't work out, because exercise, in addition to being good for you, has a tendency to be addictive. That's one obsession we can live with!

3: Be Wary of Too Much Stress

"I started writing a book when I was sick. I had to deal with all this stuff. I had to get all this garbage out. I carried all this stuff inside me and I never let it go. You carry stuff around like that, it's going to take a toll on your body."

—Vel, thyroid and ovarian cancer survivor

How much does psychological stress affect the immune system and the body's ability to resist disease? Could it be that how we process and handle fear, change, and tragedy could have a big impact on how long we stay in remission?

Researchers think so. One study showed that psychological stress prior to, during, and after surgery can impair the immune system, raising the odds of cancer recurrence.[26] A later study found that by blocking stress hormones, long-term post-operative survival rates from cancer in animal models could be increased by as much as 200-300 percent.[27]

These aren't the only studies pointing to the stress/survival connection. Scientists found that breast cancer was more likely to recur in women who had experienced severe life stresses.[28] A life event was considered severe if it had long-term threatening implications—like the death of a husband or child, or a divorce. Those women who had experienced such stresses were nine times more likely to have a relapse of the breast cancer. They added that coping behavior and social support (like methods we discussed in Chapter 4) could modify the impact of these life stressors, to reduce risk.

A more recent study by scientists at Ohio State University showed that breast cancer patients who had gone through psychological intervention had a lower risk of cancer recurrence.[29] The study followed over

200 women for eleven years and found those who were taught relaxation methods (such as muscular relaxation) had a much lower chance of the cancer coming back than did women who had only psychological assessments. The women with the lower risk of recurrence also learned problem-solving skills, identified supportive family members and friends, used assertive communication to get their needs met, improved dietary habits, and increased activities such as walking.

My default way of handling challenges, unfortunately, is to stress and worry, so I have to make a conscious effort to relax in my daily life. I meditate twenty to thirty minutes in the morning, I pray morning and night, and I try not to "sit on my stuff." In other words, if there's something I'm concerned about, I'll either write about it or call a close friend. A problem shared is half a problem, right? Having a support system is critical for me. I see a life coach weekly and make sure to reach out to close friends often.

Emotions like anxiety, anger, and isolation—especially if repressed—can impair the immune system. As we mentioned in Chapter 4, the key is to encourage positive emotions as much as possible, and to engage in daily habits like meditation, exercise, and recreation that help you de-stress and relax. Particularly after surviving cancer, it's more important than ever to schedule time every day to process emotions and center yourself.

Practice regular calming techniques that will help you cope with the stresses life inevitably throws at you. Join a support group, try the progressive muscle relaxation therapy, and regularly practice other stress-relieving exercises like walking, painting, listening to music, engaging in sports, or whatever helps you feel less stress and more good emotions.

4: Live with Fewer Toxins!

"You have control over what you put on your body and in your body. You don't always have a choice about the power lines near your house. You could decide not to use a cell phone or microwave and revert back to the twentieth century, but that's pretty drastic. Choosing better nutrition and safer personal products, and taking care of your body with exercise—these are the easier things you can do."

—Laura, breast cancer survivor

In addition to encouraging health through diet, exercise, and stress relief, as cancer survivors, we must be more aware of the toxins around us. We know that our systems are bombarded by toxins every day, from pesticides in our food to pollution in the air to dangerous chemicals in our personal care products. Now that you've gone through cancer, it's time to pay closer attention to the effects this cumulative chemical assault have on your health.

Here's a quick review of the toxins you'd be wise to avoid in your daily life. Though you may not be able to control chemicals released into the area where you live, you can do a lot to minimize what gets into your body.

- **Dry cleaning.** Traditional methods leave chemical residue on your clothes. Avoid dry cleaning altogether, or air out your clothes for at least twenty-four hours before bringing them inside.

- **Personal care products.** Read labels for ingredients like parabens, BBP, DEHP, and PEG. Check your current brands with the Cosmetic Database (www.cosmeticsdatabase.com) for safety. Even if the product says "organic" or "natural," it may still contain potentially harmful ingredients, so review my "Ingredients to Avoid" list in Chapter 3 and in Appendix V.

- **Pesticides.** Buy organic produce, wash fresh fruit and vegetables thoroughly, and be cautious of the types of pesticides you use in your garden and on your lawn.

- **Plastics.** Don't microwave in plastics, and use stainless steel water bottles.

- **Cleaning supplies.** Choose nontoxic varieties with natural cleaning components.

- **Eat wild salmon.** Farm-raised salmon are known to contain PCBs (polychlorinated bophenyls)—chemicals that have been banned in the U.S. for decades, but that still show up in ground-up fish that are fed to farm-raised salmon. Scary!

- **Avoid synthetic fragrance.** Stay away from artificial air fresheners, dryer sheets, fabric softeners, or other smelly things that could pollute the air you breathe. This includes your perfume and cologne, by the way!

- **Limit consumption of high-mercury fish.** This includes tuna. Limit your intake to one or two times a week.

- **Test your tap water.** Tap water in the U.S. is among the safest in the world. However, no matter whether you have city water or well water, it can be contaminated with small amounts of toxins. To protect yourself, use a water filter on your faucet or invest in a household drinking water purification system, which often includes reverse osmosis to trap chemicals. Beware of bottled water, as it is often no more purified than tap water and can contain harmful chemicals that have leached into the water from the plastic container.

- **Ventilate your house.** Open the windows and let in some fresh air as often as you can. Houseplants can also help reduce the level of contaminants in the atmosphere.

- **Exercise near trees.** When your heart beats faster, you breathe in more air and circulate it faster throughout your body, so try to stay away from exhaust-filled city streets. Plants naturally remove toxins from the air, so exercise in the park or along tree-lined trails.

Are You Breathing in Toxins from Household Dust?

Do you sometimes neglect to dust during your regular household cleaning chores? According to the Environmental Working Group (EWG), leaving dust around could do more than make your guests turn up their noses—it could be harmful to your health.[30]

Recent research has been delving into what exactly is in the dust that collects on our furniture, floors, and countertops. You probably already know that it contains traces of human skin, pet dander, hair, and the like. However, when scientists examined indoor air dust in 120 homes, they found phthalates, phenylphenol (disinfectant), 4-nonylphenol (detergent metabolite), and flame retardants, even the carcinogenic intermediate of a flame retardant banned in 1977.[31] (Flame retardants are now found in computers, TVs, and furniture.)

They also found twenty-seven pesticides, including DDT, and reported that the concentrations exceeded government health-based guidelines for fifteen of the compounds. These are all chemicals that have been linked to cancer, reproductive problems, and hormone disruption.

Another study conducted by health officials in Canada found lead in house dust and warned of the dangers to young children, who swallow more contaminants because they often play on the floor and tend to put their hands in their mouths more often than adults.[32]

Scientists at the University of Arizona found that around 60 percent of floor dust comes from the soil tracked in on the bottom of our shoes.[33] If someone lives or works near a contaminated site or industrial plant, the dust could contain toxins. Worse, indoor dust can contain *more* toxins than outdoor soil, because of the lack of wind, rain, and sunshine to break them down and whisk them away.

How can you cut down on the contaminants in your home? The EWG recommends you take the following actions:

- Vacuum frequently with a machine that has a HEPA filter.
- Wet mop tile and wood floors to prevent dust from accumulating. (Dry mopping kicks up dust that can resettle.)
- Buy furniture that is filled with down, wool, polyester, or cotton, as these are unlikely to contain added fire retardant chemicals.
- Regularly wipe down furniture with a wet or microfiber cloth, and stay away from synthetic sprays that only add more chemicals.
- Caulk and seal cracks and crevices in the home to prevent dust from coming in.
- Use filters on your forced-air heating and cooling systems and change them regularly.
- Regularly dust your electronic equipment.
- If you have children, pay special attention to their play areas.
- Leave your shoes at the door and use a natural doormat.
- Choose home electronics free of fire retardant chemicals; many manufacturers carry them now. Ask before you buy.
- Clean up thoroughly after any home-improvement project.
- Consider getting a high-efficiency HEPA filter air cleaner for certain rooms in your home.

5: Feed Your Soul!

"After treatment, I thought, 'Yay, I'm done! I've gone three weeks now without seeing a doctor!' But then I would go into a depression. You think you're going to be great and you are excited, but at the same time you go into a depression. That caught me a little off guard. I was like, 'Why am I depressed? I'm done with treatment.' You're kind of adrift all of a sudden. You have to refigure who you are and what your life is about."

—Laurie, breast cancer survivor

After going through cancer, you may feel more out of control of your life than ever. Maybe you did everything you could—ate a healthy diet, exercised, and practiced regular stress relief—and you got cancer anyway. Or maybe you weren't that careful about your health, but you wonder what difference it will really make now.

"Cancer doesn't run in my family," says Deb, breast cancer survivor. "I was healthy, I exercised, and I ate well, so when I got cancer, I was like, 'What's going on?' When you get shocked like that, you think, well, if that can happen, anything can happen."

We've talked a lot about thoughts and emotions throughout this book, and how powerful, or detrimental, they can be in your healing process. Once treatments are over, take the time you need to process and heal all the emotions that come up. Once you've had the time to do that, try to start directing your thoughts toward positive places. Rest assured: You probably will have worries about the cancer coming back, and that's okay. You'd have to be a robot not to wonder about it now and then.

But here is where the things we've been talking about can be so helpful. Accept all the feelings you have, unconditionally, and get the help you need to process them. Make an appointment with a counselor, take an art therapy class, get into yoga, or try any of the coping techniques mentioned in Chapter 4. Start visualizing how you want the rest of your life to be, and begin focusing on that vision. If you're still fighting cancer in some way, think back to all the positive turning points you've had, and celebrate that you're still here, still fighting, and still living.

Best of all, think about it: You have a second chance at life. Now is a great time to take stock of where you are, what you're doing, and whether or not these things fulfill you and make you happy. In other words, it's time to listen to your soul.

"I think cancer made me take a deep breath and slow down," says Laurie, breast cancer survivor. "I've always considered myself very spiritual and artistic and all that, but I race through getting all my tasks done so much that I don't take time for introspection."

A lot of us end up experiencing the same feelings as Laurie had. We jump back into life, thinking we're going to do everything we did before, but find that it just doesn't cut it anymore. Rather than feel badly about these emotions, I encourage you to celebrate them. This is your soul's way of asking you—is it time to make some changes?

"You're not a victim, no matter what has happened in your life," says

Shanda Sumpter, one of my dearest friends and founder of HeartCore Bootcamp, an organization that helps woman reconnect with what they love. "Whether you've had a divorce, suffered an injury, gotten cancer... anything that has come up in your space. It's there to guide you to what you want so badly, to what we call your 'heart drive.'"

When you survive cancer, your outlook on life often changes. You may be less concerned with material things and more interested in following your deepest desires. "Cancer gives you the gift of clearly seeing the value of life—the value of *your* life," says Shanda. "What someone with cancer has over the average Joe is the appreciation and the sense of urgency for what life really is. Whatever you've wanted to do, whatever your passion is, what is the point of holding back now?"

Connecting with what you love can be a powerful healer. Shanda teaches women around the world to stop settling for simply surviving life and start stepping into a truly empowered life. "Most of us are society robots. We do what we've been told to do, or what we think we should do. If you connect with what you love, things like illnesses, stress, and other physical problems start to reverse themselves."

Like Dr. Eva said in Chapter 7, Shanda talks about the "love frequency," a personal vibration that people have when they're truly connected to their passion. We're all made of energy, and when we're vibrating in love, there's no room for fear, worry, stress, or other negative emotions—particularly those related to cancer recurrence. "When you're faced with cancer," she says, "your frequency goes flat. You need to realign your focus and bring your vibration back up."

Just because treatment is over doesn't mean your journey is over. You need to keep pumping those positive emotions throughout your body, and what better way than going after your dreams? "Everything comes down to focus," Shanda says. "What are you focusing on? If it's only the cancer, your vibration is going to continue to spiral down."

Tapping into our dreams raises our energy in ways nothing else can. If you need a reason to get back into life after cancer, take some time to ask yourself: What have I always wanted to do? What are the dreams I haven't fulfilled?

"Let's say your dream has been to open a dessert shop," says Shanda, "but you've never done it. Now is the time. Cancer has given you the gift of realizing the value of your life and your dreams. So even if you're lying in bed after a treatment, you can create your recipe plans, or the themes around your new shop. How are you going to decorate it? What will your logo look like? If we focus on our dreams, we begin to 'think' our way into them. Watch. You'll start to get excited. You'll sketch out a few designs. Maybe you'll think of a new ingredient to spice up your grandma's chewy brownies. After a few minutes of doing this, your vibration—your energy level—will come up. You'll feel a sense of purpose again. You'll be engaged in *life*, instead of just overwhelmed by cancer. And that's going to help you heal."

The power of this engagement, according to Shanda, is that it comes from love, which is the most powerful energy in the universe. "The cancer actually encourages you to get going on your dreams, to be authentic in who you really are. When you connect to what you love, there is no fear."

Once cancer treatments are over, I hope you'll take time to reevaluate your life. What do you really want? What would give you back your passion for living? The most wondrous thing about reconnecting with your dreams or your heart's desires is that it creates a spiral effect into every part of your life. For example, if you start getting excited about opening your dessert shop, you're probably going to be more likely to want to eat right and exercise. You're going to want to fuel your new energy so you can accomplish your dreams. You're going to start thinking positively about your future, which is going to move you out of the cancer funk and into a healthier, more vibrant life.

Cancer can leave you with a lot of "stuff" to deal with. It's important to take the time you need to process it, but don't let it get you down for long. Practice daily meditation, say your affirmations in front of the mirror, do something for yourself every day, and take some time to reconsider your dreams and how you might be able to make them come true. Above all, please remember: You're still here. You've survived. And life is waiting for you. Look around you. There is much beauty, magic, and love in this world. You're done with treatment. You've received your second chance. Get out there and enjoy it!

"I live every day for today. I've been told twice that I only have a short period of time to live. I don't think about yesterday, or what's going to happen tomorrow. I live for what makes me happy. I know people who think that's selfish, but if it's not going to make me happy, I don't do it."

—Alli, ovarian cancer survivor

Goals: My Plan to Boost My Immune System and Reduce My Risk of Recurrence

Though you can't control everything about your future, you *can* regain control over your daily habits, and raise your odds of staying healthy for years to come. Write down the steps you're going to take to create your healthy, strong body, mind, and soul. I've written in some examples for each step, then left room for you to add your own thoughts. You can do it!

Category	I Used To...	Now I'm Going To...
NUTRITION	Examples: Eat a lot of fast foods, pig out on sugary treats, etc.	Examples: Eat at least five fruits and vegetables a day; choose healthier desserts like fruit and yogurt.
EXERCISE	Examples: Avoid exercising except for my daily climb up the stairs; exercise sporadically and beat myself up for lack of consistency.	Examples: Commit to a 30-minute walk five times a week; sign up at the gym and grab a workout buddy to help me stay committed.
STRESS RELIEF	Examples: Run myself ragged trying to do everything perfectly; put my needs last.	Examples: Meditate at least 15 minutes a day; do something nice for myself at least once a week.

TOXINS	Example: Expose myself to several toxins every day.	Example: Be more careful of the products I buy and use on my skin.
POSITIVE THINKING	Example: Allow negative thoughts to run rampant in my mind.	Examples: Journal at least three times a week to get my negative thoughts out; write down what I'm grateful for at least once a week.
HEART POWER	Example: Ignore the little voice inside me that encouraged me to start my own business.	Example: Start taking steps toward making my dreams come true.

Belief: I am powerless, a victim of circumstance. I must find someone else to blame.

Change to: *I'm responsible and in control of my life. I can't control circumstances, but I can control my attitude toward them. The world is not what it is, but what I believe it to be.*

Belief: Life is a struggle. Something must be wrong if it seems easy or I'm having fun.

Change to: *Life is full. Life is potential. It's good to relax. It's okay to have fun. It is safe to feel happiness in my body.*

Belief: I'm not important. My feelings and needs are of no consequence.

Change to: *I'm a valuable and important person. I'm equal to anyone, but above no one. I am deserving of all the good things that life has to offer.*

Belief: I should always look my best and be happy, no matter how I feel.

Change to: *It's okay to be who I am. I am unique and it shows. I am at my best when I am myself.*

Belief: If I worry enough it will help.

Change to: *Worrying creates a negative energy that eats the one who worries. Actions change problems. Worry is exhausting. I will create energy, not destroy my energy.*

Belief: I'm not strong enough to cope with this.

Change to: *Whatever life deals me, it also deals me the ability to overcome the situation. Balance is a fact of life. Everything can be accomplished by taking small steps.*

Let's Review

- Experiencing fear about recurrence is normal. The important thing is to practice coping techniques like therapy, journaling, and meditation, and to take action and change the things you can change to rebuild a healthy body and regain your sense of control over your life.

- Worrying about recurrence is mostly about fear. Realize that fear is raising its ugly head, and take steps to manage it by monitoring your thoughts and questioning your assumptions.

- Eating a healthy diet has shown in studies to help reduce your risk of disease. Try to eat at least five fruits and vegetables each day, and cut back on fats and sugars.

- Exercise is like a magic bullet for your health. Find one or more types of exercise that you enjoy and commit to exercising at least five days a week.

- Stress can impair the immune system and leave you vulnerable to disease. Incorporate daily stress-relief methods into your life, like meditation, journaling, therapy, or exercise, and make sure you're taking time to encourage positive, relaxed emotions.

- Cancer survivors need to be especially aware of the toxins around them. Take control and reduce your exposure by buying organic produce, choosing eco-friendly household cleansers, reading the ingredient labels and purchasing safer personal care products, and keeping the dust level down in your living area.

- Regaining passion for your life is key to a successful survival. Take the time to reconnect to your dreams, and take steps toward accomplishing the things you've always wanted to do.

Personal Affirmations

I feel my body growing stronger every day.

I have optimal health now. I release the past.

I love myself. I love my body.

I'm excited about the endless possibilities my future holds for me!

Final Thoughts

AS I HOLD THE FINISHED MANUSCRIPT IN MY HANDS, I almost can't believe it. After much soul-searching, hard work, and help from so many people, my book is done. I feel a sweet sense of accomplishment, a deep sense of gratitude, and a feeling that somehow, I have helped complete the journey my father and I both took through this disease.

Reflection now takes me into the future, to when you, as a reader, will hold the book in your hands and come to the last pages. I wonder if there is anything else I might say that would help as you walk your own path through cancer. Thinking back on my experience and my father's from the perspective of a fighter, caregiver, and survivor, I ask myself: When all is said and done, what have I learned?

I think when we're faced with any sort of difficult challenge, we long for advice from those who have been there. From our perspective at the start or middle of the journey, we fear the unknown and want some guidance as to what to expect. We also want to know what we can do to help ourselves along the way. How can we increase our chances of survival? What can we do to better handle treatments? What information will help us to avoid unnecessary hardship?

My hope is that this book answered many of your questions, but I don't presume it answered them all. I'm sure you still have some left, and I trust you will find more information in the appendices, where I've listed many helpful organizations, including one that actually connects you with others who've survived the same type of cancer you have and are happy to talk with you. (See Imerman's Angels in Appendix II.) Please take advantage of these and all resources available, and continue your quest for information, support, and encouragement.

In the end, though, as I reflect on everything, I think what I've learned, most of all, is that we must listen to that little voice inside us and always believe we are worthy of the best life has to offer. Whether you call it the subconscious, the witness, intuition, or God, your inner voice knows what's right for you. You must listen and follow where it leads. Those of us who have lived with cancer share a bond, and many of us have similarities in our lives, but at the same time, each person is unique, each diagnosis is different, and each experience unlike any other. In the end, *you* are the foremost authority on your body, your health, and your spirit. Trust yourself.

I say this not only because of my experience, or my father's, but because of the experiences relayed to me by the survivors interviewed for this book. Over and over again, people told me stories of how listening to their intuition benefited them. Some *knew* something was wrong with their bodies, but the doctors and the medical tests determined everything was fine. It was only through persistence and unflinching belief in themselves that these survivors saved their own lives.

People told me they didn't feel comfortable with a particular doctor or oncologist, so they changed, and changed again and again if they had to, to find someone they felt was right, which made all the difference in the success of their treatments and their quality of life while going through them.

People told me how their doctors discouraged them from trying supplements, but when they finally decided to listen to their own voices and seek out alternative methods of nutrition, they felt more energy and vitality for life. People told me about receiving terminal diagnoses and then moving across the nation to go to a cancer center they believed in, which helped save their lives.

People told me how they realized, after their cancer experience, that they were in the wrong relationship, with a person who wasn't right for them, and regardless of what friends and family thought, they made a change that better suited their life path.

People told me how cancer made them stop and think about how they were running their lives and how, when they were given a second chance, they listened to the dreams they had previously ignored and went on to do amazing things, like start new businesses, create helpful organizations, go back to school, or do a bit of traveling.

All these wonderful survivors may have been told a myriad of things from a plethora of "experts," but in the end, they listened to the voices inside them and heeded what they heard. For many of us, this is a difficult thing to do. We lack trust in ourselves. We think others are smarter, more experienced, or stronger than we are, so we defer to their way of thinking, whether or not it's right for us. We may hear that little voice inside us, but we look for answers elsewhere, sure that we can't *know* what's truly best for us.

Understand one thing: You *do* know what's best for you, always. You know, somewhere deep down inside, when something feels right and when it feels wrong. Sometimes you just have to slow down, be still, and listen. You know your body better than anyone, and you know what makes you feel good and what makes you feel bad. You know what helps you get through and what makes you feel defeated and hopeless.

My hope for you, as you complete this book, is that you listen to your inner voice and follow it, no matter what. If your doctor has told you your cancer is gone, yet you feel somewhere inside that something's wrong, don't be afraid to go back, and go back, until your concerns are alleviated.

If you don't feel right about a certain doctor, find another one. If a medication is tearing you up, go back and ask for something else. If your side effects are becoming more than you can stand, speak up. If you're not getting the support you need, look for it somewhere else; don't expect to get help from people who have so far disappointed you. And never, never, never allow someone to discourage you, tear you down, or make you doubt yourself.

Life is too short to be constantly questioning your own inner wisdom. I realize now, as I look back, that my father and I were lucky, both in the treatments we received and the support that surrounded us. But we also had high expectations. We expected to be treated well and to regain our health. We expected to have access to the most advanced treatments and to be cared for with dignity and respect. When we didn't have the resources we needed, we asked for help so we could find them. We never questioned whether doing something for ourselves was the right thing to do; we knew it would help us heal.

Simply put, we never questioned that we were *worthy* of the best—the best doctors, the best treatments, the best medications, the best solutions for side effects, the best alternative medicines, and the best support we could find.

Cancer will change you, but never let it make you believe you're anything but whole, precious, and worthy of the best solutions you can find. No matter what your fate, you deserve to enjoy the highest quality of life possible. Listen to yourself, follow your intuition, and never give up.

Never
give
up.

Love, strength, and survival,
Britta

Acknowledgements

THIS BOOK HAS BEEN A LABOR OF LOVE, NOT JUST FOR ME, but for all the many people who have supported me along the way, and I want to take a moment to sincerely thank everyone involved for giving so generously of their time, expertise, and compassion. Cancer is a journey shared by so many, something that brings us all together in a common bond that spans any age, distance, or background. Rest assured that if you've read this book, you've shared that journey with us, and we welcome you and hope you're feeling a little stronger now than you did when you first opened these pages.

First of all, I want to thank all the contributing experts, who were happy to spend their valuable time sharing the knowledge they have taken so many years to acquire. Through this book, their words are reaching even more people every day, and I'm so grateful for their willingness to help.

To the survivors, fighters, and caregivers who so graciously shared their experiences, strength, and hope, I offer my heartfelt gratitude and a giant hug for every one of you. Never was I so inspired than when I heard your stories of struggle, despair, and ultimate triumph as you all found your way to your best selves, despite this disease. To Alli, Chris, Deb, Dee, Heather, Hillary, Jamie, Jarrod, Joanna, Jody, Justin, Karen, Kate, Laura, Laurie, Lynn, Meghan, Rayette, Susan, Teresa, and Vel—you have confirmed my faith in the indomitable human spirit.

I feel as though the whole time I was working on this book, my father was watching over me—and smiling. He always wanted to write a book about his experiences, and I believe if he were here now, he would be ecstatic to hold this creation in his hands. Somewhere, somehow, I believe he knows it's here, and that we did it. I want to thank you, Dad, for everything you taught me, everything you gave me, and for showing me, through your courageous example, how to rise up and fight, not once, but again and again, as many times as it takes.

How do you thank a mother? My mother cared for me not only for my entire childhood, but through my own cancer journey, which I know was deeply stressful and heartbreaking for her. She was so precious in her strength and her consistent care, no matter how tough things got. I can never thank you enough, Mom, for everything you've done for me.

To Husayn, my husband, business partner, cheerleader, and voice of reason through this entire project, I thank you from the bottom of my heart! Without you, none of this would have been possible. My aunt, Chris, not only shared her cancer journey with me and allowed me to share her story in these pages, but also did me the honor of being one of my first readers—thank you! To my Uncle Raul, I very much appreciate your advice and guidance, and your belief in me and support for all my endeavors. My brother, Javier Jr., has always loaned me his shoulder to lean on and was kind enough to listen to me cry when a particular chapter brought back strong memories of my father. Thank you for continuing to encourage me and love me as we walk our life paths together. I want to thank the entire Aragon family—my aunts, uncles, and all my cousins—for always being there for me. I feel so fortunate to have such a supportive family who have always believed in me.

So many people have contributed to actually putting this book together. To my editor, Colleen Story, without whom I would not have been able to do this project—thank you for working so tenaciously and on schedule. To my lawyer, Michael Steger, thank you for taking care of any legal questions and making it all seem so easy. Alan Hebel and Ian Shimkoviak at The Book Designers turned my vision into a stunning presentation with their graphic design; thanks, guys! Katherine Stimson at Stimson Indexing put the index together beautifully. I didn't know before meeting her that indexing was a true profession! Carol Gaskin at Editorial Alchemy helped us put on the finishing touches with her editing, and Amy MacGregor and Bethany Brown of Cadence Marketing kept me laughing all the way to the bookstores while sharing great advice on the whole distrubution process.

There are other people I want to thank, for without them I might not even be here to write a book. Those are the people who helped me through my own cancer journey—my oncologist, Dr. Klimo, who fought the medical fight for me and won; all the caring nurses at Lions Gate Hospital in North Vancouver who took such good care of me and who always made my father smile; and to all my dear girlfriends—Alisa (also my cousin), Helena, Alison, Laurie, Anny, Shanda, Christine, and Carissa—who were there for me through my toughest times and who gave me strength when I couldn't get up, I love you all.

Don Wilhelm, who wrote his own book about surviving cancer, was willing to share with me what he'd learned about the writing and publishing process. Thank you, Don, and I wish you strength as you continue your journey. Jacqueline Wales, who also wrote her own book, *The Fearless Factor*, shared her journey as an author and introduced me to the girls at Cadence. My thanks, Jacqueline. Dawn Mellowship, author of *Toxic Beauty*, shares my passion about toxic chemicals in personal care products and gave me lots of tips about writing and publishing, for which I'm very grateful.

As some of you may know, Cinco Vidas was the first project in my efforts to give back to the cancer community. Thank you to the whole Cinco Vidas team for staying true to the vision, and to Liz Martin, for continuing to be my sounding board and advisor on all projects. Thank you for caring so much. And to all of you on Facebook and Twitter—I'm so blessed to have your contributions! You provide so much support to our efforts, and I hope you will continue to be involved.

Finally, I send a big hug to my life coach and dearest friend, Jennifer, who helped me stay true to who I am and who has helped me with all of my dreams, one step at a time. To Ora, an angel who came into my life four weeks before my father passed and has been by my side to support me through this whole process—thank you for reading my book in its early stages and giving me your invaluable feedback. Many blessings! I thank God for sending me the message through my dreams that this is my journey, and that this book was such an important part of it.

Above all, I thank all the people out there living with cancer. Whether it's fighting the disease, surviving it, or caring for someone who has it, you all contribute to helping us eventually find a cure for this disease, and in the meantime, find ways to support each other through it. Thank you for your compassion. It's the best gift we can give each other—the knowledge that we are not alone.

Appendix I
Contributing Experts

Judi Beerling is a Technical Research Manager who works with Organic Monitor. She regularly lectures and leads workshops on natural and organic raw materials at major worldwide industry events, such as In-Cosmetics and Organic Monitor's own Sustainable Cosmetics Summit (held both in Europe and the U.S.). She holds an MBA from the Open University Business School and is a Chartered Chemist, the Treasurer of the International Federation of Societies of Cosmetic Chemists (IFSCC), and a recent past president of the U.K. Society of Cosmetic Scientists (SCS).

Starr Carson Cleary is a certified master fitness trainer, advanced Pilates instructor, cancer-exercise specialist, and motivational speaker. A wellness educator in many facets of the fitness industry since 1999, Starr developed the StarrPower Restorative Pilates program for cancer survivors to help them regain strength and mobility after treatment. Starr is the author of *A Woman's Guide…30 Days to a Better Mind, Body and Spirit* and the producer of the "StarrPower Pilates" DVD. www.bodybystarr.com

Mórag Currin, L.A., C.M.L.T., president of Touch For Cancer Online, Mórag Currin Method of Oncology Esthetics (MCMOE), and author of *Oncology Esthetics: A Practitioner's Guide*, is originally from South Africa. Recognizing the lack of specialized skin care available for people undergoing cancer therapies, she has pioneered a Clinical Oncology Esthetics (COE) certification for licensed estheticians and has written a textbook on the subject. Her work has appeared in many national and international publications, including "Skin Inc.," "Les Nouvelle Esthetiques," "Dermascope," and others. www.touchforcanceronline.com

Alan Dattner, M.D., holistic dermatologist, is a pioneer in the field, developing natural, unique, and individual solutions for hard-to-treat skin and inflammation disorders for the past thirty years. A preceptee at Sloan-Kettering Institute for Cancer Research, investigating tumor immunology, he completed residencies at the Contra Costa Country Hospital and Albert Einstein College of Medicine. Dr. Dattner is board certified by the American Academy of Dermatology (AAD), founder and president of HolisticDermatology.com and HealthDataLink.com, and author of an upcoming book on holistic dermatology, tentatively titled *Heal Your Skin, Heal Your Life*. www.drdattner.com

Stephen H. Green, M.D., F.A.C.S., is a board certified surgeon specializing in diseases and surgery of the breast. He is currently an attending breast surgical oncologist at Brookhaven Memorial Hospital Medical Center, where he is chairman of the breast tumor board. Dr. Green lectures extensively on benign breast diseases and cancer of the breast, is a consultant for pharmaceutical companies regarding breast cancer medications, and is called upon to give expert testimony in legal issues involving breast cancer.

Fran Greenfield, a life coach specializing in mind/body medicine, has studied and taught mind/body healing for the past twenty-five years, lecturing on mind/body medicine at Columbia University's College of Physicians and Surgeons, Beth Israel Medical Center in New York, and at Dartmouth College. She has also consulted for SHARE, the Virginia Breast Cancer Foundation, and the American Infertility Association. She has co-authored a book, *Asthma Free in 21 Days*, and has also written for the *New York Times* and for *Spirituality and Health* magazine.

Laura Kupperman is a certified yoga therapist, certified yoga teacher, and life coach. For her own recovery from breast cancer, she relied heavily on her yoga practice and other holistic modalities to help her through chemotherapy and five major surgeries. She now teaches yoga classes, workshops, and private sessions to cancer survivors in Colorado, and also trains other yoga teachers wanting to work with cancer survivors. A graduate of Coach U, Laura holds a B.A. from Wellesley College and an M.A. from Stanford University. www.laurakupperman.com

Jean Lazar, energy medicine practitioner and massage therapist, has been with Hospice of South Eastern Connecticut for twelve years, working in different capacities. In the last five years with Hospice, she has been giving compassionate touch in the form of Reiki and Massage Therapy to the terminally ill, while comforting their loved ones. In addition to her Hospice caregiving, she's presently training to become a teacher at Connecticut

Center for Massage Therapy. Her book, *Their Last Painting: Stories of Life That Will Rock Your Heart*, is available at www.jeanlazar.com.

Dawn Mellowship is an author, freelance journalist, ethical stylist, and a Reiki practitioner and teacher. The Reiki work of Dawn and her partner, Andy Chrysostomou, has been featured in a range of publications, including: *Natural Health and Beauty*, *Health and Fitness*, *Healthy*, *TNT*, and *Positive Health*. Dawn's ethical styling work was recently featured on the website *Hippyshoppe* and in *New Consumer*, *The Daily Mail*, and *Natural Health Magazine*. She is the author of several books, including *Toxic Beauty*, which highlights the key chemicals you should avoid. www.dawnmellowship.com

Michelle Maniaci, licensed physical therapist, energy medicine practitioner, bellydance for healing teacher, yoga therapist, and infant massage instructor, integrates modern science with ancient energetic wisdom so individuals may learn simple and highly effective techniques to maximize self-healing and to live their life to the fullest. Michelle is founder and creator of NURTURING MOVES®, a wellness and healing approach that is also a form of birth preparation and injury prevention designed to educate, empower, awaken, and heal our world. www.nurturingmoves.com

Colleen O'Neil, R.N., has worked in various specialties, including pediatrics, maternity, emergency, ICU, and general medicine and surgery. She has spent the past fifteen years working in palliative care (end-of-life oncology practice). In 2005 she was diagnosed with breast cancer. Since her recovery she has reached out to other newly diagnosed women with breast cancer through the Canadian Cancer Society, where she performs peer counseling to help guide women through the diagnosis and treatment phase of their disease.

Eva M. Selhub, M.D., is an instructor in medicine at Harvard Medical School, having served from 1999 until the end of 2007 as Medical Director of Mind/Body Medical Institute. Now part of the world-renowned Massachusetts General Hospital, Dr. Selhub serves as Senior Clinical Affiliate Physician. She has lectured throughout the United States and in Europe and trained healthcare professionals from all over the world. She has also written several books and appeared on national television and radio programs. She currently runs a private practice and business in Integrative Medicine and Executive Coaching. www.theloveresponse.com

Donielle Wilson, N.D., C.P.M., graduated from Bastyr University in 2000 with a doctorate in naturopathic medicine and a certificate in midwifery. She was awarded the NYANP Naturopathic Physician of the Year award in 2004. Dr. Wilson works with cancer patients, helping them to identify underlying causes and to minimize the side effects of conventional therapies by using evidence-based natural therapies like diet, supplements, herbs, and homeopathy. She has presented at the annual Breast Cancer Options Conference in NY on several occasions. www.doctordoni.com

Jacqueline Wales is founder and president of the motivational company The Fearless Factor and is also the author of several books, including *The Fearless Factor,* which teaches people how to move beyond fear. Her programs have successfully helped women around the globe navigate the murky waters of change to become more confident and overcome their challenges. Jacqueline fills the hearts and minds of those she touches with the unmistakable realization that anything is possible. www.thefearlessfactor.com.

Appendix II
Contributing Organizations

4women.com
Susan Beausang is President of 4Women.com and designer of the newly patented BeauBeau® headscarf. www.4women.com

Campaign for Safe Cosmetics
Stacey Malkan is co-founder of the national Campaign for Safe Cosmetics and author of the award-winning book, *Not Just a Pretty Face: The Ugly Side of the Beauty Industry.* www.notjustaprettyface.org

Faye's Light
Vicky Weis is the founder and executive director of Faye's Light, a non-profit organization providing *Cancer Comfort Treatments* to men and women in active treatment for cancer. www.fayeslight.org

HeartCore Women
Shanda Sumpter is the founder of HeartCore Women, an organization committed to breeding a new authentic woman who lives in her authentic energy, in an environment of real support. www.heartcorewomen.com

Imerman Angels
Jonny Imerman is the founder of Imerman Angels, a nonprofit organization created on the belief that no one should have to fight cancer alone and without the necessary support. www.imermanangels.org

This Time's a Charm
Don Wilhelm is a five-time cancer survivor and author of the book *This Time's a Charm,* in which he offers up his real-life experiences for those newly diagnosed with cancer and their loved ones. www.thistimesacharm.com

Appendix III
Some of My Favorite Resources

Breast Cancer Action: Started by women in a San Francisco breast cancer support group, BCA advocates for policy change and provides information via newsletters, websites, and a toll-free number. www.bcaction.org

Breast Cancer Fund: Works to educate the public about the relationship between breast cancer and exposure to chemicals and radiation in our everyday environments. www.breastcancerfund.org

CancerCompass: Create your own personalized profile page and build your own network of friends. www.cancercompass.com

Cancer and Careers: The website, free publications, and a series of educational seminars all help employees with cancer decide what's best for them. www.cancerandcareers.org

Cancer Prevention Coalition: A nationwide coalition of leading independent experts in cancer prevention and public health, (CPC) works together with other activists and health groups to help reduce cancer rates. www.preventcancer.com

Cancer Schmancer Movement: Dedicated to saving women's lives through early detection of cancer, this organization was founded by survivor and actress Fran Drescher. www.cancerschmancer.org

Cinco Vidas: My website, so of course it's one of my favorites! Find articles here on side effects, alternative medicine, great cancer organizations, spa and wig shop directories, my Ingredients to Avoid card, survivor stories, nutrition, updates on toxic ingredients, and much more. Read, comment, and share! www.cincovidas.com

Crazy, Sexy Life: Bestselling author and motivational speaker Kris Carr inspires individuals and their families to make the link between personal and planetary health by adopting a plant-based diet and improving lifestyle choices. www.crazysexylife.com

Environmental Working Group (EWG): Founded in 1993, the EWG seeks to protect public health, particularly against problems attributed to a wide variety of toxic contaminants. www.ewg.org

Gilda's Club: Named in honor of *Saturday Night Live* comedian Gilda Radner, who died of ovarian cancer in 1989, the club develops strategies and leads activities that provide emotional and social support for people with cancer and their families and friends. www.gildasclub.org

I'm Too Young for This! Cancer Foundation: The Voice of Young Adults: Provides programs just for young adults, with loads of resources and connection possibilities. www.i2y.com

Juntos Foundation: Works with community research and treatment programs to raise awareness and promote early detection of disease. One of my good friends, Lou Moll, is on the board and works with other members to raise money and assist in research efforts to find a cure. www.juntosfoundation.org

Lance Armstrong Foundation (LAF): Founded by cancer survivor and champion cyclist Lance Armstrong, LAF empowers cancer survivors to live life on their own terms. www.livestrong.com

Let Cancer Heal Your Life: Jackie Poper, a fellow cancer survivor and a great friend, is a Certified Personal Coach who helps survivors cope with life after cancer. She offers private one-on-one coaching, as well as programs like "From Survivorship to Thrivorship," and "Building the Heart-Centered Business for Cancer Survivors." www.letcancerhealyourlife.com

Locks of Love: Provides hairpieces to financially disadvantaged children suffering from long-term medical hair loss. www.locksoflove.org

LUNGevity Foundation: Envisioning a world where no one dies from lung cancer, LUNGevity works to bring the disease to the forefront of the nation's awareness. They fund life-saving research, bring together world-class scientific minds and passionate advocates, and offer training and support for education. The organization also provides an online Lung Cancer Support Community, Ask the Experts and Link Up advocacy programs. www.lungevity.org

LYT: This is my holistic sanctuary in NYC. LYT (Love Your Transformation) offers organic, fresh-pressed juices and your choice of services, including B.E.S.T. technique (energy-balancing procedure), acupuncture, biomagnetic therapy, facial rejuvenation, massage therapy, colon hydrotherapy, and more. www.lytnyc.com

Navigating Cancer: Includes information on all different types of cancer, tools to help you navigate treatment and recovery, and helpful ways to stay connected with those you care about. www.navigatingcancer.com

Planet Cancer: Created for young adults living with cancer, Planet Cancer is an online community where participants can share with others going through the same experience. www.planetcancer.org

Think Before You Pink: A project of Breast Cancer Action, Think Before You Pink launched in 2002, calling for more transparency and accountability by companies that take part in fundraising, and encouraging consumers to ask critical questions. www.thinkbeforeyoupink.org

You Can Thrive: Founded in New York City in 2005 by breast cancer survivor Luana Halpern, this community works to ease the journey for people with cancer, opening the doors to their Integrative Wellness Center for Breast Cancer in 2007. www.youcanthrive.org

Young Survival Coalition (YSC): Dedicated to critical issues facing young women with breast cancer, YSC works to increase the quality and quantity of life for women aged forty and under who are diagnosed with breast cancer. www.youngsurvival.org

Appendix IV
My Favorites: Books, CDs, DVDs

Books

- *A New Earth: Awakening to Your Life's Purpose* (Eckart Tolle)

- *A Return to Love: Reflections on the Principles of "A Course in Miracles"* (Marianne Williamson)

- *Anti-Cancer: A New Way of Life* (Dr. Servan-Schreiber)

- *Creative Visualization: Use the Power of Your Imagination to Create What You Want in Your Life* (Shakti Gawain)

- *Exposed: The Toxic Chemistry of Everyday Products and What's at Stake for American Power* (Mark Schapiro)

- *Feel the Fear and Do it Anyway* (Susan Jeffers)

- *It's Not About the Bike: My Journey Back to Life* (Lance Armstrong)

- *Love, Medicine, and Miracles: Lessons Learned about Self-Healing from a Surgeon's Experience with Exceptional Patients* (Bernie S. Siegel)

- *Life!: Reflections on Your Journey* (Louise Hay)

- *Love is the Answer* (Gerald Jampolsky and Diane V. Cirincione)

- *No More Dirty Looks: The Truth About Your Beauty Products—and the Ultimate Guide to Safe and Clean Cosmetics* (Siobhan O'Conner and Alexandra Spunt)

- *Not Just a Pretty Face: the Ugly Side of the Beauty Industry* (Stacy Malkan)

- *Peace, Love, and Healing: Bodymind Communication & the Path to Self-Healing: An Exploration* (Bernie S. Siegel)

- *Picking Up the Pieces: Moving Forward after Surviving Cancer* (Sherri Magee and Kathy Scalzo)

- *Return to Wholeness: Embracing Body, Mind, and Spirit in the Face of Cancer* (David Simon, M.D.)

- *Slow Death by Rubber Duck: The Secret Danger of Everyday Things* (Rick Smith and Bruce Lourie)

- *The Cancer-Fighting Kitchen: Nourishing, Big-Flavor Recipes for Cancer Treatment and Recovery* (Rebecca Katz and Mat Edelson)

- *The Fearless Factor* (Jacqueline Wales)

- *The Love Response: Your Prescription to Turn Off Fear, Anger, and Anxiety to Achieve Vibrant Health and Transform Your Life* (Eva M. Selhub)

- *The Power is Within You* (Louise Hay)

- *This Time's a Charm: Lessons of a Four-Time Cancer Survivor* (Donald Wilhelm)

- *Toxic Beauty: How Cosmetics and Personal Care Products Endanger Your Health... And What You Can Do about It* (Samuel S. Epstein, M.D. and Randall Fitzgerald)

- *Toxic Beauty: The Hidden Chemicals in Cosmetics and How They Can Harm Us* (Dawn Mellowship)

- *You Can Heal Your Life* (Louise Hay)

- *Your Brain After Chemo: A Practical Guide to Lifting the Fog and Getting Back Your Focus* (Dr. Daniel Silverman)

Meditations/CDs/VIDEOS

Note: Many of these can be found at HealingJourneys.com.

- *Affirmations for Living Beyond Cancer* (Bernie Siegel, M.D.)

- *Cancer: Discovering Your Healing Power* (Louise Hay)

- *Chemotherapy* (Belleruth Naparstek)

- *Fatigue (Oncology Treatment Related)* (Belleruth Naparstek)

- *General Wellness* (Belleruth Naparstek)

- *Healthy Immune System* (Belleruth Naparstek)

- *Managing the Distress of Cancer and Its Treatment* (Carolyn Daitch)

- *Meditation to Help You Fight Cancer* (Belleruth Naparstek and Steven Mark Kohn)

- *Radiation Therapy* (Belleruth Naparstek)

- *StarrPower Restorative Pilates for Cancer Survivors* (Starr Carson Cleary)

- *The Story of Cosmetics* (online 7-minute video) www.storyofstuff.org/cosmetics

- *Successful Surgery* (Belleruth Naparstek)

- *Yoga and the Gentle Art of Healing—A Journey of Recovery After Breast Cancer* (Susan Rosen)

Appendix V
Ingredients to Avoid
in Personal Care Products

Aluminum is a chemical salt with absorbent and disinfectant properties. It's often used in deodorants and antiperspirants, and is easily absorbed into the skin. A recent study of breast cancer patients found higher amounts of aluminum in the outer regions of the breast where antiperspirant is usually applied. A study in the *Journal of Toxicology and Environmental Health* showed that aluminum accumulation in body tissues leads to impaired kidney function, bone disease, and tissue damage. [Aug 1996; 48(6):649-65] Aluminum has also been found in the brains of Alzheimer's patients.

Animal testing has left many innocent creatures maimed, diseased, and crippled. Scientists are developing new ways to test cosmetics that do not require the needless suffering of animals. We may further discourage the practice by refusing to purchase products from companies that perform animal testing.

Acetone is a strong solvent used in many nail-polish removers (as well as in some paints and varnishes). It's known to irritate the eyes and lungs, and can cause redness and irritation of skin.

Chemical sunscreens, like oxybenzone, benzophenone-3, and octyl methoxycinnamate, have been shown to disrupt endocrine activity. Oxybenzone is absorbed into the skin where it filters UV light, converting it from light to heat, which may damage growing cells. Titanium dioxide and zinc oxide are safer alternatives.

1,4-Dioxane is a chemical byproduct that's not included on many ingredient lists. Produced by the ethoxylation process in cosmetics manufacturing, it's a known animal carcinogen and penetrates readily into the skin. When ethylene oxide is added to sulfates to soften them, 1,4-dioxane is born. More than fifty-six cosmetic ingredients are associated with this chemical. Look out for "sodium myreth sulfate," "PEG," "oxynol," "ceteareth," "oleth," and "polyethylene."

Disodium-EDTA is a salt used in cosmetics and personal care products, often as a penetration enhancer, allowing other chemicals to penetrate deeper into the skin, as well as a "chelating" agent that improves the performance of cleansing products. It is found in contact solution, eye drops, shower and bath products, and more. Though approved as safe by the FDA, high doses have been shown in some studies to disrupt hormone function and mutate cells.

Ethyl acetate is a flammable liquid used as a solvent in many cosmetics, including nail polish remover, perfume, shampoo, and aftershave. (It's also used in paint remover and dishwashing liquid.) Listed on the EPA's Hazardous Waste list, it's known to be irritating to the eyes and respiratory tract and may potentially depress the nervous system. Avoid at all costs, especially on your face.

Formaldehyde is a colorless gas and a known carcinogen used in many nail polishes. The U.S. National Toxicology Program lists it as "reasonably anticipated to cause cancer." It can also cause allergic reactions, contact dermatitis, headaches, and chronic fatigue. Lab studies have shown that rats exposed to the vapors developed nasal cancer.

Fragrance (synthetic) may contain as many as 200 undeclared ingredients. Some of them can be phthalates—hormone-altering preservatives. There is often no way of knowing, since companies don't have to reveal the chemical constituents of a fragrance. They can just list it as "fragrance," when it may contain hundreds of chemicals. Potential problems include: headaches, coughing, vomiting, skin rashes, hyperpigmentation, allergies, and dizziness. Caution: Avoid the use any product with the word "fragrance" in the ingredient list, unless the label indicates it's derived from essential oils.

Hydroquinone is a lightening compound that inhibits the production of skin pigmentation and is used to lighten melasma, freckles, age spots, and other skin discolorations. It's known to increase exposure to UVA and UVB rays, and has been found to be mutagenic in laboratory studies. Hydroquinone can cause contact dermatitis as well as degeneration of collagen and elastin fibers. The Environmental Working Group has assigned a hazardous warning to this compound. Doctors advise women to avoid using it during pregnancy or nursing. In rare cases, it can cause "ochronosis," a discoloration in dark-skinned people. Studies have shown liver effects at low doses, and tests on mammal cells have shown hydroquinone to have mutation (possibly carcinogenic) properties.

Lead has been found in 61 percent of lipsticks tested by the Campaign for Safe Cosmetics. It's a proven neurotoxin that can interfere with fetal development. It's also been linked to infertility and miscarriage. It's usually not shown on the ingredient list. Check the Safe Cosmetics Database (www. cosmeticsdatabase.com) for brands without lead.

Parabens (including methyl, propyl, butyl, and ethyl parabens) are a group of preservatives used to extend the shelf life of cosmetic products. Estimates say over 90 percent of all cosmetics contain parabens. A 2006 study took urine samples from 100 adults and found two of these parabens (methyl- and n-propyl) in over 90 percent of them, with other parabens showing up in over half the samples. (*Environ Health Perspect.* 114 (12) 2006). Studies have also shown them to be estrogenic and capable of being absorbed by the body through the skin.

Petrochemicals are derived from petroleum and include mineral oil, toluene, and petroleum oil. Petroleum is an economical mineral oil used for its emollient properties in cosmetics. It has no nutrient value for the skin and can produce photosensitivity. It may also interfere with the body's own natural moisturizing mechanism, leading to dryness. Oddly enough, this ingredient often creates the conditions it claims to alleviate. Petroleum by-products coat the skin like plastic, clogging the pores. They interfere with skin's ability to eliminate toxins, promoting acne and other disorders. They also slow skin function and cell development, resulting in premature aging. Watch out on this one—it's used in many products. Even baby oil is 100 percent mineral oil. In addition, any mineral oil derivative can also be contaminated with cancer-causing PAHs (polycyclic aromatic hydrocarbons).

Phthalates are chemicals produced from oil and used to make plastics. They're also used as solvents in cosmetic products like nail polishes, perfumes, and hairsprays. (They help the product cling to the nail, hair, or skin.) These chemicals are readily absorbed by our fingernails, skin, and lungs. Animal studies with phthalates have resulted in damage to kidneys, liver, lungs, and reproductive systems. Human studies identified developmental abnormalities in male infants correlating to high phthalate levels in their mothers' bodies. These compounds can lead to liver cancer and birth defects in lab animals. Watch out for ingredients like dibutyl phthalate (DBP), butylbenzylphthalate (BBP), and di(2-ethylhexyl) phthalate (DEHP).

Propylene glycol is a synthetic petrochemical mix used as a humectant—a substance that promotes moisture retention and keeps products from drying out. It has been known to cause allergic reactions, hives, and eczema. This chemical is also drying to the skin. When you see PEG (polyethylene glycol) or PPG (polypropylene glycol) on labels, beware—these are related synthetics.

Silicone-derived emollients are derived from silica and are used as water-binding agents (moisturizers) in cosmetics. These emollients, however, are occlusive—they coat the skin and don't allow it to breathe (much like plastic wrap would do.) Recent studies have indicated that prolonged exposure of the skin to sweat, by occlusion, causes skin irritation. Some synthetic emollients are known tumor promoters and accumulate in the liver and lymph nodes. They are also non-biodegradable, negatively impacting the environment. They include dimethicone, dimethicone copolyol, and cyclomethicone.

Stearalkonium chloride is an anti-static agent used in hair conditioners and creams. It can cause allergic reactions and is known to irritate skin. Developed by the fabric industry as a fabric softener, it's a lot cheaper to use in hair-conditioning formulas than more beneficial ingredients like proteins and herbals.

Synthetic dyes are used to make cosmetics look "pretty," but are often made up of unrevealed, unsafe ingredients. They may be labeled as FD&C or D&C, followed by a color or a number (e.g., FD&C yellow No. 5). Most come from coal tar and are known to be carcinogenic. If they are on the ingredient list, do not use the product.

Sulfates (like sodium lauryl and sodium laureth) are cheap, harsh detergents used in shampoos, body washes, and face cleansers for cleansing and foam-building properties. They can cause eye irritations, skin rashes, hair loss, dry skin, and allergic reactions. Sulfates are frequently disguised with the explanation that they "come from coconut." The *Journal of the American College of Toxicology* concluded that through skin absorption, sulfates enter and maintain residual levels in the heart, lungs, and the brain. It also noted that sodium lauryl sulfate has a degenerative effect on the cell membranes because of its protein-denaturing properties. High levels of skin penetration may occur at even low-dose concentration.

Talc is a mineral widely used as talcum powder. According to the American Cancer Society, talcum powder particles applied to the genital area, on sanitary napkins, or on condoms may migrate to the ovaries, where they can cause damage. Studies have found a higher risk of ovarian cancer among talc users. Talc can also be found in antacids, garden pesticides, some deodorants, and baby powders. Because the particles are ground to such a small size, they are easily carried in the air, like dust, and can get into the lungs.

TEA, MEA, DEA are ammonia compounds often used in cosmetics as emulsifiers and/or foaming agents. DEA can also be found in some pesticides and is listed by the World Health Organization as an unclassified carcinogen. These chemicals contain ammonia compounds and can cause allergic reactions, eye irritation, and dryness of hair and skin. Any of the three can be toxic if absorbed into the body for a long period of time. If they come in contact with nitrates, they can form harmful nitrosamines, which can be carcinogenic.

Toluene is used in nail polishes to make the polish form a smooth color across the nail. It affects the nervous system and can cause fatigue, mental confusion, dizziness, nausea, and headaches. Toluene may also negatively affect reproduction and fetal development.

Triclosan is an antibacterial and antifungal agent present in all kinds of personal care, home care, and dental products—even though the FDA has reported that there is no evidence that antibacterial products protect people any better than regular soap. Triclosan has a chemical structure similar to dioxin—a class of toxic chemicals formed as by-products of the manufacture of chlorine-containing products. This similarity could lead to contamination of triclosan with dioxins. The agent has also been shown to be an endocrine disruptor and is accumulating in our soils and farm fields. Because of its widespread use, it may result in germs resistant to it.

Ureas are synthetic ingredients widely used as preservatives as well as water-binding and exfoliating ingredients. (Also known as diazolidinyl urea, imidazolidinyl urea, or DMDM hydantoin and sodium hydroxymeth-ylglycinate.) The American Academy of Dermatology has found them to be a primary cause for contact dermatitis. Urea has also been shown to release formaldehyde. Non-synthetic forms are derived from animal urine.

Sources include:
Cosmetic Dictionary, Campaign for Safe Cosmetics, and the Environmental Working Group (EWG).

Appendix VI
Ingredients to Avoid in Foods

Artifical Colorings like Blue 1, Blue 2, Green 3, and Yellow 6 create color in foods like candy, soda pop, baked goods, fruit snacks, and many others. These are synthetic, man-made chemicals, and all four of these have been linked to cancer in various animal studies. Results are inconclusive, but further tests have yet to be completed. Some artificial colorings are also known to cause allergy-like hypersensitivity reactions, and to trigger hypersensitivity in some children.

Artificial Sweeteners like acesulfame-K, aspartame, and saccharine are found in all sorts of sweetened foods and beverages. Acesulfame-K is found in baked goods, chewing gum, diet soda, and gelatin desserts. Animal studies have suggested it may cause cancer. Aspartame (NutraSweet) is a chemical combination of two amino acids and methanol, and has been linked to brain tumors in animals. Saccharine is 350 times sweeter than sugar and used in diet foods or as a tabletop sugar substitute. Many animal studies have shown saccharin to cause cancer of the urinary bladder, and an epidemiology study done by the National Cancer Institute found that the use of artificial sweeteners like saccharin was associated with a higher incidence of bladder cancer.

BHA and BHT are antioxidant compounds that retard rancidity in fats, oils, and oil-containing foods. Results are inconclusive, but some studies show that they cause cancer in rats, mice, and hamsters.

BPA is a chemical used to make plastics, as well as an ingredient in the material used to line metal food and drink cans. It's been linked to breast cancer because of its ability to mimic female hormones, as well as to prostate cancer, and has been shown to have adverse effects on childhood development. A recent study found that levels of BPA in many good-for-you foods like vegetables and fruits are as high as those found to cause harm in animal studies.

Carmine (Cochineal Extract) is an artificial coloring obtained from the cochineal insect, which lives in Peru, the Canary Islands, and other locations. Carmine is a more purified coloring made from cochineal. These colorings appear to be safe, but can cause allergic reactions in some people, including hives and even anaphylactic shock. Some products hide the actual preservative on the ingredient label as "artificial coloring" or "color added," but the FDA has ordered that by 2011, products are supposed to list the source to help people identify this possible source of allergic reactions.

Caramel Coloring in dark-colored colas like Coca-Cola and Pepsi has recently come under scrutiny because of its possible connection to a very rare type of cancer. The Center for Science in the Public Interest (CSPI) filed a petition with the FDA early in 2011 stating that this caramel coloring should be banned because its made by reacting sugars with ammonia and sulfates under high pressure and temperatures.[2] Chemical reactions in the process produce 2-methylimidazole and r-methylimidazole, which in government conducted animal studies, caused cancer. More studies need to be done, but for those who drink a lot of dark-colored soda, it's good to know about the possible risk.

Enriched (or Bleached) Flour is flour that has been stripped of many of the nutrients and fiber found in natural wheat and other grains, making it a low-nutritional-value food that's little more than empty carbs and calories.

High Fructose Corn Syrup (HFCS) is a manmade sweetener made from corn and enzymes. Because it extends the shelf life of processed foods and is cheaper than sugar, HFCS became the sweetener of choice starting in the 1980s. Today, it's present in so many of our foods that the U.S. Department of Agriculture estimates our consumption increased by 1,000 percent between 1970 and 1990. The evidence against HFCS is inconclusive. Some studies say the real danger is that fructose is not metabolized by the body the same as regular sugar (sucrose). It fails to signal hormones that help us feel full, so it's converted to fat, and we keep eating it.[3] Other studies have failed to duplicate these results. In addition, one study found mercury in almost half the tested samples of commercial high-fructose syrup, and in nearly a third of tested beverage products.[4] Until we know more, the main issue now is that HFCS is in so many of our food products—breads, soft drinks, desserts, processed foods, fruit-flavored drinks, baked goods, ketchups, soups, yogurts, granola bars, cereals, and much more—that we ingest far too much of it, contributing to our obesity epidemic.

Monosodium Glutamate (MSG) is a flavor enhancer used in many soups, salad dressings, chips, frozen foods, and restaurant foods. Studies have shown that some people are sensitive to large amounts, and can have reactions like headaches, nausea, weakness, and wheezing.

Olestra is a fat substitute used in potato chips. It can cause diarrhea, abdominal cramps, flatulence, and other adverse effects.

Partially Hydrogenated Oil (Trans Fat) is an altered vegetable oil found in frozen foods and bakery items, margarine, crackers, and microwave pop-corn. It contains trans fats, which promote heart disease. Harvard School of Public Health researchers confirmed in their study that intake of partially hydrogenated vegetable oils may contribute to the risk of heart attack.[5]

Potassium Bromate is an additive long used in bread to produce a find-crumb structure. Most rapidly breaks down into innocuous forms, but bro-mate itself has shown in studies to cause cancer in animals. Bromate has been banned in most countries except Japan and the U.S.

Preservatives are added to foods to help them stay fresh while on store shelves. They help prevent the food from spoiling during shipment while killing microbes like bacteria and fungi. Several preservatives, however, are linked to health effects like allergies, digestive problems, headaches, and birth defects, and others—like BHA, BHT, and mono- and di-glycer-ides—have been linked to cancer in animal studies. More research needs to be done, but buying fresh and frozen foods without preservatives can help safeguard your health.

Propyl Gallate is a preservative added to meat products, chicken soups, vegetable oils, and chewing gum. Results are inconclusive, but some animal studies have suggested it may cause cancer.

Sodium Nitrate and Sodium Nitrite are preservatives, colorings, and flavorings that enhance meat products like hot dogs, bacon, sausages, and lunchmeats. It helps cured meat show a consistent healthy-looking red color and gives it a characteristic flavor. Nitrites can break down into cancer-causing nitrosamines in the stomach, so many manufacturers now add ascorbic acid to bacon to inhibit this reaction. The use of these preservatives has decreased over the decades, but it's still found in fatty, salty foods.

References

1. No Silver Lining: An Investigation into Bisphenol A in Canned Foods. National Workgroup for Safe Markets. 2010. www.contaminatedwithoutconsent.org.

2. FDA Urged to Prohibit Carcinogenic "Caramel Coloring." Center for Science in the Public Interest. February 16, 2011. http://www.cspinet.org/new/201102161.html.

3. Mattes RD. *Physiol Behav* 1996;59:179-87.

4. "Study Finds High-Fructose Corn Syrup Contains Mercury," Jan 28, 2009, Washingtonpost.com.

5. Ascherio A, et al. Trans-fatty acids intake and risk of myocardial infarction. *Circulation* 1994 Jan;89(1):94-101.

Other Sources

Center for Science in the Public Interest (CSPI): http://www.cspinet.org/reports/chemcuisine.htm.

Appendix VII
Where to Find Safe Products

We think if we go to health food stores or places that claim to sell "natural" or "organic" products, we'll be able to pull most anything off the shelf and feel good about it, but unfortunately, even these stores can sometimes have products with toxic ingredients. Rule of thumb: Always read product labels, no matter what the claims are. If you start with locations like these listed below, you'll have better luck finding what you need, but always check the ingredient list just to be safe.

Skin Deep Database: Whatever product you choose, you can always check it out at the Skin Deep Database, which will list the ingredients for you and give you toxicity scores on each. www.cosmeticsdatabase.com

Health Food Stores: Though you must still be careful and always read labels, health food stores typically have more safe personal care products than will your typical department store. Try Whole Foods Markets, Vitamin Cottages, natural health stores, organic shops, and the like.

Organic Departments in Grocery Stores: Many grocery stores now have organic sections that carry organic and natural brands of personal care products. You may find what you're looking for there.

Beautorium: www.beautorium.com

Bella Floria: www.bellafloria.com

Best in Beauty: www.bestinbeauty.com

Caren Online: www.carenonline.com

Cathy's Organic Super Store: www.cathysorganicsuperstore.com

Edible Nature: www.ediblenature.com

Fig and Sage: www.figandsage.com

Future Natural: www.futurenatural.com

Good Earth Beauty: www.goodearthbeauty.com

Mint & Berry: www.mintandberry.com

Natural Solutions: www.bewellstaywell.com

Nature of Beauty (The): www.natureofbeauty.com

Nimli: www.nimli.com

Pristine Planet: www.pristineplanet.com

Saffron-Rouge: www.saffronrouge.com

Spirit Beauty Lounge: www.spiritbeautylounge.com

References

Forward by Donald F. Richey, M.D.

1. A. C. Haley, C. Calahan, M. Gandhi, D. P. West, A. Rademaker, M. E. Lacouture, "Skin Care Management in Cancer Patients: an Evaluation of Quality of Life and Tolerability," *Support Care Cancer*, 2010.

2. Heidary Noushin, Naik Haley, Burgin Susan, "Chemotherapeutic Agents and the Skin: an Update," *Journal of American Academy of Dermatology* 58 (4): 545-570 (April 2008).

3. "Depression Associated with Reduced Cancer Survival," The Australasian Gastro Intestinal Trials Group study, *Clinical Oncological Society of Australia News Release*, accessed 3/28/2011: http://www.cosa.org.au/media-releases/depression.html.

Introduction

1. Jane Hamilton, "515 Chemicals a Day on a Woman's Face." *The Sun*, Nov 19, 2009.

CHAPTER 1

1. Leslie A. Zebrowitz and Joann M. Montepare, "Social Psychological Face Perception: Why Appearance Matters," *Social and Personality Psychology Compass* 2 (3): 1497-1517 (2008).

2. H. Frith, D. Harcourt, A. Fussell, "Anticipating an Altered Appearance: Women Undergoing Chemotherapy Treatment for Breast Cancer," *European Journal of Oncology Nursing* 11 (5): 385-391.

3. N. Avis, S. Crawford, J. Manuel, "Quality of Life Among Younger Women with Breast Cancer," *Journal of Clinical Oncology* 23 (15) :3322-3330 (2005).

4. M. R. Katz, G. Rodin, G. M. Devins, "Self-esteem and Cancer: Theory and Research," *Canadian Journal of Psychiatry* 40 (10): 608-15 (December 1995).

5. J. S. Carpenter, D. Y. Brockopp, M. A. Andrykowski M.A, "Self-transformation as a Factor in the Self-esteem and Well-being of Breast Cancer Survivors," *Journal of Advanced Nursing* 29 (6): 1402-1411 (June 1999).

6. The Environmental Working Group, "Have You Ever Counted How Many Cosmetic or Personal Care Products You Use in a Day? Chances Are It's Nearly 10." http://www.cosmeticsdatabase.com/research/whythismatters.php.

7. The Cancer Prevention Coalition. Letter to Congress, June, 2009.

8. Mellowship, Dawn. *Toxic Beauty: How Hidden Chemicals in Cosmetics Harm You*. Great Britain: Gaia, a division of Octopus Publishing Group Ltd., 2009.

CHAPTER 2

1. *Chemical Hazards Handbook*, Section 2: Chemicals and Chemistry/Toxicity/Routes of Exposure. © 1999 London Hazards Centre Trust, Interchange Studios, Hampstead Town Hall Centre, 213 Haverstock Hill, London NW3 4QP, UK.

2. Rebecca Sutton, Ph.D, "Adolescent Exposures to Cosmetic Chemicals of Concern," September 2008. Environmental Working Group. http://www.ewg.org/reports/teens.

3. Xiaoyun Ye, Amber M. Bishop, John A. Reidy, Larry L. Needham, and Antonia M. Calafat, "Parabens as Urinary Biomarkers of Exposure in Humans," *Environ Health Perspect.* 114 (12): 1843-1846 (December 2006).

4. Hanne Frederiksen, Niels Jorgensen, and Anna-Maria Andersson, "Parabens in Urine, Serum and Seminal Plasma from Healthy Danish Men Determined by Liquid Chromatography-tandem Mass Spectrometry (LC-MS/MS)," *Journal of Exposure Science and Environmental Epidemiology*, March 10, 2010.

5. J. D. Meeker, T. Yang, X. Ye, A. M. Calafat, and R. Hauser, "Urinary Concentrations of Parabens and Serum Hormone Levels, Semen Quality Parameters, and Sperm DNA Damage," *Environmental Health Perspectives* 119: 252-257 (2010).

6. Fourth National Report on Human Exposure to Environmental Chemicals: Phthalates. Centers for Disease Control and Prevention. www.cdc.gov/exposurereport/data_tables/chemical_group_12.html.

7. Dana B. Barr, Manori J. Silva, Kayoko Kato, John A. Reidy, Nicole A. Malek, Donald Hurtz, Melissa Sadowski, Larry L. Needham, and Antonia M. Calafat, "Assessing Human Exposure to Phthalates Using Monoesters and Their Oxidized Metabolites as Biomarkers," *Environmental Health Perspectives* 111 (9): July 2003.

8. S. Sathyanarayana, C. Karr, P. Lozano, E. Brown, A.M. Calafat, F. Liu, and S.H. Swan. "Baby Care Products: Possible Sources of Infant Phthalate Exposure," *Pediatrics* 121: e260-e268 (2008).

9. "Vitamin Supplement Use During Breast Cancer Treatment and Survival: A Prospective Cohort Study," *Cancer Epidemiol Biomarkers Prev* 20: 262-271 (February 2011).

10. Trimmer, Casey, et al., "Caveolin-1 and Mitochondrial SOD2 (MnSOD) Function as Tumor Suppressors in the Stromal Microenvironment: A New Genetically Tractable Model for Human Cancer Associated Fibroblasts," *Cancer Biology & Therapy*, 11 (4): February 15, 2011.

11. "Cancer Tumors Shown to Consume Large Amounts of Vitamin C. Researchers are Cautious About Cancer Patients Taking Vitamin C

Supplements," Memorial Sloan-Kettering Cancer Center, 1999. http://www.mskcc.org/mskcc/html/1166.cfm.

12. Williamson D, "Study: Avoiding Vitamins A, E Might Improve Cancer Therapy," University of North Carolina News Services, December 13, 1999, www.unc.edu/news/newsserv/research/dec99/salganik121399.htm.

13. J.W. Fluhr, M. Miteva, G. Primavera, M. Ziemer, P. Elsner, E. Berardesca, "Functional Assessment of a Skin Care System in Patients on Chemotherapy," *Skin Pharmacology and Physiology* 20: 253-259 (2007).

14. The Food and Drug Administration, "Product and Ingredient Safety: Selected Cosmetic Ingredients, Parabens," Updated October 31, 2007. www.fda.gov/Cosmetics/ProductandIngredientSafety/SelectedCosmeticIngredients/ucm128042.htm.

15. The Food and Drug Administration, "FDA Authority Over Cosmetics," March 3, 2005. www.fda.gov/Cosmetics/GuidanceComplianceRegulatoryInformation/ucm074162.htm.

CHAPTER 3

1. J. Gray, N. Evans, B. Taylor, J. Rizzo, M. Walker, (2009), "State of the Evidence, The Connection Between Breast Cancer and the Environment," *International Journal of Occupational Environmental Health* 15:43 78 (2009).

2. National Report on Human Exposure to Environmental Chemicals. Fact Sheet. Centers for Disease Control and Prevention. www.cdc.gov/exposurereport/General_FactSheet.html.

3. J. R. Byford, L. E. Shaw, M. G. Drew, G. S. Pope, M. J. Sauer, P. D. Darbre, "Oestrogenic Activity of Parabens in MCF7 Human Breast Cancer Cells," *Journal of Steroid Biochemistry and Molecular Biology* 80 (1): 49-60 (January 2002).

4. 1,4-Dioxane. U.S. Environmental Protection Agency, Air Toxics Web Site. www.epa.gov/ttn/atw/hlthef/dioxane.html.

5. National Cancer Institute (NCI). *Bioassay of 1,4-Dioxane for Possible Carcinogenicity.* CAS No. 123-91-1. NCI Carcinogenesis Technical Report Series No. 80. NCI-CG-TR80. National Institutes of Health, Bethesda, MD. 1978.

6. Environmental Working Group (2007). Impurities of Concern in Personal Care Products. www.cosmeticsdatabase.com/research/impurities.php.

7. "Cancer-Causing Chemical Found in Children's Bath Products." Campaign for Safe Cosmetics Press Release, February 8, 2007. www.safecosmetics.org/article.php?id=64.

8. Landgren et al., "Pesticide Exposure and Risk of Monoclonal Gammopathy of Undetermined significance...," *Blood* 113: 6386-6391 (2009).

9. W. Lee and D. Sandler, "Pesticide Use and Colorectal Cancer Risk in the Agricultural Health Study," *International Journal of Cancer* (March 27, 2007).

10. M. C. R. Alavanja, C. Samanic, M. Dosemeci, J. Lubin, R. Tarone, C. F. Lynch, C. Knott, K. Thomas, J. A. Hoppin, J. Barker, J. Coble, D. P. Sandler, A. Blair, "Use of Agricultural Pesticides and Prostate Cancer Risk in the Agricultural Health Study cohort," *American Journal of Epidemiology* 157: 800-814 (2003).

11. Chensheng Lu, Kathryn Toepel, Rene Irish, Richard A. Fenske, Dana B. Barr, and Roberto Bravo, "Organic Diets Significantly Lower Children's Dietary Exposure to Organophophorus Pesticides," *Environmental Health Perspectives,* The National Institute of Environmental Health Sciences, Online September 1, 2005. www. organicconsumers.org/organic/ehpstudy.pdf.

12. Asphalt Fumes Hazard Recognition. Occupational Safety & Health Administration (OSHA). www.osha.gov/SLTC/asphaltfumes/recognition.html.

13. Health Concerns: Roofing Projects. The Department of Environmental Health & Safety (DEHS) at the University of Minnesota. www.dehs.umn.edu/iaq_hcrp.htm.

14. Peter C. Van Metre, Barbara J. Mahler, and Jennifer T. Wilson, "PAHs Underfoot: Contaminated Dust from Coal-Tar Sealcoated Pavement is Widespread in the United States," *Environmental Science and Technology* 43 (1): 20-25 (2009).

15. Alison Cohen; Sarah Janssen, M.D., Ph.D., M.P.H.; Gina Solomon, M.D., M.P.H.; "Clearing the Air, an NRDC Issue Paper," September 2007. www.nrdc.org/health/home/airfresheners/airfresheners.pdf.

16. Julie Fleming, MCS-Global Georgia State Coordinator, "Let's Clear the Air About Air Fresheners and Plug-Ins," The Global Campaign for Recognition of Multiple Chemical Sensitivity. www.mcs-america.org/airfresh.pdf.

17. A. Soto, H. Justicia, J. Wray, and C. Sonnenschein. "Nonylphenol: An Oestrogenic Xeniobiotic Released from Modified Polystyene," *Environmental Health Perspectives* 92: 167 (1991).

18. IARC (International Agency for Research on Cancer), "IARC Monographs on the Evaluation of Carcinogenic Risks to Humans," *Tetrachloroethylene* 63: 159–221 (1995).

19. Jing Ma, et al, "Association Between Residential Proximity to PERC Dry Cleaning Establishments and Kidney Cancer in New York City," *Journal of Environmental and Public Health* 2009, Article ID 183920.

SIDEBARS

Stay Away from Synthetic Fragrance

• Neurotoxins: At Home and the Workplace, Report by the Committee on Science & Technology, U.S. House of Representatives, Sept. 16, 1986. (Report 99-827).

Dioxins Could be Present in Your Tampons
- Dioxins and Furans. The Environmental Protection Agency. Last updated April 22, 2010. www.epa.gov/pbt/pubs/dioxins.htm.

- S. E. Rier, W. E. Turner, D. C. Martin, R. Morris, G. W. Lucier, G. C. Clark, "Serum Levels of TCDD and Dioxin-like Chemicals in Rhesus Monkeys Chronically Exposed to Dioxin: Correlation of Increased Serum PCB Levels with Endometriosis," *Toxicological Sciences* 59 (1): 147-59 (January 2001).

- Michael J. DeVito and Arnold Schecter, "Exposure Assessment to Dioxins from the Use of Tampons and Diapers," *Environmental Health Perspectives* 110 (1): 23–28 (January 2002).

Pesticides and Childhood Cancer
- Offie P. Soldin, PhD, MBA, et al., "Pediatric Acute Lymphoblastic Leukemia and Exposure," *Therapeutic Drug Monitoring* 31 (4): 495-501 (August 2009).

- Y. Shim, S.P. Mlynarek, and E. van Wijngaarden, "Parental Exposure to Pesticides and Childhood Brain Cancer: United States Atlantic Coast Childhood Brain Cancer Study," *Environmental Health Perspectives* 117 (6): 1002-1006 (2009).

Dangers in Plastics
- Indiana University, "Suspicion Lingers Over Bisphenol and Breast Cancer," *ScienceDaily*, August 2009. www.sciencedaily.com/releases/2006/08/060826171235.htm.

- S. Ho, W. Tang, J. Belmonte De Frausto, G. Prins, "Developmental Exposure to Estradiol and Bisphenol A Increases Susceptibility to Prostate Carcinogenesis and Epigenetically Regulates Phosphodiesterase Type 4 Variant 4," *Cancer Research* 66 (11): 5624–5632 (2006).

- National Institutes of Health. "Since You Asked: Bisphenol A (BPA)." www.niehs.nih.gov/news/media/questions/sya-bpa.cfm.

- Antonia M. Calafat, Xiaoyun Ye, Lee-Yang Wong, John A. Reidy, and Larry L. Needham, "Exposure of the U.S. Population to Bisphenol A and 4-*tertiary*-Octylphenol: 2003–2004," *Environmental Health Perspectives* 116 (1): 39–44 (January 2008).

Candles Can Be Toxic
- "Romantic, Candle-Lit Dinners: An Unrecognized Source of Indoor Air Pollution," *American Chemical Society Press Release,* August 19, 2009.

Household Cleaners Double Risk for Breast Cancer?
- Ami R. Zota, Ann Aschengrau, Ruthann A. Rudel, and Julia Green Brody, "Self-reported Chemicals Exposure, Beliefs About Disease Causation, and Risk of Breast Cancer in the Cape Cod Breast Cancer Environment Study: a Case-Control Study," *Environmental Health* 9 (40): 20 July 2010.

CHAPTER 4

1. J. C. Coyne, T. F. Pajak, J. Harris, A. Konski, B. Movsas, K. Ang, D. Watkins Bruner, "Emotional Well-being Does Not Predict Survival in Head and Neck Cancer Patients: a Radiation Therapy Oncology Group Study," *Cancer* 110 (11): 2568-75 (December 1, 2007).

2. P. Rainville, Q. Bao, P. Chrétien, "Pain-related Emotions Modulate Experimental Pain Perception and Autonomic Responses," *Pain* 118 (3): 306-318.

3. David H. Zald, Dorothy L. Mattson, and José V. Pardo, "Brain Activity in Ventromedical Prefrontal Cortex Correlates with Individual differences in Negative Affect," *Proceedings of the National Academy of Sciences* 99 (4): 2450-2454 (February 19, 2002).

4. Yeur-Hur Lai, Joseph Tung-Chien Chang, Francis J. Keefe, Chung-Fong Chiou, Shu-Ching Chen, Shu-Chin Feng, Su-Jene Dou, Mei-Nan Liao, "Symptom Distress, Catastrophic Thinking, and Hope in Nasopharyngeal Carcinoma Patients," *Cancer Nursing* 26 (6): 485-493 (December 2003).

5. Dorthe Kirkegaard Thomsen, Mimi Yung Mehlsen, Marianne Hokland, Andrus Viidik, Frede Olesen, Kirsten Avlund, Karen Munk, and Robert Zachariae, "Negative Thoughts and Health: Associations Among Rumination, Immunity, and Health Care Utilization in a Young and Elderly Sample," *Psychosomatic Medicine* 66:363-371 (2004).

6. Yumi Iwamitsu, Kazutaka Shimoda, Hajime Abe, Tohru Tani, Masako Okawa, and Ross Buck, "Anxiety, Emotional Suppression, and Psychological Distress Before and After Breast Cancer Diagnosis," *Psychosomatics* 46:19-24 (February 2005).

7. J. M. Smyth, "Written Emotional Expression: Effect Sizes, Outcome Types, and Moderating Variables," *Journal of Consulting and Clinical Psychology* 66 (1): 174-84 (February 1998).

8. A. L. Stanton, S. Danoff-Burg, C. L. Cameron, M. Bishop, C. A. Collins, S. B. Kirk, L. A. Sworowski, R. Twillman, "Emotionally Expressive Coping Predicts Psychological and Physical Adjustment to Breast Cancer," *Journal of Consulting and Clinical Psychology* 68 (5): 875-82 (October 2000).

9. Jeong Yeob Han, "Expressing Positive Emotions within Online Support Groups by Women with Breast Cancer," *Journal of Health Psychology* 13 (8): 1002-1007 (2008).

10. Lee S. Berk, Stanley A. Tan, and James Westengard, "Beta-Endorphin and HGH Increase are Associated with both the Anticipation and Experience of Mirthful Laughter," 12:30 p.m.- 3 p.m. Sunday April 2, APS Behavioral Neuroscience & Drug Abuse Section Abstract 233.18/board #C706.

11. L. S. Berk, S. A. Tan, W. F. Fry, B. J. Napier, J. W. Lee, R. W. Hubbard, J. E. Lewis, W. C. Eby, "Neuroendocrine and Stress Hormone Changes During Mirthful Laughter," *American Journal of Medical Science* 298 (6): 390-6 (December 1989).

12. Jeffrey J. Froh, William J. Sefick, and Robert A. Emmons, "Counting Blessings in Early Adolescents: An Experimental Study of Gratitude and Subjective Well-being," *Journal of School Psychology* 46 (2): 213-233 (April 2008).

13. Emmons, Robert. *Thanks!: How the New Science of Gratitude Can Make You Happier.* Houghton Mifflin, 2007.

14. P. Lamanque, S. Daneault, "Does Meditation Improve the Quality of Life for Patients Living with Cancer?" *Canadian Family Physician* 52: 474-5 (April 2006).

15. Mary Jane Ott, Rebecca L. Norris, Susan M. Bauer-Wu, "Mindfulness Meditation for Oncology Patients: A Discussion and Critical Review," *Integrative Cancer Therapies* 5 (2): 98-108 (2006).

16. Morris L, Linkemann A, Kroner-Herwig B, "Writing Your Way to Health? The Effects of Disclosure of Past Stressful Events in German Students." In: Abelian ME, editor. *Trends in Psychotherapy Research.* Hauppauge (NY): Nova Science Publishers; 2006.

17. Joshua M. Smyth, Arthur A. Stone, Adam Hurewitz, Alan Kaell, "Effects of Writing About Stressful Experiences on Symptom Reduction in Patients with Asthma or Rheumatoid Arthritis," *Journal of American Medical Association* 281: 1304-1309 (1999).

18. Nancy P. Morgan, Kristi D. Graves, Elizabeth A. Poggi, Bruce D. Cheson, "Implementing an Expressive Writing Study in a Cancer Clinic," *The Oncologist* 13 (2): 196-204 F(ebruary 2008).

19. I. Oster, A. C. Svensk, E. Magnusson, K. E. Thyme, M. Sjodin, S. Astrom, J. Lindh, "Art Therapy Improves Coping Resources: a Randomized, Controlled Study Among Women with Breast Cancer," *Palliative and Supportive Care* 4 (1): 57-64 (March 2006).

20. K. E. Thyme, E. C. Sundin, B. Wiberg, I. Oster, S. Astrom, J. Lindh, "Individual Brief Art Therapy can be Helpful for Women with Breast Cancer: a Randomized Controlled Clinical Study," *Palliative and Supportive Care.* 7 (1): 87-95 (March 2009).

21 Charlotte van Oyen Witvliet, Thomas E. Ludwig, and Kelly L. Vander Laan, "Granting Forgiveness or Harboring Grudges: Implications for Emotion, Physiology, and Health," *Psychological Science* 12 (2): 117-123.

22. Everett L. Worthington Jr, Charlotte vanOyen Witvliet, Andrea J. Lerner, Micahel Scherer. *Forgiveness in Health Research and Medical Practice* 1 (3): 169-176 (May 2005).

23. Elisabeth Westerdahl, et al., "Deep-breathing Exercises Reduce Atelectasis and Improve Pulmonary Function After Coronary Artery Bypass Surgery," *Chest* 128 (5): 3482-3488 (November 2005).

24. David Rykel. *Integrative Medicine.* Second edition. Saunders Publishing, 2007.

25. Bernardi L et al., "Effect of Rosary Prayer and Yoga Mantras on Autonomic Cardiovascular Rhythms: Comparative Study," *British Medical Journal* 323 (7327):1446-1449 (2001).

26. Wenjuan Wu, Takeshi Yamaura, Koji Murakami, Jun Murata, Kinzo Matsumoto, Hiroshi Watanabe, and Ikuo Saiki, "Social Isolation Stress Enhanced Liver Metastasis of Murine Colon 26-L5 Carcinoma Cells by Suppressing Immune Responses in Mice," *Life Sciences* 66 (19): 1827-1838 (March 31 2000).

27. H. Liu, Z. Wang, "Effects of Social Isolation Stress on Immune Response and Survival Time of Mouse with Liver Cancer," *World Journal of Gastroenterology* 11 (37): 5902-4 (October 7 2005).

28. R. Gray, M. Fitch, C. Davis, C. Phillips, "A Qualitative Study of Breast Cancer Self-help Groups." *Psychooncology.* 6 (4): 279-89 (December 1997).

Music Therapy

• S. J. Burns, M. S. Harbuz, F. Hucklebridge, L. Bunt, "A Pilot Study into the Therapeutic Effects of Music Therapy at a Cancer Help Center," *Alternative Therapies in Health and Medicine* 7 (1): 48-56 (January 2001).

• M. Good, et al., "Relaxation and Music Reduce Pain after Gynecologic Surgery," *Pain Management Nursing* 3 (2): 61-70 (2002).

Pet Therapy

• I. J. Muschel, "Pet Therapy with Terminal Cancer Patients," *Social Casework* 65 (8): 451-458 (1989).

CHAPTER 5

1. Yao-Ping Lu, et al., "Tumorigenic Effect of Some Commonly Used Moisturizing Creams When Applied Topically to UVB-Pretreated High-Risk Mice," *Journal of Investigative Dermatology* 129: 468-475 (2009).

2. John Knowland, Edward A. McKenzie, Peter J. McHugh, and Nigel A Cridland, "Sunlight-induced Mutagenicity of a Common Sunscreen Ingredient," *FEBS Letters* 324 (3): 309-313 (June 21, 1993).

3. Cedric F. Garland, et al., "Could Sunscreens Increase Melanoma Risk?" *American Journal of Public Health* 82 (4): 614-15 (April 1992).

4. Tomoharu Suzuki, et al., "Estrogenic and Antiandrogenic Activities of 17 Benzophenone Derivatives Used as UV Stabilizers and Sunscreens," *Toxicology and Applied Pharmacology* 203 (1): 9-17 (February 15, 2005).

5. R. Jiang, M.S. Roberts, D. M. Collins, and H. A. E. Benson, "Absorption of Sunscreens Across Human Skin: an Evaluation of Commercial Products for Children and Adults," *British Journal of Clinical Pharmacology* 48 (4): 635-637 (October 1999).

6. Press Release. Boom in Nanotechnology Growing, But Safety Studies Lag. NRDC Press Archive. www.nrdc.org/media/pressreleases/061127.asp.

CHAPTER 6

1. A. M. Courtens, F. C. J. Stevens, H. F. J. M. Crebolder, H. Philipsen, "Longitudinal Study on Quality of Life and Social Support in Cancer Patients," *Cancer Nursing* 19 (3): 162-169 (June 1996).

2. J. J. Guidry, L. A. Aday, D. Zhang, R. J. Winn, "The Role of Informal and Formal Social Support Networks for Patients with Cancer," *Cancer Practice* 5 (4): 241-6 (July-August 1997).

3. Candyce H. Kroenke, Laura D. Kubzansky, Eva S. Schernhammer, Michelle D. Holmes, Ichiro Kawachi, "Social Networks, Social Support, and Survival After Breast Cancer Diagnosis," *Journal of Clinical Oncology* 24 (7): 1105-1111 (March 1, 2006).

4. "A Poison Kiss: The Problem of Lead in Lipstick. The Campaign for Safe Cosmetics. October, 2007. www.safecosmetics.org.

Makeup Counters Harbor Germs

*   Alene Dawson, "Handle Those Store Makeup Testers with Care," *Los Angeles Times,* April 18, 2010.

CHAPTER 7

1. Margot E. Kurtz, Jay C. Kurtz, Charles W. Given, Barbara A. Given, "Patient Optimism and Mastery—Do They Play a Role in Cancer Patients' Management of Pain and Fatigue?" *Journal of Pain and Symptom Management* 36 (1): 1-10 (July 2009).

2. E. Ernst, M. H. Pittler, "Efficacy of Ginger for Nausea and Vomiting: a Systematic Review of Randomized Clinical Trials," *British Journal of Anaesthesia* 84 (3): 367-71 (March 2000).

3. T.J. Gan, S. Parrillo, J. Fortney, G. Georgiade, "Comparison of Electraacupuncture and Ondansetron for the Prevention of Postoperative Nausea and Vomiting," *Anesthesiology* 95: A22 (2001).

4. J. M. Ezzo, M. A. Richardson, A. Vickers, et al., "Acupuncture-point Stimulation for Chemotherapy-induced Nausea or Vomiting," *Cochrane Database Systematic Reviews* 19 (2) (April 2006).

5. A. Morganti, C. Digesu, S. Panunzi, A. De Gaetano, G. Macchia, F. Deodato, M. Cece, M. Cirocco, A. Di Castelnuovo, L. Iacoviello, "Radioprotective Effect of Moderate Wine Consumption in Patients with Breast Carcinoma," *International Journal of Radiation Oncology Biology Physics* 74 (5): 1501-1505.

6. Paul Okunieff, Weimin Sun, Wei Wang, Jung Kim, Shammin Yang, "Anti-cancer Effect of Resveratrol is Associated with Induction of Apoptosis via a Mitochondrial Pathway Alignment," *Advances in Experimental Medicine and Biology* 614: 179-86 (2008).

7. C. Kerr, "Curry Ingredient Protects Skin Against Radiation," *The Lancet Oncology* 3 (12): 713-713.

8. M. K. Garcia, J. S. Chiang, L. Cohen, M. Liu, J. L. Palmer, D. I. Rosenthal, Q. Wei, S. Tung, C. Wang, T. Rahifs, M. S. Chambers, "Acupuncture for Radiation-induced Xerostomia in Patients with Cancer: a Pilot Study," *Head Neck* 31 (10): 1360-8 (October 2009).

9. B. Miljanovic, K. A. Trivedi, M. R. Dana, J. P. Gilbard, J. E. Buring, D. A. Schaumberg, "Relation Between Dietary n-3 and n-6 Fatty Acids and Clinically Diagnosed Dry Eye Syndrome in Women," *American Journal of Clinical Nutrition* 82 (4): 887-93 (October 2005).

10. "Herbal Medicines for Menopausal Symptoms," *Evidence Based Nursing* 13: 29-33 (2010). Doi:10.1136/dtb.2008.12.0031.

11. J. Hervik, O. Mjaland, "Acupuncture for the Treatment of Hot Flashes in Breast Cancer Patients, a Randomized, Controlled Trial," *Breast Cancer Research and Treatment* 116 (2): 311-6 (July 2009).

12. "Breast Cancer Patients Taking Arimidex May Get Pain Relief from Vitamin D," News Release, St. Louis: Washington University in St. Louis School of Medicine, March 30, 2006. http://mednews.wustl.edu/news/page /normal/6902.html.

SIDEBARS

Could Your Toothpaste Encourage Mouth Sores?

• B. B. Herlofson, P. Barkvoll, "Sodium Lauryl Sulfate and Recurrent Aphthous Ulcers. A Preliminary Study," *Acta Odontologica Scandinavica* 52 (5): 257-9 (October 1994).

• B. B. Herlofson, P. Barkvoll, "The Effect of Two Toothpaste Detergents on the Frequency of Recurrent Aphthous Mouth Ulcers," *Acta Odontologica Scandinavica* 54 (3): 150-3 (June 1996).

Deodorant Linked with Breast Cancer?

• Christopher Exley, Lisa M Charles, Lester Barr, Claire Martin, Anthony Polwart, and Philippa D Darbre, "Aluminum in Human Breast Tissue," *Journal of Inorganic Biochemistry* 101 (9): 1344-1346 (September 2007).

• K. G. McGrath, "An Earlier Age of Breast Cancer Diagnosis More Frequent Use of Antiperspirants/Deodorants and Underarm Shaving," *European Journal of Cancer Prevention* 12 (6): 479-485 (December 2003).

Homeopathy Relieve Dermatitis?

• Society of Homeopaths. www.homeopathy-soh.org.

• S. Kassab, M. Cummings, S. Berkovitz, R. van Haselen, P. Fisher, "Homeopathic Medicines for Adverse Effects of Cancer Treatments," *Cochrane Database of Systematic Reviews* 2009, Issue 2. Art. No.: CD004845.

Metal Taste

- J.H. Hong, P. Omur-Ozbek, B.T. Stanek, A.M. Dietrich, S.E. Duncan, Y.W. Lee, and G. Lesser, "Taste and Odor Abnormalities in Cancer Patients," *Journal of Supportive Oncology* 7: 58-65 (2009).

CHAPTER 8

1. B. R. Cassileth, A. J. Vickers, "Massage Therapy for Symptom Control: Outcome Study at a Major Cancer Center," *Journal of Pain Symptom Management* 28 (3): 244-9 (September 2004).

2. Curties, Debra. *Massage Therapy and Cancer* 1999, Curties Overzet Publications.

3. N. Stephenson, J. A. Dalton, J. Carlson, "The Effect of Foot Reflexology on Pain in Patients with Metastatic Cancer," *Applied Nursing Research* 16 (4): 284-6 (November 2003).

4. N. L. Stephenson, S. P. Weinrich, A. S. Tavakoli, "The Effects of Foot Reflexology on Anxiety and Pain in Patients with Breast and Lung Cancer," *Oncology Nursing Forum* 27 (1): 67-72 (January-February 2000).

5. H. Hodgson, "Does Reflexology Impact on Cancer Patients' Quality of Life?" *Nursing Standard* 14 (31): 33-8 (Apr 19-25, 2000).

6. L. Grealish, A. Lomasney, B. Whiteman, "Foot Massage: A Nursing Intervention to Modify the Distressing Symptoms of Pain and Nausea in Patients Hospitalized with Cancer," *Cancer Nurse* 23 (3): 237-43 (June 2000).

7. Andrew Sparber, "State Boards of Nursing and Scope of Practice of Registered Nurses Performing Complementary Therapies," *Online Journal of Issues in Nursing* 6, Manuscript 10. August 31, 2001.

8. K. Olson, J. Hanson, "Using Reiki to Manage Pain: a Preliminary Report," *Cancer Prevention and Control* 1 (2): 108-13 (June 1997).

9. National Institutes of Health. *Acupuncture. Consensus Development Conference statement, November 3-5, 1997.* Available at http://consensus.nih.gov/1997/1997Acupuncture107html.htm.

10. Andrew J. Vickers, David J. Straus, Bertha Fearon, Barrie R. Cassileth, "Acupuncture for Postchemotherapy Fatigue: A Phase II Study," *Journal of Clinical Oncology* 22 (9): 1731-1735 (May 1, 2004).

11. D. Alimi, C. Rubino, E. Pichard-Léandri, S. Fermand-Brulé, M. L. Dubreuil-Lemaire, C. Hill, "Analgensic Effect of Auricular Acupuncture for Cancer Pain: a Randomized, Blinded, Controlled Trial," *Journal of Clinical Oncology* 21 (22): 4120-6 (November 15, 2003).

12. E. D. Borud, T. Alraek, A. White, V. Fonnebo, A. E. Eggen, M. Hammar, L. L. Astrand, E. Theodorsson, S. Grimsgaard, "The Acupuncture on Hot Flushes

Among Menopausal Women (ACUFLASH) Study, a Randomized Controlled Trial," *Menopause* 16 (3): 484-93 (May-June 2009).

13. E. M. Walker, A. L. Rodriguez, B. Kohn, R. M. Ball, J. Pegg, J. R. Pocock, R. Nunez, E. Peterson, S. Jakary, R. A. Levine, "Acupuncture Versus Venlafaxine for the Management of Vasomotor Symptoms in Patients with Hormone Receptor-positive Breast Cancer: a Randomized Controlled Trial," *Journal of Clinical Oncology* 28 (4): 634-40 (February 1, 2010).

14. C. D. Joseph, "Psychological Supportive Therapy for Cancer Patients," *Indian Journal of Cancer* 20: 268-270 (1983).

15. S. Culos-Reed, L. E. Carlson, L. M. Daroux, et al., "Discovering the Physical and Psychological Benefits of Yoga for Cancer Survivors," *International Journal of Yoga Therapy* 14: 45-52 (2004).

16. M. Speca, L. E. Carlson, E. Goodey, et al., "A Randomized, Wait-list Controlled Clinical Trial: the Effect of a Mindfulness Meditation-based Stress Reduction Program on Mood and Symptoms of Stress in Cancer Outpatients," *Psychosomatic Medicine* 62: 613-622 (2000).

17. S. C. Danhauer, S. L. Mihalko, G. B. Russell, C. R. Campbell, L. Felder, K, Daley, E. A. Levine, "Restorative Yoga for Women with Breast Cancer: Findings from a Randomized Pilot Study," *Psychooncology* 18 (4): 360-8 (April 2009).

18. Tai Chi: An Introduction. National Institutes of Health. NCCAM Publication No. D322. Created June 2006. Updated April 2009. http://nccam.nih.gov/health/taichi/#research.

19. K. M. Mustian, J. A. Katula, H. Zhao, "A Pilot Study to Assess the Influence of Tai Chi Chuan on Functional Capacity Among Breast Cancer Survivors," *Journal of Supportive Oncology* 4 (3): 139-45 (March 2006).

20. C. E. Matthews, S. Wilcox, C. L. Hanby, C. Der Ananian, S. P. Heiney, T. Gebretsadik, A. Shintani, "Evaluation of a 12-week Home-based Walking Intervention for Breast Cancer Survivors," *Supportive Care in Cancer* 15 (2): 203-11 (February 2007).

21. C. M. Friendenreich, K. S. Courneya, "Exercise as Rehabilitation for Cancer Patients," *Clinical Journal of Sport Medicine* 6 (4): 237-44 (October 1996).

22. K. Griffith, J. Wenzel, J. Shang, C. Thompson, K. Stewart, V. Mock, "Impact of a Walking Intervention on Cardiorespiratory Fitness, Self-reported Physical Function, and Pain in Patients Undergoing Treatment for Solid Tumors," *Cancer* 115 (20): 4874-84 (October 15, 2009).

23. M. L. Winningham, "Walking Program for People with Cancer. Getting Started," *Cancer Nursing* 14 (5): 270-6 (October 1991).

24. M. D. Holmes, W. Y. Chen, D. Feskanish, C. H. Kroenke, G. A. Colditz, "Physical Activity and Survival After Breast Cancer Diagnosis," *Journal of American Medical Association* 293 (20): 2479-86 (May 25 2005).

Benefits of Hand Massage
- S. Y. Chang, "Effects of Aroma Hand Massage on Pain, State Anxiety and Depression in Hospice Patients with Terminal Cancer," *Taehan Kanho Hakhoe Chi* 38 (4): 493-502 (August 2008).

CHAPTER 9

SIDEBAR

Phthalates In Your Hair Spray?
- Bis (2-ethylhexyl) Phthalate (DEHP) Hazard Summary. Environmental Protection Agency. http://www.epa.gov/ttn/atw/hlthef/eth-phth.html.

- M. C. Kohn, S. A. Masten, C. J. Portier, M. D. Shelby, J. W. Brock, L. L. Needham, et al., "Human Exposure Estimates for Phthalates [Letter]," *Environmental Health Perspectives* 108: A440-442 (2000).

CHAPTER 10

1. Azadeh Tavoli, Ali Montazeri, Rasool Roshan, Zahra Tavoli, and Mahdiyeh Melyani, "Depression and Quality of Life in Cancer Patients With and Without Pain: the Role of Pain Beliefs," *BMC Cancer* 8: 177 (2008).

2. H. J. Gerbershagen, E. Ozgur, K. Straub, O. Dagtekin, K. Gerbershagen, F. Petzke, A. Hidenreich, K. A. Lehmann, R. Sabatowski, "Prevalence, Severity, and Chronicity of Pain and General Health-related Quality of Life in Patients with Localized Prostate Cancer," *European Journal of Pain* 12: 339-350 (2008).

3. I. E. Lamé, M. L. Peters, J. W. Vlaeyen, M. Kleef, J. Patijn, "Quality of Life in Chronic Pain is More Associated with Beliefs about Pain, Than with Pain Intensity," *European Journal of Pain* 9 (1): 15-24 (February 2005).

4. C. J. Fabian, R. Molina, M. Slavik, S. Dahlberg, S. Giri, R. Stephens, "Pyridoxine Therapy for Palmar-plantar Erythrodysesthesia Associated with Continuous 5-fluorouracil Infusion," *Investigational New Drugs* 8 (1): 57-63 (February 1990).

5. R. A. Beveridge, A. N. Kales, R. A. Binder, J. A. Miller, S. G. Virts, "Pyridoxine (B6) and Amelioration of Hand/Foot Syndrome," *Proc American Society of Clininical Oncology* 9: 102 (1990).

6. L. Mollart, "Single-Blind Trial Addressing the Differential Effects of Two Reflexology Techniques Versus Rest, on Ankle and Foot Oedema in Late Pregnancy," *Complementary Therapies in Nursing and Midwifery* 9, (4): 203-8 (2003).

7. S. Schroder, J. Liepert, A. Remppis, J. H. Greten, "Acupuncture Treatment Improves Nerve Conduction in Peripheral Neuropathy," *European Jounral of Neurology* 14 (3): 276-81 (March 2007).

8. B. B. Abuaisha, J. B. Costanzi, A. J. Boulton, "Acupuncture for the Treatment of Chronic Painful Peripheral Diabetic Neuropathy: a Long-term Study," *Diabetes Research and Clinical Practice* 39 (2): 115-21 (February 1998).

SIDEBAR

Triclosan
- Triclosan: What Consumers Should Know. The Food and Drug Administration. http://www.fda.gov/ForConsumers/ConsumerUpdates/ucm205999.htm.

- M. Lores, M. Llompart, L. Sanchez-Prado, C. Garcia-Jares, R. Cela, "Confirmation of the Formation of Dichlorodibenzo-p-dioxin I the Photodegradation of Triclosan by Photo-SPME," *Analytical and Bioanalytical Chemistry* 381 (6): 1294-8 (March 2005).

- Antonia M. Calafat, Xiaoyun Ye, Lee-Yang Wong, John A. Reidy, and Larry L. Needham, "Urinary Concentrations of Triclosan in the U.S. Population: 2003-2004," *Environmental Health Perspectives* 116 (3): 303-307 (March 2008).

- N. Veldhoen, R. C. Skirrow, H. Osachoff, H. Wigmore, D. J. Clapson, M. P. Gunderson, G. Van Aggelen, C C. Helbing, "The Bactericidal Agent Triclosan Modulates Thyroid Hormone-associated Gene Expression and Disrupts Postembryonic Anuran Development," *Aquatic Toxicology* 80 (3): 217-27 (December 1, 2006).

CHAPTER 11

1. P. Joseph, A. J. Klein-Szanto, A. K. Jaiswal, "Hydroquinones Cause Specific Mutations and Lead to Cellular Transformation and In Vivo Tumorigenesis," *British Journal of Cancer* 78 (3): 312-20 (August 1998).

2. Silverman D.H., Dy CJ, Castellon S.A., et al. Altered frontocortical, cerebellar, and basal ganglia activity in adjuvant-treated breast cancer survivors 5-10 years after chemotherapy. *Breast Cancer Research and Treatment* 2007 Jul;103(3):303-11.

CHAPTER 12

1. Timothy J. Key, Naomi E. Allen, Elizabeth A. Spencer, Ruth C. Travis, "The Effect of Diet on Risk of Cancer," *The Lancet* 360: September 14, 2002.

2. World Cancer Research Fund. Food, nutrition, and the prevention of cancer: a global perspective. Washington DC: American Institute for Cancer Research, 1997.

3. Palli D., "Epidemiology of Gastric Cancer: an Evaluation of Available Evidence," *Journal of Gastroenterology* 35 (suppl): 84–89 (2000).

4. T. Norat, A. Lukanova, P. Ferrari, E. Riboli, "Meat Consumption and Colorectal Cancer Risk: Dose-response Meta-analysis of Epidemiological Studies," *International Journal of Cancer* 98: 241–56 (2002).

5. T. J Key, P. K. Verkasalo, E. Banks, "Epidemiology of Breast Cancer," *Lancet Oncology* 2: 133–40 (March 2001).

6. International Agency for Research on Cancer. "Overweight and Lack of Exercise Linked to Increased Cancer Risk." In: *IARC Handbooks of Cancer Prevention* Volume 6. Lyon: IARC Press, 2002.

7. U.S. Department of Health and Human Services: The Surgeon General's Report on Nutrition and Health, DHHS (PHS) Publ. No. 88-50210. Washington, DC: Dept. of Health and Human Services, Public Health Service, 1988. And National Research Council, Committee on Diet and Health, Food and Nutrition Board, Commission on Life Sciences. Diet and Health: Implications for Reducing Chronic Disease Risk. Washington, DC: National Academy Press, 1989.

8. Noel T. Mueller, Andrew Odegaard, Kristin Anderson, Jian-Min Yuan, Myron Gross, Woon-Puay Koh, and Mark A. Pereira, "Soft Drink and Juice Consumption and Risk of Pancreatic Cancer: The Singapore Chinese Health Study," *Cancer Epidemiology, Biomarkers and Prevention* 19: 447 (February 2010).

9. E. Lanza, S. Shankar and B. Trock, "Dietary Fiber." In *Macronutrients: Investigating Their Role in Cancer.* ed Micozzi MS, Moon TE. New York: Marcell Dekker, Inc., 293-319, 1992.

10. D. Feskanisch, R. G. Ziegler, D. S. Michaud, E. L. Giovannucci, F. E. Speizer, W. C. Willett, G. A. Colditz, "Prospective Study of Fruit and Vegetable Consumption and Risk of Lung Cancer Among Men and Women," *Journal of the National Cancer Institute* 92 (22): 1812-23 (November 13, 2000).

11. Gregory L. Austin, Linda S. Adair, Joseph A. Galanko, Christopher F. Martin, Jessie A. Satia and Robert S. Sandler, "A Diet High in Fruits and Low in Meats Reduces the Risk of Colorectal Adenomas," *American Society for Nutrition Journal of Nutrition* 137: 999-1004 (April 2007).

12. "Two Studies Find High-Fiber Diet Lowers Colon Cancer Risk," *CA Cancer Journal for Clinicians* 53:201 (2003).

13. A. Lindsay Frazier, Catherine Tomeo Ryan, Helaine Rockett, Walter C. Willett, and Graham A. Colditz, "Adolescent Diet and Risk of Breast Cancer," *Breast Cancer Research* 5: R59-R64 (2003).

14. G. A. Saxe, C. L. Rock, M. S. Wicha, D. Schottenfeld, "Diet and Risk for Breast Cancer Recurrence and Survival," *Breast Cancer Research and Treatment* 53(3): 241-53 (February 1999).

15. Marilyn L. Kwan, Erin Weltzien, Lawrence H. Kushi, Adrienne Castillo, Martha L. Slattery, Bette J. Caan, "Dietary Patterns and Breast Cancer Recurrence and Survival Among Women with Early-Stage Breast Cancer," *Journal of Clinical Oncology* 27 (6): 919-926 (February 20, 2009).

16. R. T. Chlebowski, G. L. Blackburn, C. A. Thomson, D. W. Nixon, A. Shapiro, M. K. Hoy, M. T. Goodman, A. E. Giuliano, N. Karanja, P. McAndrew, C. Hudis, J. Butler, D. Merkel, A. Kristal, B. Caan, R. Michaelson, V. Vinciguerra, S. Del Prete, M. Winkler, R. Hall, M. Simon, B. L. Winters, R. M. Elashoff, "Dietary Fat Reduction and Breast Cancer Outcome: Interim Efficacy Results from the Women's Intervention Nutrition Study," *Journal of the National Cancer Institute* 98 (24): 1767-1776 (2006).

17. L. Holmberg, E. Lund, R. Bergström, H. O. Adami, O. Meirik, "Oral Contraceptives and Prognosis in Breast Cancer: Effects of Duration, Latency, Recency, Age at First Use and Relation to Parity and Body Mass Index in Young Women with Breast Cancer," *European Journal of Cancer* 30A(3): 351-354 (1994).

18. Alfred I. Neugut, Gail C. Garbowski, Won Chul Lee, Todd Murray, Jeri W. Nieves, Kenneth A. Forde, Michael R. Treat, Jerome D. Waye, and Cecilia Fenoglio-Preiser, "Dietary Risk Factors for the Incidence and Recurrence of Colorectal Adenomatous Polyps: a Case-Control Study," *Annals of Internal Medicine* 118 (2): 91-95 (January 15, 1993).

19. P. Wallstrom, E. Wirfait, L. Janzon, I Mattisson, S. Elmstahl, U. Johansson, G. Berglund, "Fruit and Vegetable Consumption in Relation to Risk Factors for Cancer; a Report from the Malmo Diet and Cancer Study," *Public Health Nutrition* 3 (3): 263-71 (September 2000).

20. Mark Toles and Wendy Demark-Wahnefried. "Nutrition and the Cancer Survivor: Evidence to Guide Oncology Nursing Practice," *Seminars in Oncology Nursing* 24 (3): 171-179 (August 2008).

21. Haibo Liu, et al., "Fructose Induces Transketolase Flus to Promote Pancreatic Cancer Growth," *Cancer Research* 70: 6368 (August 1, 2010).

22. Lee W. Jones, Wendy Demark-Wahnefried, "Diet, Exercise, and Complementary Therapies After Primary Treatment for Cancer," *Lancet Oncology* 7: 1017–26 (2006).

23. J. A. Meyerhardt, D. Heseltine, D. Niedzwiecki, D. Hollis, L. B. Saltz, R. J. Mayer, J. Thomas, H. Nelson, R. Whittom, A. Hantel, R. L. Schilsky, C. S. Fuchs, "Impact of Physical Activity on Cancer Recurrence and Survival in Patients with Stage III Colon Cancer: Findings from CALGB 89803," *Journal of Clinical Oncology* 24 (22): 3535-41 (August 1, 2006).

24. M. D. Holmes, W. Y. Chen, D. Feskanish, C. H. Kroenke, G. A. Colditz. "Physical Activity and Survival After Breast Cancer Diagnosis," *Journal of American Medical Association* 293: 2479–86 (2005).

25. Margaret L. McNeely, Kristin L. Campbell, Brian H. Rowe, Terry P. Klassen, John R. Mackey and Kerry S. Courneya, "Effects of Exercise on Breast Cancer Patients and Survivors: a Systematic Review and Meta-analysis," *Canadian Medical Association Journal* 175 (1) (July 4, 2006).

26. S. Ben-Eliyahu, G. G. Page, R. Yirmiya, G. Shakhar, "Evidence That Stress and Surgical Interventions Promote Tumor Development by Suppressing Natural Killer Cell Activity," *International Journal of Cancer* 80 (6): 880-8 (March 15, 1999).

27. Ella Rosenne, Guy Shakhar, Rivka Melamed, Yossi Schwartz, Anat Erdreich-Epstein, and Shamgar Ben-Eliyahu, "Inducing a Mode of NK-Resistance to Suppression by Stress and Surgery: a Potential Approach Based on Low Dose of Poly I-C to Reduce Postoperative Cancer Metastasis," *Brain, Behavior and Immunity* 21(4): 395-408 (May 2007).

28. A. Ramirez, T. Craig, J. Watson, I. Fentiman, W. North, R. Rubens, "Stress and Relapse of Breast Cancer," *BMJ* 298: 291-293 (1989).

29. B. L. Andersen, H-C. Yang, W. B. Farrar, D. M. Golden-Kreutz, C. F. Emery, L. M. Thornton,D. C. Young, W. E. Carson III, "Psychological Intervention Improves Survival for Breast Cancer Patients: A Randomized Clinical Trial," *Cancer* 113: 3450-3458 (2008).

30. "Tip 9: Get Rid of That Toxic Dust," Environmental Working Group. http://www.ewg.org//healthyhometips/toxicchemicalsinhousedust#whytoxic.

31. R. A. Rudel, D. E. Camann, J. D. Spengler, L. R. Korn, J. G. Brody, "Phthalates, Alkylphenols, Pesticides, Polybrominated Diphenyl Ethers, and Other Endocrine-disrupting Compounds in Indoor Air and Dust," *Environmental Science and Technology* 37 (20): 4543-53 (October 15, 2003).

32. Bob Weinhold, "Metals: Fresh Track on Indoor Dust," *Environmental Health Perspectives* 116 (5): A198 (May 2008).

33. David W. Layton and Paloma I. Beamer, "Migration of Contaminated Soil and Airborne Particles to Indoor Dust," *Environmental Science and Technology* 43 (21): 8199-8205 (2009).

SIDEBARS

Six Immune Power Foods

- B. B. Ray, A. Raychoudhuri, R. Stee, P. Nerurkar, "Bitter Melon (Momordica charantia) Extract Inhibits Breast Cancer Cell Proliferation by Modulating Cell Cycle Regulatory Genes and Promotes Apoptosis," *Cancer Research* 70 (5): 1925-31 (March 1, 2010).

- Christine B. Ambrosone, Susan E. McCann, Jo L. Freudenheim, James R. Marshall, Yeushang Zhang and Peter G. Shields, "Breast Cancer Risk in Premenopausal Women is Inversely Associated with Consumption of Broccoli, a Source of Isothiocyanates, but is Not Modified by GST Genotype," *Journal of Nutrition* 134:1134-1138 (May 2004).

- M. Inoue, K. Tajima, M. Mizutani, et al., "Regular Consumption of Green Tea and the Risk of Breast Cancer Recurrence: Follow-up Study from the Hospital-based Epidemiologic Research Program at Aichi Cancer Center (HERPACC), Japan," *Cancer Letters* 167 (2): 175-182 (2001).

- L. S. Adams, S. Phung, X Wu, L. Ki, S. Chen, "White Button Mushroom (Agaricus bisporus) Exhibits Antiproliferative and Proapoptotic Properties and Inhibits Prostate Tumor Growth in Athymic Mice," *Nutrition and Cancer* 60 (6): 744-56 (2008).

- Arshi Malik, Farrukk Afaq, Sami Sarfaraz, Vaqar M. Adhami, Deeba N. Syed, and Hasan Mukhtar, "Pomegranate Fruit Juice for Chemoprevention and Chemotherapy of Prostate Cancer," *Proceedings of the National Academy of Sciences* 102 (41): 14813-14818 (October 11, 2005).

- W. E. Hardman, G. Ion, "Suppression of Implanted MDA-MB 231 Human Breast Cancer Growth in Nude Mice by Dietary Walnut," *Nutrition and Cancer* 60 (5): 666-74 (2008).

Herbs to Reduce Your Risk of Recurrence

- Ralph W. Moss, Ph.D. Cancer Treatment with Essiac. www.world-mysteries.com/sci_essiac.htm.

- Artemisia Annua. Memorial Sloan-Kettering Cancer Center. About Herbs. www.mskcc.org/mskcc/html/69126.cfm.

- Mistletoe Extracts (PDQ®). Overview. National Cancer Institute. Updated 3/26/2010. www.cancer.gov/cancertopics/pdq/cam/mistletoe.

- Scutellaria barbata. Memorial Sloan-Kettering Cancer Center. About Herbs. www.mskcc.org/mskcc/html/69367.cfm.

- S. K. Yadav, S. C. Lee, "Evidence for Oldenlandia Diffusa-evoked Cancer Cell Apoptosis Through Superoxide Burst and Caspase Activation," *Zhong Xi Yi Jie He Xue Bao* 4 (5): 485-9 (September 2006).

Do You Need Supplements?

- Nutrition and Physical Activity During and After Cancer Treatment: Answers to Common Questions. Revised 3/20/08. American Cancer Society. www.acsevents.org/docroot/mbc/content/MBC_6_2x_FAQ_Nutrition_and_Physical_Activity.asp?sitearea=MH.

- Cedric F. Garland, Edward D. Gorham, Sharif B. Mohr, Frank C. Garland, "Vitamin D for Cancer Prevention: Global Perspective," *Annals of Epidemiology.* 19 (7): 458-483 (July 2009).

- J. Lin, J. E. Manson, I. M. Lee, N. R. Cook, J. E. Buring, S. M. Zhang, "Intakes of Calcium and Vitamin D and Breast Cancer Risk in Women," *Archives of Internal Medicine* 167 (10): 1050-9 (May 28, 2007).

Index

About the Author

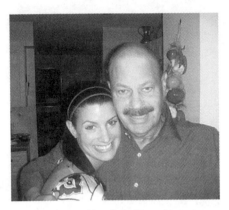

Britta Aragon and her father, Javier Aragon.

Britta Aragon, entrepreneur, natural beauty expert, and author, discovered her passion for promoting safe self care through her experience as a caregiver during her father's eight-year battle with cancer. A survivor herself of Hodgkin's disease at the age of 16, she hoped to help find solutions for the difficult side effects her father experienced on his hair, skin and nails, but was disheartened by the lack of quality information or safe products. Inspired and determined to help others, she founded Cinco Vidas in 2008, and dedicated her work to her father's legacy.

A lifestyle brand of products and services, Cinco Vidas provides expert resources and safe solutions to those going through side effects from chemotherapy, radiation, or medications, or who experience skin conditions like eczema, rosacea and chronic dryness. With the goal of fostering prevention and encouraging change, the organization also works to increase awareness of potential carcinogens in food, personal care products, and the environment.

As a result of years of working with people living with cancer and as a makeup artist and skincare expert, Britta specializes in compromised skin and lectures on Safe Self-Care for Compromised Skin in the New York area. In addition to her book *When Cancer Hits*, she is the creator of a unique skin care line that provides safe, non-toxic solutions to soothe and repair damaged skin without harmful chemicals. Additional copies of her book are available at Amazon.com, and her book and products can be found at www.cincovidas.com. Britta lives in New York, NY.

For more information or feedback, email info@cincovidas.com or connect on Facebook: Cinco Vidas, and on Twitter: @Britta_Aragon or @WhenCancerHits.